# LESSONS
## *from* THE
# MIRACLE
# DOCTORS

*A Step-by-Step Guide to Optimum Health
and Relief from Catastrophic Illness*

## JON BARRON

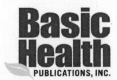
Basic Health
PUBLICATIONS, INC.

The statements found within the pages of this book have not been evaluated by the Food and Drug Administration. If a product or treatment is recommended in these pages, it is not intended to diagnose, treat, cure, or prevent any disease. The information contained herein is meant to be used to educate the reader and is in no way intended to provide individual medical advice. Medical advice must only be obtained from a qualified health practitioner.

All information contained in this book is received from sources believed to be accurate, but no guarantee, express or implied, can be made. Readers are encouraged to verify for themselves, and to their own satisfaction, the accuracy of all information, recommendations, conclusions, comments, opinions or anything else contained within these pages before making any kind of decisions based upon what they have read herein.

**Basic Health Publications, Inc.**
www.basichealthpub.com

**Library of Congress Cataloging-in-Publication Data**

Barron, Jon.
    Lessons from the miracle doctors : a step-by-step guide to optimum
    health and relief from catastrophic illness / Jon Barron. — Expanded ed.

   p. cm.
   Includes bibliographical references and index.
   ISBN 978-1-59120-224-0 (Hardback)
   ISBN 978-1-68162-744-1 (Pbk.)

   1. Alternative medicine. 2. Holistic medicine. 3. Herbs—Therapeutic use.
4. Naturopathy. I. Title.

   R733.B275     2008
   615.5—dc22

                           2008026129

Editor: John Anderson
Typesetting/Book design: Gary A. Rosenberg
Cover design: Mike Stromberg

# Contents

*Medicine is, and always should be, considered a vast field of service, constantly pioneering to improve the well-being of us all. From the beginning of my education in health and nutrition, I have known many healers whose efforts and service to humanity could be described as nothing less than heroic. It is with these heroes (and that perspective) in mind that I offer this book to any and all who read it. This book is for all those who have fought ignorance and prejudice, for those who have paid the price to keep this information alive and available for the rest of us. Among a whole host of others, these include Dr. John Christopher, Dr. Richard Schultz, Dr. David Williams, Dr. Jonathan Wright, and my wife, Kristen.*

# Preface

It has been almost ten years since I wrote the first draft of *Lessons from the Miracle Doctors*. That's a lot of time in the world of health and nutrition, and although I have periodically updated it in subsequent printings, I have never really done a full rewrite—until now. This is the first major update since I published that first edition in 1999, and it contains a significant amount of new material.

Why is a rewrite needed? The amazing thing is that virtually nothing involved with the core of the program is in need of updating or correction. A decade has passed, and yet the basic principles are as valid now as when I first wrote them. Actually, it shouldn't be that much of a surprise when you consider that the principles mirror concepts used by some of the greatest alternative healers of the last fifty years. The step-by-step instructions or methodologies involved in the program have also remained largely unchanged over the last ten years. So, if the core principles and methodologies of the Baseline of Health Program haven't changed, what's the need for a new edition?

The answer is that although the core of the Baseline of Health hasn't changed, there has indeed been tremendous change in the environment surrounding the program:

- The availability of "new" ingredients and "new understandings" of some old favorite ingredients.

- New areas of interest. We receive over 10,000 e-mails a month at the Baseline of Health Foundation. Every day, people from all over the world let us know the "hot" or "new" major health issues they want to know more about, everything including anti-aging, bird flu, antibiotic-resistant bacteria, and extreme drug-resistant tuberculosis (XDR-TB).

- Also, as evidenced by the questions coming in, there is a profound need to expand on some specific health issues, such as cholesterol and diabetes, that were only touched on in the previous editions.

- Finally, the world of medicine is catching up (well, maybe just a little) with the Baseline of Health Program. Many "new" areas of exploration in medicine (such as using the immune system to combat cancer) now echo the principles and techniques of the Baseline of Health detailed over a decade ago, and that's certainly worth exploring.

Now, keep in mind that the effective response to all of these new issues still lies in the same core principles and methodologies of the Baseline of Health Program. But it is useful and reassuring to know in detail why the program works, not only for old threats such as cancer but equally well for new ones such as bird flu and the exploding diabetes epidemic. The old saying, "The more things change, the more they stay the same" applies to the Baseline of Health over the last ten years. There have indeed been many changes and much new information to deal with in revising *Lessons from the Miracle Doctors*, but, again, when it comes to the core principles and step-by-step techniques of the book, they are unchanged. If anything, much of their validity has been confirmed by medical research (within limits).

In the pages that follow, I have tried to illuminate for you the barriers to obtaining good health, and I have presented practical, proven step-by-step methods for breaking down those barriers and seizing (for yourself and your family) health, energy, and mental and spiritual well-being. A lot of what you will learn here will fly in the face of so-called "conventional wisdom," but just because something is commonly accepted does not necessarily make it true. Our modern society has invested trillions of dollars in the ideas, equipment, research, facilities, and promises of our present health-care system, and it is almost unbearable to consider that much of it may be a waste. It will take great courage to accept responsibility for your own health, but I believe you, and millions like you, can and will do just that.

It has often been said that this is the only body you will ever get, and it must last a lifetime. The only question is how long and healthy that lifetime will be. The simple fact is that you absolutely can live well into your seventies, eighties, and beyond, in great health and with great vitality—but you need to make the right decisions now for that to happen. If you want to live a full and satisfying life, then you must take back control of your own health today. And the Baseline of Health Program can show you how to do just that.

# Introduction

hirty years ago, diseases such as colon cancer, diabetes, prostate cancer, Alzheimer's disease, osteoporosis, and diverticular disease were virtually unknown. Today, they are almost a certainty if you live long enough. This fact alone should be enough for any rational person to question the state of health care in the world today, but when you also consider how much we pay for this privilege, the doubt looms even larger. Every year we dump more money into pharmaceutical drugs, doctors, hospitals, ever more expensive medical devices, and insurance, but with what result? We certainly aren't getting any healthier.

## WHAT WE PAY FOR HEALTH CARE

In 1960, total health expenditures in the United States amounted to $27 billion; in 2003, the figure stood at nearly $1.7 trillion (a 63-fold rise) and is projected to reach an almost unimaginable $3.5 trillion by 2014. In contrast, the U.S. population grew by only 51 percent. During that same period, health expenditures per person rose from $143 to $5,670 (a 40-fold rise), while general inflation, as a point of reference, showed only a fivefold increase.[1] The bottom line is that, according to the World Health Organization, the U.S. spends more on health care than any other country in the world—more than twice as much per person as Britain and Japan and nearly 30 percent more than second-ranking Monaco. And the amount has risen steadily. Annual medical spending in the U.S. stood at more than $6,000 per person in 2005.[2] And while the United States certainly spearheads this trend (we spend more on health care than the entire gross national product of almost every other country in the world), we are hardly alone. Britain, Germany, Canada, and France all now spend upwards of $2,000 to $3,000 per person.[3]

1

## WHAT VALUE HAVE WE RECEIVED?

The main argument in support of this vast expenditure is that we are all living longer. During the millennium celebrations in 2000, medical experts in the media touted a 28-year increase in life expectancy over the last century. Life expectancy at birth in the United States in 1901 was forty-nine years, and at the end of the century it was seventy-seven years—an increase of 57 percent. This increase, however, is the result of a statistical game. The low life expectancy in the early 1900s is distorted by the extremely high infant and childhood mortality experienced back then. Anyone surviving childhood tended to last well into their sixties. Much of the gain in life expectancy we've seen in the last century has very little to do with advancements in medical care. It results largely from the eradication and control of numerous infectious diseases and from non-sustainable advances in agriculture (fewer people are starving to death).

In 2006, an article in the *New England Journal of Medicine* claimed a more modest increase in life expectancy of just seven years in the last forty.[4] The study's lead author acknowledged that as much as half of that gain, though, is the result of declines in rates of smoking and fatal accidents. And critics point out that, as previously referenced, a decline in infant mortality accounts for even more. So, now we're down from a seven-year increase in life expectancy in the last century to a mere two to three years, and when you consider that for many of those people those extra two to three years are spent incapacitated in a rest home, or dying miserably from chemotherapy and cancer, or hooked up to an intravenous feeding tube in a hospital, that modest increase in life expectancy somehow seems worth even less.

So, what benefits have we received for the trillions of dollars the world spends?

- The United States leads the developed world in deaths from heart disease, prostate cancer, breast cancer, colorectal cancer, and diabetes.[5]

- Cancer rates are up 400 percent (using ultraconservative numbers from the Centers for Disease Control or CDC) in the last hundred years.[6]

- Digestive diseases are the leading cause of hospitalization and surgery in the U.S. and cost nearly $107 billion in direct health-care expenditures in 1992. They result in nearly 200 million sick days, 60 million visits to physicians, 16.9 million days lost from school, 14 million hospitalizations, and nearly 250,000 deaths per year.[7]

- Diabetes is now a worldwide epidemic,[8] with the incidence increasing by over 40 percent in the U.S. in the seven-year span from 1997 to 2004 alone.[9]

- New strains of viral and bacterial infections, including bird flu, methicillin-resistant staph (MRSA) infections, and XDR tuberculosis, that are totally drug resistant have started to emerge.[10]

- Male sperm counts are down 50 percent in the last century, with counts in the U.S. continuing to drop at the rate of 1.5 percent per year, while those in European countries are declining at the rate of 3.1 percent per year.[11]

- The average age of puberty for young girls in the developed world has dropped from fifteen or sixteen to an astonishing eight years old, with one in a hundred girls now showing signs of puberty by the age of three.[12]

- The incidence of birth defects worldwide is soaring. Every year, an estimated 8 million children—6 percent of total births worldwide—are born with a serious birth defect of genetic or partially genetic origin.[13]

## AND IT'S GETTING WORSE

The incidence of diabetes in the U.S. has doubled in just the last five years! In 2005, the National Diabetes Information Clearinghouse estimated that nearly 21 million people had diabetes. The same study also estimated that some 54 million Americans were pre-diabetic—based on 2006 data.[14] And it's not just the United States—diabetes is exploding everywhere.

Fifty years ago, diverticular disease (herniations of the colon) was virtually unknown, afflicting less than 10 percent of the American population. Today, according to the American Society of Colon and Rectal Surgeons, virtually 100 percent of Americans will have many, if they live long enough.[15]

The number of Americans who suffer from asthma, according to the CDC, rose by an astounding 75 percent between 1980 and 1994.[16] And rates among children in some parts of North America are up a mind-boggling 400 percent in the last twenty years.[17]

Breast cancer rates are up 30 percent in just the last fifteen years. The American Cancer Society estimated that in 2005 alone, some 211,000 women in the U.S. were diagnosed with invasive breast cancer (stages I–IV).[18] Cancer is also the leading cause of death by disease in children under the age of fourteen.[19] And even though we spend $100 billion a year on cancer treatment and research in the U.S. alone, the overall survival rate for cancer patients is virtually unchanged over the last 100 years.[20] And on, and on, and on.

## THE MOST SHOCKING FACT OF ALL

As it turns out, the very people and medications we turn to for protection against this onslaught may be doing more harm than good. The *Journal of the American Medical Association* reported that there are more than 2 million drug "reactions" annually in the U.S., and more than 100,000 of those reactions are fatal.[21] This makes prescription drugs the fourth leading cause of death in America.[22] But the reality is actually much worse. These numbers do not include:

- Patients who are given the wrong drugs or who are given those drugs at the wrong dosage or in the wrong combination.

- Patients who have fatal reactions to the drugs, but whose death is mistakenly (or deliberately) attributed to other causes. A patient is prescribed a painkiller and dies from a heart attack. How is that recorded on the death certificate—reaction to the drug or heart attack? Both are true, but only one is the truth.

Add these circumstances to the aforementioned "official" count and you find that deaths from adverse reactions to drugs may number as high as 700,000 a year. Actually, the U.S. Food and Drug Administration (FDA) estimates that only 1 percent of all adverse reactions are reported,[23] which, if true, would make 700,000 an incredibly conservative estimate. Now, combine those 700,000 deaths with the number of people who die from misdiagnosis, inappropriate treatment, secondary infections received in hospitals, or just plain physician error,[24] and the startling fact you're left with is that modern medicine, despite all the great things it may have accomplished, is arguably the single leading cause of death in the United States.

It is not a coincidence that time after time, when doctors go on strike, mortality rates drop dramatically in those cities or countries. In 1976, in Bogota, Columbia, medical doctors went on strike for fifty-two days, with only emergency care available. The death rate dropped by 35 percent. In 1976, in Los Angeles County, a similar doctors' strike resulted in an 18 percent drop in mortality. As soon as the strike was over, the death rate went back to previous levels. A 50 percent decrease in mortality occurred in Israel in 1973 when there was a thirty-day doctors' strike—with similar results seen in doctor strikes in 1983 and 2000![25] This should not be surprising when you also note the Institute of Medicine's report entitled *To Err is Human*, which states that medical errors cause as many as 98,000 deaths each year in the U.S. alone, more than traffic accidents, breast cancer, or AIDS. Right behind prescription drugs, medical error is the fifth leading cause of death.[26]

Understand, this is not an attack on medical doctors, the vast majority of whom are extremely competent, highly dedicated, and often even heroic. Nevertheless, it is important to realize that when it comes to the major diseases of our time, the modern medical paradigm of searching for "magic bullets" and managing symptoms with drugs has failed miserably.

## THERE HAS TO BE AN ALTERNATIVE

There is a network of elite herbalists, holistic healers, and renegade medical doctors throughout the world performing miracles on a daily basis. The network is not only elite, it is also extremely difficult to penetrate because it is technically illegal to diagnose or treat people for major diseases unless you use the government-approved modalities such as cutting, burning, and poisoning (surgery, radiation, and chemotherapy). Thousands of people throughout the world have come to these "miracle doctors" certain that they were terminally ill, and thousands have left perfectly healthy—not everyone, to be sure, but a surprisingly high percentage. And now the secrets of these miracle doctors are revealed in this book.

In the following chapters, I will share with you those things that I have learned in over forty years of working with, studying with, and sharing with these remarkable healers. By the time you have finished, you will have learned everything you need to know (in precise detail) to optimize your own health (and the health of those you love) so that you all may live long and happy lives.

In Chapter 1, we will explore exactly how your health has been stolen from you and who is responsible. In Chapter 2, I will outline the principles of the Baseline of Health Program. If you read no other chapter in this book, the heart of everything I have to say is located here. The rest of the book addresses all of the different body systems you need to concern yourself with in order to optimize your health—and provides protocols for maximizing the health of each of those systems. Finally, I will help you make sense of all that you have read and offer specific summary guidelines for how to take back your health.

Keep in mind that good health really comes down to "playing the odds." For example, if you smoke cigarettes, there's no guarantee that you're going to get sick and die. We've all heard stories of the man who smoked and drank like a fiend for eighty years, was never sick a day in his life, but died at the hands of a jealous husband who shot the old letch when he discovered him in bed with his twenty-year-old wife. These things happen, or so I've been told. On the other hand, there's no question that your odds of having emphysema or lung cancer or of having parts of your mouth, lips, and tongue surgically removed increase dramatically if you smoke. It's all a question of odds.

In the same way, if you follow the program in this book, your odds of having good health and long life are significantly increased—not guaranteed, but significantly increased. Oh yes, and you're going to feel a whole lot better, have more energy, alertness, sexuality, youthfulness, and radiance in the process. As they say in corporate boardrooms, it's a win/win scenario.

# PART ONE
## *Overview*

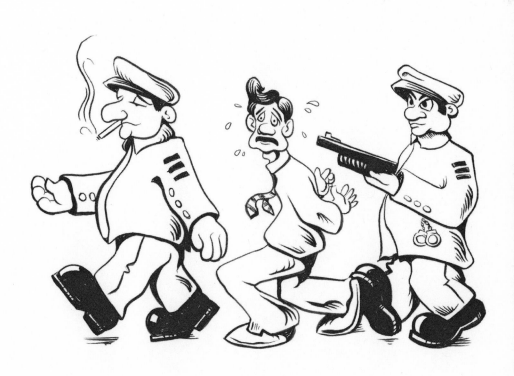

**I just wanted to buy some Vitamin C!**

# CHAPTER 1

## *The Thieves of Health*

- **The Modern Medical Paradigm**
- **Creating the "Disease Industry"**
- **The Medical Fraternity**
- **Government Regulators—The U.S. Food and Drug Administration (FDA)**
- **Drug Companies**
- **Supporting Players**
- **What Can Be Done?**

*L*et me begin by saying that, unlike some in the alternative health community, I am not anti-doctor. I was, in fact, a pre-med student for several years. I understand that sometimes there is no substitute for a doctor. In terms of surgical technique (the cutting apart and repair of the human body), modern medicine has made remarkable advances. In terms of identifying the germs that play a role in causing many diseases and improving sanitation to prevent those diseases, once again modern medicine has made remarkable advances. In terms of burns, trauma, and emergency room care, modern medicine is nothing short of miraculous. But in terms of treating and preventing most catastrophic illness, particularly the major scourges of the modern era—heart disease, cancer, diabetes, osteoporosis, and Alzheimer's—modern medicine stands an abject failure . . . to this point.

Despite all of the games played with statistics, the numbers referenced in the Introduction are undeniable. But more to the point, all of the above scourges are modern diseases, at least in terms of their emergence as epidemics. In the early 1900s, these diseases were almost unheard of. There is actually a documented conversation, from the beginning of the twentieth century, from a group of doctors standing around a patient with cancer. "Take a good look," remarked the senior physician, "for this is the last time you will see this illness in your lifetime."[1] Yet, today, that remark is inconceivable. The important point to understand is that these diseases are not "natural," not "normal." They have only appeared en masse in our lifetimes.

As for arguments that higher numbers just represent better detection and an aging population, that's self-evident nonsense! Obesity, diabetes, and sky-rocketing cancer rates (breast cancer rates in England, for example, are up 80 percent in just the last thirty years[2]) are not only afflicting more people, they are afflicting younger people. Adult-onset diabetes has been renamed type 2 diabetes, not because of better detection but because so many children are now getting it. Despite trillions of dollars spent on medical care worldwide, the incidence of these diseases is accelerating year by year, a fact only occasionally acknowledged by the mainstream media.[3]

Despite its abject failure in the treatment of these diseases (mortality rates are virtually unchanged for all of them), the modern medical machine has actually made it illegal for you, in many areas of United States and Europe, to seek out alternative therapies. For example, in 2005, Assembly Bill 2393 and Senate Bill 1691, which were written to allow doctors in California to legally prescribe alternative medicine in place of, or in combination with, conventional treatments for cancer, were crushed in committee and never even voted on. California's physicians are still at risk of losing their licenses if they prescribe anything other than surgery, radiation, and chemotherapy for treating cancer. How did this happen? How did we reach this point?

## THE MODERN MEDICAL PARADIGM

As Michael Culbert, in his book *Medical Armageddon*, describes it, modern medicine likes to claim Hippocrates and the ancient Greeks as its founding fathers, but the fact is that Isaac Newton and the seventeenth-century philosophers and scientists—who defined the universe as a giant machine ruled by the laws of mechanical physics and math—are probably much better candidates for the title.[4] Physicians of that era likewise began to define the human body as a machine that ran smoothly until acted upon by some outside agent. Accordingly, the human body could be studied, documented, medicated, and tweaked as required. This viewpoint became more and more dominant as time went by, until by the nineteenth century:

- The human body was no longer viewed as a holistic entity but rather as a grouping of separate parts and pieces.

- Disease was no longer viewed as an imbalance in the body but rather as a set of symptoms.

- Medical research was defined as the observation and classification of both the body's parts and its various sets of symptoms.

Based on the above, the physician's job was now defined as eliminating (or at least managing) those symptoms. In other words, disease or injury manifests as symptoms entirely separate from the body as a whole. Eliminate the symptoms, and you eliminate the problem.

As it turns out, this paradigm works extremely well when it comes to surgical repair. If you break an arm, the doctor works with that part of the body and repairs the arm. If you're shot by a bullet, the doctor removes the bullet and repairs all of the separate parts of your body damaged by the bullet. It's a direct one-to-one correlation. Unfortunately, the paradigm proves far less successful when it comes to many of our most feared degenerative diseases.

## Modern Medicine and Heart Disease

Consider how the medical community handles heart disease. Say you have clogged arteries. This eventually causes your blood pressure to rise, so your doctor prescribes blood pressure medication to eliminate the symptom—but not the problem, the clogged arteries. To reduce blood pressure, doctors have essentially four classes of medication.

1. Diuretics, which reduce pressure by making you eliminate water from your body. Reduce the volume of fluid in the blood, and you reduce the pressure. Unfortunately, side effects can include dizziness, weakness, and impotence. (Not to worry, there are more medications to alleviate these side effects.)

2. Calcium channel blockers, which work to relax and widen the arteries, thus reducing blood pressure. Unfortunately, a major side effect of channel blockers is a 60 percent increased risk of heart attack.

3. Beta blockers, which work by weakening the heart so it won't pump as strongly, thereby reducing blood pressure. What genius thought this one up? One of the major problems with beta blockers is the increased risk of

congestive heart failure. Nevertheless, despite the increased risk of heart failure, leading doctors have recommended putting every heart attack survivor on beta blockers.[5]

4. ACE inhibitors (the new drug of choice), which like the calcium channel blockers also work to relax and widen the arteries, but with fewer side effects (just "minor" things such as kidney impairment, upper respiratory problems, headache, dizziness, and congenital "anomalies").[6]

Keep in mind that, in addition to all of the side effects that these drugs cause (which require further medication), there is a fundamental flaw in your doctor's treatment. All the doctor has done is treat the "manifest" symptom—high blood pressure—but has done nothing to deal with the underlying problem—clogged or hardened arteries. So, eventually, as your arteries continue to clog and harden to the point where even the medication no longer helps, you start getting the inevitable chest pains. Your doctor then chases the next set of symptoms and performs a coronary bypass or angioplasty to relieve those symptoms—until the next, even more radical, intervention.

As a side note, a study published in 2007 found that angioplasties did not save lives or prevent heart attacks in non-emergency patients.[7] In fact, the study showed angioplasties only give slight and temporary relief from chest pain, and by five years, there was no significant difference in symptoms. Oh yes, we spend $48 billion a year on angioplasties in the U.S. alone.

Then again, in addition to all of the side effects, complications, and dangers of surgery, we are once more presented with a fundamental flaw in your doctor's treatment. If all your doctor does is bypass or clear the arteries supplying blood to your heart, doesn't that mean that all of the other arteries in your body are still clogged, including the arteries that supply blood to your brain? You bet it does. Isn't that going to be a problem? Since the arteries are narrowed, won't it be more likely that a small blood clot will get lodged in your brain and cause a stroke? Absolutely! But that's a different "symptom." At this point your doctor, once again prescribes another drug or more dangerous surgery to deal with this problem. . . .

## CREATING THE "DISEASE INDUSTRY"

The bottom line is that the average number of prescriptions per senior citizen has grown from 19.6 in 1992 to 28.5 in 2000, an increase of 45 percent.

And it is projected to grow to 38.5 by 2010, an additional increase of 35 percent. From 1992 to 2010, then, the average number of prescriptions per senior will grow by 96 percent.[8] Stunningly, only the first one or two drugs actually deal with the symptoms presented by the original medical problem. The other drugs are all required to deal with the negative side effects of the original drugs, plus the interactions of all the other drugs steadily being added to the mix. And the really sad fact is that in most cases, the original problem could have been resolved by merely changing diet and lifestyle, with no side effects.

Somehow, along the way, we have created a major industry centered on disease and manipulating the symptoms of those diseases, and everyone wants a piece of the action—from insurance companies to doctors, administrators to state legislatures, lobbyists to hospitals, drug companies to researchers, medical device companies to universities, and even all the nonprofits that collect millions of dollars to support this massive system of dysfunction. Make no mistake, this is not a wellness industry—as Paul Pilzer states in *The Wellness Revolution*, it is a "disease industry," designed not to eliminate disease but to perpetuate the management of symptoms.

So, we've looked at the problem and the paradigm that created it. Now, let's take a look at some of the players—the medical fraternity, government regulators, pharmaceutical companies, and the insurance industry—that actually make it all happen.

## THE MEDICAL FRATERNITY

I know a lot about doctors. As I mentioned earlier, I was pre-med myself in college, and there are many doctors in my family. I both respect them for the dedicated service they provide and, at the same time, am very angry with them for the needless suffering they inflict. The problem is that doctors are only human, and as such, they have all of the brilliance, stupidity, nobility, greed, dedication, flaws, and ego traits that plague each and every one of us. None of this would be a problem, except for one fact: despite their human frailties and lack of divine insight, they have set themselves up as the only authoritative dispensers of health care in the developed world and have set up political action groups such as the American, British, and German Medical Associations to protect their positions. These associations use all means at their disposal to prevent any contrary points of view from being heard.

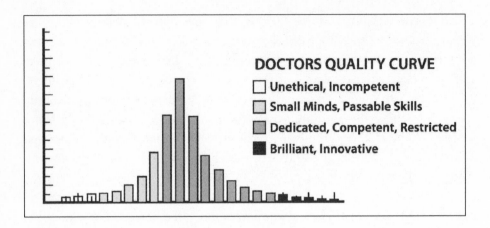

Against healers outside of their fraternity, they are particularly ruthless. There are numerous examples, but three stand out:

- First, most people are not aware that the American Medical Association (AMA) was not actually formed to promote health, but to combat homeopathic medicine—or as characterized in the AMA's original charter, "An enemy who has many strongholds upon the affection of the people; and one who in many places rivals us in their esteem."

- Second, in 1980, the U.S. Court of Appeals upheld a 1978 Federal Trade Commission (FTC) ruling that found the AMA guilty of "conspiracy to restrain competition" in regard to chiropractic care. The AMA fought this decision for seven years, when in 1987, Judge Susan Getzendanner ruled that the AMA had engaged in "systematic, long-term wrongdoing and the long-term intent to destroy a licensed profession." The AMA continued to fight these rulings, and it wasn't until 1990 that it finally lost for good (for now).

- On June 8th, 2004, AMA trustee Dr. Ronald M. Davis testified before Congress that the AMA calls for the "pre-market approval by the FDA of all dietary supplements." Dr. Davis also stated, "The AMA has been concerned for years about the use and abuse of dietary supplements. Congress must provide the FDA with greater regulatory power over dietary supplements to bring needed oversight to the industry and to protect the health of America's consumers." And this from the people (organized medicine) that, according to its own figures, may be the single leading cause of death in the United States today.

But what's going on here? Certainly, not all doctors accept this absurd view of alternative health? Why do we never hear from the rebels? How are members of the medical community kept in line?

## Why the System Never Changes

**Lack of Information**—Many doctors become so busy "practicing" medicine once they graduate from medical school that they no longer have time to study their art. They then rely on "trusted" sources to keep up to date. In fact, for most doctors, their sole source of information, once they start practicing, is the "party line" provided by the associations they belong to and the drug companies promoting their drugs or paying for "peer reviewed" studies that appear in their associations' journals or, even worse, on the sensationalized reports of those studies in the media. The net result is that, over time, they become ill-informed or misinformed—merely parroting the party line.

**The Wrong Paradigm**—We've already discussed the modern medical paradigm, which focuses on body parts and symptoms, but what we haven't discussed is how this paradigm determines how doctors filter reality. A few examples:

- Doctors complain that alternative healing is based on anecdotal evidence, not science like "real" medicine. Nevertheless, they remain blind to the fact that 85 percent of all medical procedures they rely on are also untested and based purely on anecdotal evidence.[9] They've even developed a euphemism to describe the process: *off-label use*, the practice of prescribing drugs for a purpose outside the scope of the drug's approved label. That's right, once the FDA approves a drug for prescription use, there is no regulation as to what it's used for, and so physicians can make decisions based on anecdotal evidence—or even their own best guess. In other words, large numbers of drugs are used for diseases for which their efficacy and safety have never been tested. And that's called "science."

- Doctors say that many alternative healing procedures and herbal remedies are dangerous. In fact, fewer than five people die (theoretically) each year in the U.S. from complications resulting from overdosing on vitamins or an allergic reaction to herbal remedies. That matches up quite well with the 106,000 (conservatively) who die from the pharmaceuticals that doctors prescribe.

- Doctors say that even when people aren't being harmed by alternative health care, they're being fleeced. "Millions of dollars are wasted each year on megadoses of vitamins that are peed down the toilet and on useless herbal concoctions." Somehow, though, these same doctors don't seem too concerned about the billions of dollars that have been spent on the "war on cancer," only to see cancer rates soar to epidemic proportions, or about the $48 billion spent on useless angioplasties each year.

**Fear**—There is a saying in the medical community that goes, "It is better to die than to go against the faculty of medicine." We've all seen prison movies—*Cool Hand Luke, Papillon,* and *The Shawshank Redemption*—where the evil warden keeps his prisoners in line by brutally and publicly punishing any who break any rules. Amazingly, these movies could just as easily have been stories about how the medical establishment keeps its ranks in line. Every doctor knows about the "renegade" doctors who have been harassed, raided, arrested, and driven from their practices for "going against the established order." This tends to keep the rest in line. In 1979, for example, the Florida First District Court of Appeal reversed an order by the Florida Board of Medical Examiners placing Dr. Robert Rogers on probation, accusing him of "quackery under the guise of scientific medicine," and directing him to stop using chelation therapy (a detoxification therapy for removing heavy metals). The district judges not only disagreed with the examiner's ruling, but also declared that Dr. Rogers was a scientific and medical innovator comparable to Freud, Pasteur, and Copernicus. There are literally thousands of such stories—unfortunately, 99 percent of them end less happily.

**Self-Validation**—This is the ultimate expression of the doctor as God. It is total closed-mindedness to anything the medical community does not already know. Almost an attitude of "Well, if it were so good, don't you think I'd already know about it and be doing it?" It is also reflected in a superiority complex that is dismissive of anyone or anything that is not part of the same "superior" fraternity. Examples of this include the near total dismissal of chiropractic treatment, oriental medicine, and nutritional therapy—which is only now beginning to change.

**Economic Pressure**—The medical community creates its own treatment biases. For example, several thousand cardiologists and cardiovascular surgeons are produced by the medical community every year. These doctors have a vested interest (unconscious, to be sure) in favoring high-cost, high-risk invasive techniques for the treatment of your heart disease. After all, their careers are invested in it. What do you think the odds are that someone trained to make their living opening up your body will recommend a low-cost non-invasive treatment—administered by someone outside the medical fraternity at that?

These same economic pressures influencing your doctor's behavior can be found in hospitals too. The new expensive equipment for open heart surgery, the computerized multi-million-dollar MRI machine, and the high-tech neo-natal intensive care unit all need to be paid for through extensive patient utilization. Do you have any doubt that this affects at least some of the treatment decisions that are made concerning your illness?

And then, of course, there's greed. The unnecessary surgeries and treatments that doctors in the trade refer to as "boat payments." Fortunately, the number of doctors who base your treatment on their financial self-interest is small. Unfortunately, because those few each do it multiple times (such as the doctor who performed several thousand unnecessary hysterectomies before he was identified), the numbers of patients who are brutalized is quite large.

**Patient Demand**—To be fair, there are a number of doctors who do try to get their patients on a healthy regimen of diet and exercise, but many patients have abrogated personal responsibility for their own health and have bought into the principle espoused in so many drug commercials that one can simply "pop a pill" to cure all ills—everything from colds to cancer. For the most part, we get the health care we ask for.

## Two 800-Pound Gorillas

So, where do we go from here? I believe that medical doctors are now in a very difficult position. It is as though they are locked in a room with two 800-pound gorillas. One of those gorillas is managed health care, whose sole goal is to restrict the way these doctors practice medicine and to limit the amount of money they make doing it. The other gorilla is alternative health, which has become a multi-billion-dollar industry despite the best efforts of the medical community to stop it. If you are indeed in a room with two huge gorillas, there is one place you don't want to be—between them. At some point, you are going to have to get behind one of them or you will be crushed in the middle. And since, by definition, managed health care is dedicated to crushing the individual doctor, there is only one option—doctors will have to step in behind supplements and herbs. But therein lies my greatest fear. I believe that when that happens, doctors will try to turn alternative medicine into another branch of organized medicine, available only by prescription and only through their members. In business terms (and with billions of dollars at stake), we're talking about a hostile takeover.

## GOVERNMENT REGULATORS—
## THE U.S. FOOD AND DRUG ADMINISTRATION (FDA)

It doesn't matter what country you live in, you have an FDA-type regulatory authority promoting questionable pharmaceutical solutions while at the same time limiting your access to far safer alternatives. A 2006 article in *The Washington Post* brings home the point that FDA approval (actually, any government approval) does not guarantee safety.[10] It also makes it clear that approved pharmaceuticals, over-the-counter medications, medical devices, and even food products are not what you think they are.

This article highlights the findings of a 15-month investigation of the FDA following a worldwide flu vaccine shortage. In the process, investigators documented profound and disturbing indications of much more far-reaching and deep-seated problems. While the motivation for the investigation was undoubtedly political, the results are inarguable. First, consider the trends revealed in the investigation:

- In the previous five years, the number of warning letters that the FDA issued to drug companies, medical device makers, etc., dropped 54 percent to 535 in 2005 from 1,154 in 2000.

- The seizure of mislabeled, defective, and dangerous products dipped 44 percent.

- The biggest decline was found at the agency's device center, where enforcement actions decreased 65 percent in the five-year period of the study, despite a wave of problems with devices including implantable defibrillators and pacemakers. The most disturbing indicator in these statistics is that the research found no evidence that such declines could be attributed to increased compliance with regulations. Investigators at the FDA continued to uncover about the same number of problems at drug and device companies during the study as during comparable time periods before the study. The inquiry found instead that top officials at the

FDA increasingly overruled the investigators' enforcement recommendations.

## FDA Missteps

In 2006, the Union of Concerned Scientists published the results of a survey of 1,000 doctors who work for the FDA.[11] The results were disturbing to say the least:

- Almost one in five (18 percent) responded, "I have been asked, for non-scientific reasons, to inappropriately exclude or alter technical information or my conclusions in an FDA scientific document."

- More than three in five (61 percent) knew of cases in which "Department of Health and Human Services or FDA political appointees have inappropriately injected themselves into FDA determinations or actions."

- Three in five (60 percent) also knew of cases "where commercial interests have inappropriately induced or attempted to induce the reversal, withdrawal, or modification of FDA determinations or actions."

- Fifty percent also felt that nongovernmental interests (such as advocacy groups) had induced or attempted to induce such changes.

- Less than half of them (49 percent) agreed that "FDA leadership is as committed to product safety as it is to bringing products to the market."

## More Conflicts of Interest

Many FDA managers have conflicts of interest, from holding stock in the pharmaceutical industries they regulate to holding jobs at these same pharmaceutical companies either before or after they work for the FDA. Yes, top FDA officials frequently end up with top positions at the same drug companies they were entrusted to regulate. Does this automatically mean that these positions are improper or that "improper" decisions were made as a result? No, of course not. But sometimes the appearance of impropriety is so overwhelming that it's more than enough to convict.

Consider too that the FDA admits this failure. In a July 2006 article entitled "FDA Pledges Conflict Reforms," the FDA issued a preemptory mea culpa.[12] The agency said it would clarify rules on advisory panel members with ties to drug companies. But the proposed reforms are unlikely to stop many doctors and researchers with such conflicts from serving on panels whose recommendations can determine the fate of drugs worth billions of dollars in corporate profits—but that may endanger consumers at the same time. The FDA has about fifty advisory panels that are supposed to provide impartial technical advice on issues such as over-the-counter allergy medicines, silicone breast implants, and chemotherapy drugs with toxic side effects. A study published in 2006 found that 28 percent of panel members disclosed financial conflicts, but only 1 percent recused themselves.[13]

To be fair, there are many, many good, conscientious people working for the FDA. I've talked to a number of them. The problem is that the nice people don't control the agenda.

## Government Regulation around the World

For those of you living outside the United States, don't feel smug. Remember, you have your own government agencies—in most cases, even worse than the FDA. Just look at the European Health Initiative and Codex, or look at how Canada treats naturally occurring substances such as DMAE as drugs, or how Australia's new rules require massive amounts of documentation for the importation of even the most innocuous natural health supplements. Don't think for one moment that what happens in the U.S. with the FDA doesn't matter to you, or that what happens in your country vis-à-vis alternative health regulation doesn't matter to those of us in the United States. It most assuredly does. To paraphrase Ben Franklin: "We must all stand together [regarding our health rights], or assuredly we shall all hang separately."

## DRUG COMPANIES

The relationship of the drug industry to doctors is no less prevalent or obscene than is the relationship of political action committee (PAC) money to politicians or the influence of defense contractors to the U.S. military. Money buys votes; money buys defense contracts; and money buys doctors' treatment choices. As I've already mentioned, for many doctors their sole source of information about drugs and treatments comes from drug company representatives. In a very real sense, the drug companies take an active role in your treatment. How often have you been to a doctor's office and been given free samples of medications? Those samples were given to your doctor by the drug company reps, and he has given them to you as part of your treatment.

But there is even more—and worse. The major drug companies have frequently been investigated for, and found guilty of, gross ethical violations in influencing doctors by doing things such as awarding free travel and kickbacks to doctors who convert prescriptions written for generic drugs or competitors' drugs to prescriptions written for their products. It is important to note that, in almost every case where the drug companies have been called to task for these illegal acts, the call has come from outside the medical community.

By their very nature, prescription drugs are the perfect product for a monopoly. Drugs are patented and available from only one manufacturer for a number of years, and prices can be increased at the discretion of the company with few consumer complaints. How many people who are terminally ill question the cost of drugs prescribed by their doctor, particularly when it's paid for by health insurance? During the 1980s, inflation rose 58 percent, and yet pharmaceutical companies managed to triple their prices.[14] In 2001, as the economy reeled and corporate profits sank for the average Fortune 500 company, drug companies in the top 500 list saw their profits soar by 33 percent over the previous year. Quite simply, the drug industry is one of the most profitable industries in world, with annual profits of 18.9 percent—more than five times the average Fortune 500 company. In 2000, worldwide sales reached an astronomical $365 billion. The nine largest pharmaceutical giants netted $30.6 billion in 2001 profits.

Drug companies now spend, on average, over twice as much on advertising as on research. And since 1997 the industry has spent nearly $478 million lobbying the federal government. Also, during that same period, the top twenty-five pharmaceutical companies and trade groups contributed $48.6 million to federal election campaigns. Well over $100 million more went to pay for issue ads, hiring academics, funding non-profits, and other activities to promote the industry's agenda in Washington. All told, the drug industry has spent nearly $650 million on political influence in the last six years.

And has all this lobbying had any impact? You be the judge: U.S. regulators have sharply cut the number of warnings sent to drugmakers for false or misleading advertising. The FDA, which monitors drug promotions, issued more than 250 letters to companies about problems in their ads between January 1999 and December 2001, according to Representative Henry Waxman, a California Democrat. However, from December 2001 through August

2002, the agency sent only nineteen such letters, a 70 percent drop.[15] "It appears that FDA is now granting major drug manufacturers virtually a free pass," Waxman wrote in a letter to Health and Human Services Secretary Tommy Thompson.

And it's not just in the United States. The major pharmaceutical companies have managed to exert undue influence in worldwide attempts to shut down the alternative health industry. For example, the underlying proposal to establish the Codex guidelines for worldwide standards for foods, drugs, and supplements has been guided by the three German companies: Hoechst, Bayer, and BASF.

And what about the millions of dollars spent on "buying" the good opinion of medical doctors? In September 2000, both Reuters and USA Today reported that 54 percent of the experts that the FDA asks for advice on which medicines should be approved had a direct financial interest in the drugs or topics they were evaluating. These financial conflicts of interest typically included stock ownership, consulting fees, and/or research grants. Understand, these experts are hired (that is, paid) by the FDA to advise on which medicines should be approved for sale, what the warning labels should say, and how studies of drugs should be designed. The experts are supposed to be independent, but over half the time they have a direct financial interest.

And for achieving such results and establishing such influence in the government decision-making process, the major executives of the pharmaceutical companies are obviously well rewarded. In fact, the five most highly paid drug company executives pocketed more than $183 million in compensation in 2001. But that doesn't count stock options. In 2000, the chairman and CEO of Bristol-Myers Squibb, for example, held unexercised options valued at an additional $227.9 million.[16]

## Who Pays for This?

Everybody in every country is a victim, but because the U.S. is the only major industrialized nation that does not regulate the prices or profits of drug companies, prescription drugs generally cost 25 to 40 percent more than in other countries. With the exception of health insurance premium payments, prescription drug expenses represent the single largest component of out-of-pocket spending on health care (17 percent of the total health care dollar, on average). Prescription drug expenses account for as much as those spent on physician care, vision care services, and medical supplies combined.[17] For 75 percent of elderly Americans, prescription drugs are their single biggest expense.

There's the cost in health to consider as well. In 2002, there were approximately 3.34 billion prescriptions filled—about eleven drugs for every man, woman, and child in the U.S. No human being or computer program can keep track of all the possible side effects of this many drugs. The problem is that each drug affects the body chemistry in multiple (hundreds, even thousands) of ways. As soon as you add a second drug, the interaction between the two drugs increases the possibilities to tens (or even hundreds) of thousands of possible chemical interactions in the body. Add a third drug, and you're into the millions. Make that ten or fifteen drugs and you're dealing with numbers beyond comprehension. In one study, an alarming one-in-four patients suffered observable side effects from prescription drugs.[18]

Don't despair—a new field of expertise called polypharmacy is being created to "deal" with this problem. What a joke!

## SUPPORTING PLAYERS

There is no question but that the three biggest players in keeping the current system in place and ruthlessly suppressing any dissenting voices are the medical establishment, the FDA (and its international equivalents), and the pharmaceutical industry. Nevertheless, there are some supporting players worthy of honorable mention.

### The Insurance Industry

Insurance carriers have forced some of the most financially counterproductive decisions. Their fear of "open-ended" procedures has led them to support high-cost and largely ineffective "closed-end" procedures. For example, insurance carriers for years were among the strongest resisters of chiropractic care. Why? Because chiropractic treatment didn't end in one visit; rather, it took multiple sessions. It was for this reason that insurance companies preferred to pay for one expensive back operation rather than ten $50 trips to the chiropractor. Only now are insurance companies beginning to realize that a back operation costs them thousands (and in close to 80 percent of cases does not resolve the problem) whereas ten trips to a chiropractor will cost them only a few hundred dollars and is statistically more effective. Nevertheless, the insurance companies still "force" some

300,000 people a year into heart bypass operations rather than support the use of simple supplements such as proteolytic enzymes and omega-3 fatty acids that actually help eliminate the problem throughout the entire body.

## The Processed Food Industry

Here's to the people who have brought us refined carbohydrates, massive amounts of sugar and caffeine, hydrogenated oils, petrochemical additives, xenoestrogens, pesticides, irradiated foods, animal growth hormones, and, of course, the omnipresent high-potency antibiotics. And then, without batting an eye, they jumped onto the low-fat bandwagon (pumping us with trans-fatty acids in the process) and, again without batting an eye, onto the low-carb craze. What next?

## The U.S. Department of Agriculture (USDA)

And special praise must go to the U.S. Department of Agriculture, which, early in 1998, proposed changing the definition of "organic" to include foods that have been genetically modified, irradiated, injected with antibiotics, and grown with sewage sludge (with its incredibly high levels of toxic metals and waste) as fertilizer. It makes you wonder whose side these guys are on. Then again, maybe it doesn't.

## WHAT CAN BE DONE?

It's worth mentioning one more time that just because the policies of the medical establishment, government regulators, and pharmaceutical giants are bad doesn't mean that the people involved are bad. As I've said repeatedly, on a one-on-one basis, most of the individuals involved are good people trying to do the best job they can. It's only in group think (and when hundreds of billions of dollars are on the line) that their better instincts are co-opted. But the bottom line is that these players and the rest of the system get away with this nonsense because we let them.

- We need to take back control of our own health. The rest of this book will show you how to do that. Understand, all of the aforementioned agencies and organizations only exercise the power over our health that we have allowed them to take, inch by inch, over the years. We share in the responsibility for what has happened to us. We have contributed to our own bad health with every unwise choice we make at the supermarket, in fast food restaurants, and in the voting booths. Ultimately, it is up to us, as individuals and citizens, to take back control of our own health.

- We need to stop equating health with the temporary elimination of symptoms—and insist that our health-care providers do the same. The first injunction of the Hippocratic Oath, which all doctors swear to, is: "First, do no harm." We need to insist that our health-care system adheres to that injunction.

- Hamlet may have been addressing doctors when he said, "There is more in heaven and earth than is dreamt of in your philosophy." Doctors are dedicated practitioners of merely one branch of the healing arts—they are not gods. We need to take back the god-like powers we have granted them over our health. In most states and in many parts of the world, it is illegal to treat cancer with anything other than the three "approved" modalities: surgery, radiation, and chemotherapy. This is unconscionable and intolerable.

- We need to demand fairness from the medical powers that be. If only 15 percent of all medical procedures have been scientifically validated, why does alternative health care carry a 100 percent requirement? If drugs that kill over 100,000 people a year can legally be sold, why then are herbs (which may be responsible for one or two deaths a decade, when severely overdosed) under attack? We must demand a level playing field.

- There is certainly a need to control the use of pharmaceutical drugs. Some agency needs to be in charge, but government regulatory agencies need to be totally restructured and put on a leash, with their cozy ties to the pharmaceutical industry severed.

- And, yes, there needs to be some agency in charge of alternative healing. An examination of alternative health practitioners will find the same kind of quality curve you see for physicians: a small percentage of charlatans and incompetents, those practicing with merely passable skills, the dedicated and competent healers, and the brilliant "miracle doctors." Somebody needs to regulate them, along with the potions, lotions, and devices that are used. But that someone is most assuredly not the FDA, its international equivalents, or any physician-dominated group. Asking medical doctors to oversee alternative healing is like asking executives from the National Football League to oversee professional soccer in the United

States. The medical establishment doesn't like alternative healing; they have no feel for it and they view it as competitive. Certainly, there are individual doctors who support alternative medicine, but as a whole the medical establishment is extremely hostile to all forms of complementary medicine. The AMA and the FDA repeatedly demonstrate their antipathy toward alternative healing, so there's no way they can function as overseers. The only solution is to create new agencies staffed and run by alternative healers to oversee the practice of the alternative healing arts—and then in ten years, after these agencies have been infiltrated by the financial interests that back alternative healing, throw everyone out and start again.

## IN THE MEANTIME . . .

But what do we do in the meantime while waiting for these changes to take place? That's what the rest of this book is about. I'm going to lay out a different paradigm for you, based on the concept that your health has been stolen from you. I'm going to provide you with a step-by-step program that will allow you to take back control of your health and well-being.

There is nothing new or innovative about this program. As I mentioned earlier, variations of it have been used by the great healers for many decades. The results are not problematic, because they have been proven over and over, and have stood the test of time. The only thing new is that you will see it all in one place—a program that integrates all of your body's biological systems into a cohesive whole. All that's required of you is to read it and put it into practice.

# CHAPTER 2

## The Baseline of Health

- **Your Personal Health Line**
- **Basic Principles of the Baseline of Health Program**
- **A Road map to Optimum Health**

Over the years, I've lectured to thousands of people, and several hundred thousand more have read my newsletters. Even though my message is always based on the same principle espoused by all of the great miracle doctors—that the body is a holistic system and needs to be treated as such—I nevertheless receive dozens of requests from people desperately looking for that "magic" herb or supplement to "cure" themselves or their loved ones of some dreaded disease. The problem is that health does not work like that. First, the concept of the magic bullet is a myth, and second, the legal system takes a dim view of anyone espousing specific "cures" that do not fall within the mainstream of modern medicine.

The good news is that it doesn't matter. Everything you need to know is laid out in the Baseline of Health Program. Getting rid of disease is not the big problem (doctors do it all the time). The problem is making sure the disease doesn't return (something doctors don't do quite as well). And this is where the Baseline of Health Program comes in. This program is the synthesis of all the best that is taught by today's miracle doctors. It is designed to empower your own body to throw off illness and keep the illness from returning. And for those of you who are already healthy, it is designed to keep you that way—to maximize your body's defense and repair mechanisms so that you never get sick in the first place. It can even help maximize athletic performance. Variations of this program have proven so effective that thousands of people have experienced remarkable healings by using it.

## YOUR PERSONAL HEALTH LINE

Before we can understand the program itself, we first have to understand what the baseline of health actually is. For purposes of our discussion, we will use a simple chart to represent the state of our health. The Y axis represents the level of our health. On the X axis, we have all the systems and organs that affect our health. These actually number in the hundreds (if not thousands), but to keep things simple on our chart, we'll list just three: the immune system, the circulatory system, and control of mutated cells. For all these systems and organs, there are only three lines that we are concerned with:

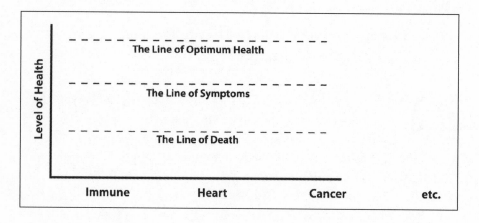

- The Line of Optimum Health—In a perfect world, our Personal Health Line would match the Line of Optimum Health. In reality, that's not achievable, so what we try to do is keep everything as close to Optimum Health as possible.

- The Line of Symptoms—As long as all our organs and systems function above this line, we have no problems. But the moment any part of our Personal Health Line dips below the Line of Symptoms, problems begin to manifest. Sometimes, the problems are so slight that we don't notice them at first, such as the early warning signals of heart disease and cancer. But at a certain point, if the symptoms persist long enough, and if our Personal Health Line dips below the Line of Symptoms far enough, we take notice.

- The Death Line—If any part of our Personal Health Line touches the Death Line, we die.

Now let's take a look at this concept in action. As an example, we'll track the case history of Jim, an average forty-year-old. Below is Jim's Personal Health Line at birth:

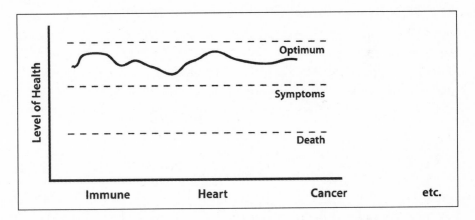

As we can see from Jim's line, he was born with a slight weakness (either genetic or as a result of his parents' lifestyle and environment) in his circulatory system. Note also that, at birth, Jim is in relatively good health and is symptom free (since no point on his Personal Health Line dips below the Line of Symptoms). Over the forty years of his life, however, Jim has contributed to that weakness in his heart and circulatory system because of a diet high in hydrogenated oils (trans-fats) and refined carbohydrates, a folic acid deficiency, a low pH (acidic body fluids and tissues), and heavy free radical damage, to the point where his Personal Health Line has dipped below the Line of Symptoms and he has begun to experience symptoms such as shortness of breath and minor chest pains.

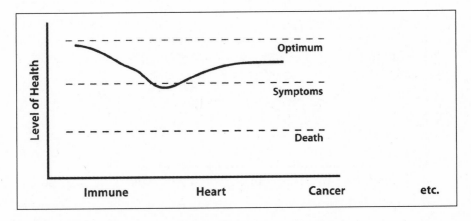

A friend of Jim's suggests that he try an antioxidant supplement. Since the antioxidant addresses one of Jim's problems (free radical damage), Jim's Personal Health Line once again rises above the Line of Symptoms (even if just by a little bit) and all of Jim's visible symptoms disappear.

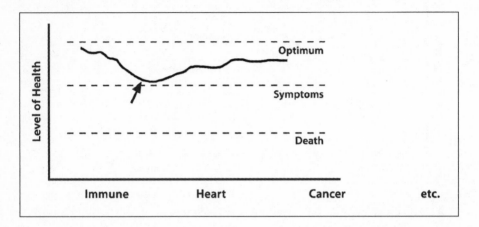

"It's a miracle! All of my symptoms are gone. I'm cured. If you have any heart problems or any health problems at all, you must try this supplement." Jim is so excited, he decides to promote the antioxidant company as a network marketing distributor and proceeds to sell his miracle cure to everyone he meets. One day, he talks to Mary, who also has heart problems. Like Jim, Mary was also born with a predilection to heart problems, and like Jim she has managed to exacerbate that problem through folic acid deficiency, low pH, and a high-stress work environment on Wall Street.

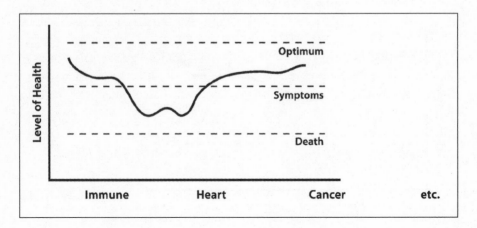

Jim convinces Mary to buy a supply of his "miracle" antioxidant and, as recommended by Jim, Mary starts gulping down handfuls of her daily dose. But unlike Jim, Mary has very little free radical damage because she eats a Mediterranean diet with olive oil and red wine—two foods that, over the years, have mitigated any free radical damage. The net result is that Mary notices no change in her condition.

Mary now proceeds to tell Jim that he's crazy, that whatever benefit he got from the antioxidant was purely a placebo effect, and that it's a waste of money. Of course, later on, when Mary enters a stress management program, or has heart bypass surgery, she tells everyone that she's found the *real* cure for heart disease and recommends to all her friends that they do the same. It's worth noting that the antioxidant did, in fact, significantly improve the overall level of her Personal Health Line, but since Mary didn't feel any difference, she incorrectly assumed that she had received no benefit.

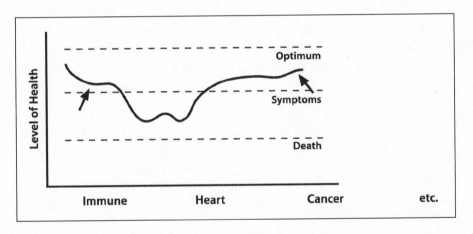

The bottom line is that the same supplement used by two different people for the same condition produced two entirely different results. What does that mean? It means that gulping down "miracle" herbs and supplements to treat disease is like trying to hit a clay pigeon in the sky with a 22-caliber rifle . . . while blindfolded. The odds are very much against you.

The secret to health, the secret to all the success that the great alternative healers share, is that they look to raise every inch of a person's Personal Health Line. If you do that, if you raise the entire line, the odds are in your favor. In fact, it's almost impossible to miss.

## BASIC PRINCIPLES OF THE BASELINE OF HEALTH PROGRAM

1. Your body is composed of a series of integrated systems—some large (such as your organs, immune system, and hormonal systems) and some small (such as your cellular energy system, the blood/brain barrier, and various enzyme systems). Your body is the sum of those systems, and it is only as strong as the weakest of them. You can have the strength of a Hercules, but if the smallest of blood clots manages to get lodged in an artery leading to your brain, you can drop dead in the blink of an eye. Again, you are only as strong as your weakest link.

2. Your body is designed to be healthy. It has intelligent, built-in mechanisms to repair damage, optimize performance, and keep you going—provided you don't damage those mechanisms. So, what can damage them?

   • An accumulation of toxins and harmful substances, including heavy metals, industrial chemicals, xenoestrogens (synthetic substances such as some pesticides and food additives that mimic the action of hormones), too many free radicals, unrelieved stress, excessive circulating immune complexes, etc., steadily degrades function. If these substances accumulate beyond the body's ability to eliminate them, the degradation of your internal organs and systems will be both rapid and catastrophic.

   • An insufficient supply of essential nutrients also degrades function. Quite simply, you cannot build the same body out of pepperoni pizza, beer, and Ding Dongs® as you can out of live foods.

3. Since you don't know everything affecting your body at any point in time, you've got to do the entire program all at once. You can't look for magic bullets—if there were a magic bullet for what ails you, your doctor would have given it to you already. Or to state it another way: suppressing symptoms is not actually the same thing as eliminating the cause of a disease. Magic bullets and drugs are basically symptom suppressors. The Baseline of Health Program can actually eliminate the causes of many diseases, even if we don't know exactly what those causes are!

That's the Baseline of Health Program. Everything else in this book is commentary, but that commentary is important. It provides the step-by-step instructions that allow you to attain these three principles. For the most part, these instructions are presented in a defined sequence. For example, intestinal cleansing comes before diet so that you end up maximizing the nutrition you draw from your food. Enzymes come before rebuilding your immune system, because eliminating circulating immune complexes (CICs) with enzymes frees up a massive burden on your immune system, thus making it that much easier to rebuild your immune response. Yes, you can jump right to a specific topic of interest, but your results will be far better if you start at the beginning and rebuild your body systems one by one, in sequence.

## A ROAD MAP TO OPTIMUM HEALTH

The body systems and topics that we're going to address throughout the rest of this book are as follows.

### Cleansing and Detoxification

- Intestinal Cleansing—Digestive disorders are responsible for over 50 million physician visits and more hospitalizations than any other category of medical problem. Cleaning out the elimination channels is fundamental to any health building program.

- Intestinal Rebuilding with Probiotics—As a result of chlorinated/fluorinated/treated water and antibiotics and pesticides in our food, we have virtually eliminated an essential component of health and well-being: the friendly bacteria in our gut. There can be no true health or relief from disease until we rebuild those beneficial bacteria with probiotics.

- Your Mouth is Killing You—Aluminum in your cookware, mercury in your fillings, and root canals from your dentist can all be deadly. Avoiding these potential hazards is essential to the program.

- Cleansing Your Liver, Blood, and Kidneys—Our liver is the primary filter of our body. Over time, we so abuse it and overtax it that illness is the inevitable result. Our blood is filled with many impurities, including everything from an overabundance of artificial fats to toxic heavy metals. These must be removed for optimum health. And kidney disease, the consequence of ill-advised dietary and lifestyle choices, is approaching epidemic levels. Detoxification and rebuilding programs, such as a kidney flush or liver/gallbladder/blood flush, as well as chelation therapy for heavy metals, can produce a profound improvement in your health.

## Diet, Water, and Supplements

- Diet, the Slow Killer—Every cell, organ, and system in our bodies is produced from the food we eat. Sorry, but you can't make a healthy body from a diet predominantly comprised of potato chips and diet soda. We'll address five key areas: healthy and unhealthy fats, refined and complex carbohydrates, good and bad sources of protein, poor quality food, and Frankenfoods (genetic engineering, irradiation, and microwaves).

- Dying of Thirst—Clean water for drinking, bathing, and growing food is one of the most precious commodities on the planet. Unknowingly, virtually everyone in the world now drinks tap water that is polluted by pharmaceutical residues, biofilm, and other contaminants—not to mention adulterated with known carcinogens such as chlorine and fluoride. Why is clean water so important? Quite simply, it's essential for life. And the sad fact is that most people just don't get enough. We will explore both how to optimize the quality of the water you drink and bathe in and how to maximize its bioavailability in your body.

- Vitamins, Minerals, and Phytochemicals—You often hear doctors say that there's no need to supplement if you eat a balanced diet. Unfortunately, the food we eat today is not as nutritious as the food available even fifty years ago. We have to compensate for the loss of "value" in our food. Supplementation of some kind is mandatory. I'll discuss how to differentiate between good and bad supplements and how to determine which supplements you should take.

- Free Radicals and Antioxidants—Scientists now know that free radicals play a major role in the aging process as well as in the onset of cancer, heart disease, stroke, arthritis, possibly allergies, and a host of other ailments. But which antioxidants work best for you and how much should you take? I'll provide you with a formula for finding the best antioxidant.

- Enzymes = Life—Modern man is the only animal that eats a diet almost entirely devoid of live enzymes. As a result, virtually every American has an enlarged pancreas by the time he or she is forty and a significantly diminished life expectancy. Oral enzymes can help eliminate this problem.

- Miracle Herbs—Herbs are an important part of any healthy lifestyle. While herbs are currently a hot topic in the health world, they are also under siege by business and government entities interested in controlling their use. The Baseline of Health Program provides tips on finding the best herbal products and how to guarantee optimal results.

## Balancing the Body's Systems

- Balancing Hormone Levels in the Body—Every day, we are exposed to thousands of chemicals that work to destroy the hormonal balance of our bodies, with disastrous effects. Diet, stress, and environmental factors are constantly working to throw our bodies out of balance. Correcting these imbalances can save our health and our sanity! Advice for supplementing with bio-identical hormones, as well as safe natural alternatives, is provided.

- Optimizing Your Immune System—Your immune system is the most awesome system in your body, easily rivaling your brain in terms of complexity, subtlety, and self-awareness. Yet we seem to do everything in our power to destroy it. For example, just one can of cola can depress parts of your immune system by some 50 percent for as long as six hours. There is no chance for good health, or the elimination of disease, until your immune system has been optimized. We will discuss how to use natural immune system builders, pathogen destroyers, and immunomodulators to take your immune system to the next level.

- It's All About Energy—All life is energy. Optimize that energy and you optimize your health. The proper use of energy in the healing arts has a long and significant history. Charge your body with the right frequencies and you can prevent, and in many cases even reverse, disease.

- The Thought That Kills—For years, stress and depression have been suspected of increasing the risk of contracting numerous infectious diseases and even cancer. What we think (and how we think) absolutely (and unequivocally) does affect our health. You'll learn how to alleviate stress and depression with natural alternatives, including vitamins and minerals, herbs, breathing exercises, and meditation.

- Exercise: Move or Die—Exercise fundamentally changes every system and function in your body. Regular exercise does everything from improving the health of the heart to building up your bones and speeding up the elimination of toxins from your body. The Baseline of Health Program helps you optimize your exercise routine to maximize the whole range of health benefits.

## Specific Conditions

- The Cholesterol Myth and Other Cardiovascular Stories—Would you like to drive your doctor crazy? Just ask him or her, "If cholesterol is responsible for clogging my arteries, why doesn't it clog my veins too?" The answer is that cholesterol is guilty primarily by being found at the scene of the crime, not because it actually commits the crime. We'll take a look at the real causes of cardiovascular disease and how diet, exercise, and other options can lower your risk.

- Let's Talk About Cancer—The incidence of cancer is soaring: it is up between 800 and 1,700 percent in the last 100 years (depending on whose statistics you look at). We'll look at the real reasons behind this alarming trend and look at your options for avoiding becoming another statistic.

- The Plagues of Our Time—The incidences of Alzheimer's disease, osteoporosis, multiple sclerosis (MS), and diabetes are all rising rapidly. They are monsters of our own creation—largely the result of inapt choices. We'll explore each of these conditions and natural options for prevention and treatment.

- Aging: It's Not Just for the Old—We may not have any choice about getting older, but we sure have a choice about how we age. While there may not be a single magic bullet you can take, there are definitely steps that you can implement that will not only help retard the aging process but will also keep you more youthful and energized for longer than you ever thought possible.

Once you've learned the hows, whys, and wherefores of health, I will detail specific recommendations on what you can do to build your baseline of health, day by day. I will outline a step-by-step program (based on all that has been learned from the miracle doctors and from over thirty years of my own work in the development of cutting-edge nutritional products) for optimizing your health and eliminating disease from your body.

So with that in mind, let's look, step-by-step, at how we maximize our Personal Health Line. Let's begin by looking at how we clean out and purify the body.

# PART TWO

# *Cleansing and Detoxification*

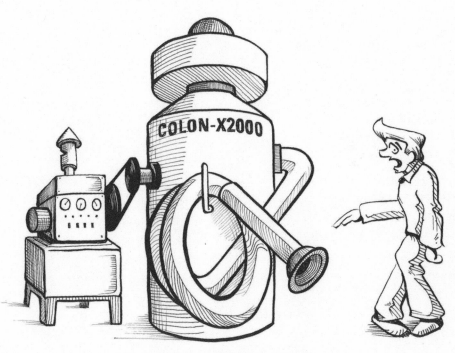

*And that's going up my what?!?*

# CHAPTER 3

# *Intestinal Cleansing*

- **Problems in the Digestive System**
- **What's Gone Wrong?**
- **Health Begins with the Intestinal Tract**
- **Ways to Cleanse the Intestines**

T here is an old saying that "death begins in the colon." This is an oversimplification, to be sure, but more accurate than not. In fact, the road to health begins with intestinal cleansing and detoxification—no matter what the disease or problem. Unfortunately, most people confine their understanding of intestinal cleansing to its effect on fecal matter. And while it is true that cleansing programs do draw old fecal matter out of the colon, limiting the discussion to this misses the big picture.

The digestive system in humans is essentially a continuous tube from the mouth to the anus. (Don't think about that the next time you kiss someone.) As a system, it performs several critical functions, ranging from digestion to immune support, with each part of the tube performing a specific function:

- Digestion of the food we eat.

- Transferring the nutritional value of that food into the body.

- Processing the waste from that food and eliminating it from the body.

- Serving as a drain pipe for waste produced as a result of metabolic functions within the body itself.

- Serving as a drain for toxic substances absorbed through our lungs and skin.

- Functioning as a first line of defense in the body's immune system by identifying and eliminating viruses and unhealthy bacteria ingested with our food and water.

As you can see from this list, the digestive system is critical to your health and well-being. Any program of intestinal cleansing and detoxification, therefore, must address all of these aspects. Specifically, it must serve to:

- Remove all old fecal matter and waste from the colon (to clear the drain, if you will).

- Help remove all the heavy metals and drug residues that have accumulated in the body as a result of having your drain plugged.

- Strengthen the colon muscle so that it works again.

- Repair any damage, such as herniations and inflammations of the colon and small intestine.

- Eliminate the presence of polyps and other abnormal growths that have been allowed to flourish because of an unhealthy intestinal environment.

- Rebuild and replenish the various "friendly" bacteria cultures that ideally should line virtually every square inch of the tube—again, from mouth to anus.

## PROBLEMS IN THE DIGESTIVE SYSTEM

Diseases of the digestive system have reached an all time high in the United States and are still on the rise. In 1985, 60–70 million Americans were affected by digestive disorders.[1] Today, it's over 100 million. The number two cancer among men and women combined is colorectal cancer, trailing only lung cancer. The incidence of diverticulosis has increased dramatically from just 10 percent of the adult population over the age of 45 who had this disease in 1952 to an astounding "every person has many" diverticuli, according to the 1992 edition of the *Merck Manual.* In other words, according to the latest medical studies, virtually all American adults will eventually have diverticulosis of the large intestine if they live long enough.

Digestive disorders are responsible for over 50 million physician visits and more hospitalizations than any other category of medical problem in the United States.[2] The total cost to the American public for all aspects of digestive disease is well over $100 billion per year.[3] The most prevalent digestive diseases include:

- Constipation and the attendant symptoms of self-toxification
- Diverticular disease (herniations of the colon)

- Polyps
- Hemorrhoids
- Irritable bowel syndrome

- Ulcerative colitis
- Crohn's disease
- Colorectal cancer

It is worth noting that many other diseases that at first glance appear to have no connection with the digestive tract have actually been related by many doctors to functional bowel disorder. These include diabetes, gallstones and kidney stones, gout, hypertension, varicose veins, rheumatoid arthritis, psoriasis, and obesity.

As if that were not enough, it has been estimated that as many as 80 percent of Americans are afflicted with intestinal parasites. Many health professionals would dispute this number, calling it far too high, and if you limit your discussion of parasites to things such as tapeworms and Chinese liver flukes, they are correct. But as soon as you open up to the true nature of the problem and include the lesser known, but far more prevalent, parasites such as *Fasciolopsis buskii*, the 80 percent figure begins to fall into line. And if you include pathogenic *E. coli* and *Candida* yeast overgrowths, then the 80 percent figure is decidedly conservative.

Symptoms of parasites include nervousness, grinding of the teeth at night, aches and pains that move from place to place in the body, mimicked appendicitis, ulcers and various digestive pain, nausea or diarrhea, itching, acne, foul breath, furred tongue, jaundice, fatigue, menstrual irregularities, and insomnia.

More doctors are becoming aware of how endemic yeast infections such as *Candida albicans* truly are. Symptoms include chronic fatigue (especially after eating), depression, bloating and gas, cramps, chronic diarrhea or constipation, rectal itching, allergies, severe premenstrual syndrome (PMS), impotence, memory loss, severe mood swings, recurrent fungal infections (such as athlete's foot), extreme sensitivity to chemicals (perfumes, smoke, odors, etc.), and lightheadedness or drunkenness after minimal wine, beer, or sugar ingestion.

## WHAT'S GONE WRONG?

Our modern lifestyle has taken its toll on our digestive and elimination organs. Refined, processed, low-fiber foods, animal fats, a lack of exercise, and an ever increasing level of stress all contribute to our current gastrointestinal health crisis.

Consider that a sluggish bowel can retain pounds of old toxic and poisonous fecal matter (2–3 pounds is common, 10–20 pounds is not as unusual as you might think, and up to 65 pounds has actually been reported in exceptional cases). Often, the real cause behind sickness and disease is this retention and reabsorption of built-up toxic waste. Now, doctors who perform colonoscopies dispute these numbers, saying that they never see any sign of this mythical accumulated fecal matter. But then it has to be remembered that they have their patients drink a purgative the day before a colonoscopy to "blow out" any trace of fecal matter, so that it doesn't interfere with the colonoscopy. Duh!

In the U.S., the average frequency of stool passage is just over three bowel movements per week.[4] Individuals with colonic inertia (a condition of the colon when muscles do not work properly, causing constipation) often do not pass a stool for 7–10 days at a time. There has been a great misconception among the public and most medical professionals about how often a healthy person should move their bowels. For years, doctors have thought that anywhere between one bowel movement a day and one a week was normal. (Unfortunately, that's probably the norm of the doctors who think it.) What we have learned is that it is normal, and *necessary*, to have one bowel movement a day for each major meal you ate the day before. If you eat three meals, you should have three bowel movements the next day.

A sluggish bowel also has a major health impact on another body system: your lymph system. Think for a moment, if you will, of your colon as your body's drain pipe—the drain that removes waste from your body. If the drain is clogged, not only will waste not be eliminated, but when you flush the toilet, the drain backs up and spills over. And that's exactly the point which leads us to a discussion of waste removal from the body and the lymph system.

The lymph vessels are a network of capillaries that filter blood impurities; they contain a clear, colorless fluid called lymph. Lymph passes from capillaries to lymph vessels and flows through lymph nodes that are located along the course of these vessels. Cells of the lymph nodes phagocytize, or ingest, impurities such as bacteria, old red blood cells, and toxic and cellular waste. Lymph fluid can also collect other impurities such as heavy metals, pesticides, and drug residues stored in bodily tissue.

Once loaded with toxic waste, the compromised lymph must exit your body. What can't be eliminated in your urine must pass out through your colon. What do you think happens to all this waste if the plumbing is plugged up or sluggish? It backs up into your bloodstream. Is it any wonder we get sick and keep on getting sicker? Is it any wonder that the incidence of lymph cancer is doubling every twenty years?

## HEALTH BEGINS WITH THE INTESTINAL TRACT

The foundation of any health or healing program must begin with the intestinal tract—not necessarily because it is inherently more important than any other system or organ in the body, but because it's the area of the body upon which we focus our greatest abuse, and because it impacts virtually every other system in the body.

Your intestinal tract is the source of all nutrient access to your body. If it isn't working properly, you have two major problems. First, you have a hard time digesting food properly—breaking it down sufficiently so that your body can use it. And then, even if you can digest it properly, if the intestinal wall is covered with hardened waste and colonies of hostile bacteria, you'll end up absorbing only a fraction of the nutritional value of the food you eat.

In addition, the colon is the main elimination channel of the body. It is the means by which we eliminate the toxic waste of the digestive process, including massive amounts of *E. coli* bacteria and parasite larvae. If that waste hangs around longer than necessary, its impact on the body is profound. We've already discussed how waste from the lymph system passes out through the colon, but so too does waste from the liver. The liver filters out dangerous drug residues and poisons from the blood and passes them out of the body through the colon via the bile duct. Plug the colon and everything backs up—the net result is sickness and disease. The important point to remember here is that you can't even begin to cleanse and repair the other systems in the body until you clean out the colon so that the toxic material will have a path out of the body.

Physically, the colon is not designed to store large amounts of old fecal matter. If you have pounds of extra garbage in there, there's only one thing that can happen; the colon must distend and expand. This causes the walls of the colon to thin out (like blowing up a balloon more and more). As the walls extend out, they press on and compress other organs in the abdominal cavity. Also, old fecal matter is an ideal breeding ground for harmful bacteria and dangerous parasites.

Any program, then, designed to improve our health or to eliminate disease from our bodies must begin with intestinal cleansing and detoxification. It is the *sine qua non* of health (literally, "without which, there is not").

## WAYS TO CLEANSE THE INTESTINES

In order to clean and detoxify the colon, it is mandatory that you address several key areas. To be effective, any intestinal rebuilding program must:

- Help bring the colon back to life by stimulating the muscle movement of the colon, encouraging matter to move forward through the system and halting putrefaction.

- Draw old fecal matter off the walls of the colon and out of any bowel pockets.

- Disinfect.

- Draw out poisons and toxins, leach out heavy metals such as mercury and lead, remove chemicals, drug residues, and even radioactive material such as strontium 90.

- Soothe and promote the healing of the mucous membrane lining the entire digestive tract.

- Help stimulate the body to begin the healing and repair of herniated areas.

- Increase the flow of bile to help clean the gallbladder, bile ducts, and liver.

- Optimize the growth of beneficial bacteria, which are a fundamental component of intestinal health.

- Destroy and expel parasites and inhibit *Candida albicans* overgrowth.

- Maintain regularity.

- Decrease straining.

- Speed up the transit time of feces through the large intestine.

Once you look at the requirements of a good intestinal program, it's easy to see that no one formula or magic pill can accomplish it all.

### Thoughts on Enemas and Colonics

During an enema, water is inserted into the rectum through a tube, causing the emptying of the lower bowel. Enemas are useful for a quick fix, particularly when you are "temporarily" backed up. However, they only flush loose fecal matter in the lower part of the colon, and they do nothing to restore normal functioning to the colon.

A colonic is a type of enema that injects large amounts of water, under controlled pressure, through the rectum and high into the colon for cleansing purposes. Some treatments add ingredients to the water, such as peroxide, herbs, or coffee, to bolster the cleansing action. Think of the colonic as a powered enema—it still only captures loose fecal matter, but goes higher into the colon and is more thorough.

Colonics do work to flush loose waste and sediment from the rectum and lower intestine, but they have several drawbacks. They can actually weaken bowel muscles over time. Colonics don't draw toxins from bowel pockets or from tissue. They do, however, flush all bacteria out—the good as well as the bad. Colonics can also disrupt natural pH (acid/alkaline) balance. Finally, you run the risk that some water retained in the equipment from another patient's previous use may be injected into your colon. Yech!

However, if you are so inclined, periodic colonics are not necessarily a bad thing. They can definitely improve your health and sense of well-being. Regular colonics, on the other hand, may be too much of a good thing.

## GENERAL RECOMMENDATIONS

The Baseline of Health Program uses a four-pronged approach.

1. A good source of soluble fiber to compensate for all of the fiberless processed foods, meat, and dairy that we eat. The two best sources of fiber are psyllium seed husks and freshly ground organic flaxseed meal. (It should be freshly ground, or at the very least stabilized, so that it does not go rancid.) One tablespoon of psyllium each day or 1.5 tablespoons of ground flax in the morning and evening with juice will keep you regular. Flax also provides you with healthy omega-3 essential oils. In addition, the sulfur-rich proteins and lignans present in the seeds work hand in hand with the omega-3 oils to reverse mutated cells and cancer in the body.

2. Most people will need a stimulating herbal colon-activator formula that provides both cleansing and healing to the entire gastrointestinal system (at least until their colons rebuild).

   Look for a formula that contains all organic herbs such as cape aloe, senna, cascara sagrada, barberry, ginger root, *Terminalia cherbula*, African bird pepper, and fennel. This formula will serve as an intestinal detoxifier to loosen and draw out old fecal matter, waste, and toxins. It will stimulate peristalsis (the muscular movement of the colon), halt putrefaction, and disinfect, soothe, and heal the mucous membrane lining of your entire digestive tract. These herbal formulas can also help improve digestion, relieve gas and cramps, increase the flow of bile (which in turn cleans the gallbladder, bile ducts, and liver), destroy *Candida albicans* overgrowth and expel intestinal parasites, and promote a healthy intestinal flora.

3. Periodically (approximately every three months), you will need a strong purifier and intestinal vacuum to help draw old fecal matter off the walls of your colon and out of any bowel pockets and to also draw out poisons, toxins, and heavy metals from your body. Such a formula will also remove over 2,000 known drug residues as well as radioactive residues.

    Look for a formula that contains all organic herbs such as apple fruit pectin, pharmaceutical-grade montmorillonite clay, slippery elm bark, licorice root, marshmallow root, fennel seed, pau d'arco, activated willow charcoal, and psyllium seeds and husks. The natural mucilaginous properties of this formula will soften old hardened fecal matter for easy removal. This also makes it an excellent remedy for any inflammation or irritation in the stomach and intestines. This formula is helpful in irritable bowel syndrome, diverticular disease, hemorrhoids, and even food poisoning or stomach flu.

4. Consistent use of a good probiotic formula is essential to promote the growth of beneficial bacteria colonies in the intestinal tract. (We will talk more about this in the next chapter.) Also, for some people, a good probiotic formula alone will serve to wake up their colon and get it working again.

Regular use of this four-part program will help keep your body in optimal health and vitality for as long as you live.

Okay, we've now learned how to clean out and purify the intestinal tract. Let's explore in detail how we can repopulate it with beneficial bacteria for digestive health.

# CHAPTER 4

# Intestinal Rebuilding with Probiotics

- **The Probiotic Miracle**
- **What Harms the Beneficial Bacteria?**
- **The Benefits of Friendly Bacteria in the Intestinal Tract**

Cleaning out the bad stuff in the digestive tract is merely the first step in cleansing and detoxification. A crucial next step is to rebuild your intestinal tract and help it recover from any harm that's been done. Probiotics, supplements containing friendly bacteria, can rebalance your intestinal tract with healthy bacteria, which is critical for proper digestion and as a first line of defense in fighting disease.

## THE PROBIOTIC MIRACLE

Before you were born, your intestines were free of microorganisms. They were virtually sterile. From the moment you passed through the birth canal swallowing flora on your way out, however, bacteria (both beneficial and harmful) began a fight for dominance destined to continue until the day you die. If you were breast-fed, somewhere between days four and seven after you were born the "good guys" won the battle and staked their claim to virtually every square inch of your digestive tract.

It's a battle that's never totally won, however, as the harmful bacteria are never completely eliminated. But in a healthy body, the bad guys never get a chance to gain a foothold to colonize and reproduce exponentially. One of the problems, of course, is that every second of every single day, we are constantly exposed to billions of potentially harmful microorganisms, with every breath that we take, bite of food that we swallow, or swig of water that we drink.

Researchers now realize that one of the chief reasons breast-fed babies get so many fewer infections than formula-fed babies is that mother's milk tends to promote the growth of beneficial bacteria in the gastrointestinal tract, whereas store-bought formulas have no such beneficial effect. In fact, the primary role of colostrum, the fluid in the breasts that nourishes the baby until the breast milk becomes available, is to "launch" the baby's immune system. The net result is that, in a breast-fed baby, beneficial bacteria (such as acidophilus and bifidobacteria) control over 90 percent of the intestinal tract. These microorganisms, in turn, produce a large amount of essential byproducts in the intestines, which act as a barrier to the growth of pathogenic microbes that can cause disease and infection. When you're healthy, over 100 trillion microorganisms from some 400 species flourish in your intestinal tract. They cover virtually every square inch of available surface space from your mouth to your anus, thus crowding out all harmful bacteria—allowing them no place to gain a foothold. They also aid in digestion, absorption, and the production of significant amounts of B vitamins, vitamin K, and enzymes.

## WHAT HARMS THE BENEFICIAL BACTERIA?

Unfortunately, the levels of beneficial bacteria decline dramatically as the human body ages. Some of the reasons for this decline include:

- Over time, the colonies of friendly bacteria naturally age and lose their vitality.

- Disruptions and changes in the acid/alkaline balance of the bowels can play a major role in reducing the growth of beneficial bacteria. In addition, these changes tend to favor the growth of harmful viral and fungal organisms as well as putrefactive, disease-causing bacteria.

- Nonsteroidal anti-inflammatory drugs (NSAIDs) such Advil, Motrin, Midol, etc., are destructive to intestinal flora.

- Chlorine in the drinking water not only serves to kill bacteria in the water, it is equally devastating to the colonies of beneficial bacteria living in the intestines. In fact, drinking even one glass of chlorinated water can destroy much of your intestinal flora.

- Radiation and chemotherapy are particularly harmful to your inner bacterial environment.

- Virtually all meat, chicken, and dairy that you eat (other than organic) is loaded with antibiotics, which destroy all of the beneficial bacteria in your gastrointestinal tract.

- A diet high in meats and fats—because they take so long to break down in the human body—promotes the growth of the harmful, putrefying bacteria.

- Constipation, of course, allows harmful bacteria to hang around longer, which allows them to proliferate.

- Cigarettes, alcohol, and stress are also major culprits.

- Some antibiotic herbs, such as goldenseal, are detrimental if taken in sufficient quantity and/or used too frequently. Colloidal silver presents the same problems.

- And if you've ever been subjected to a round of "medicinal" antibiotics, you can kiss your beneficial bacteria good-bye. The problem is that antibiotics indiscriminately destroy both bad and good bacteria, allowing virulent, mutant strains of harmful microorganisms to emerge and run rampant inside the body. Antibiotics (both medicinal and in our food supply) are the number one culprit in the overgrowth of harmful pathogens in the gastrointestinal tract (a condition called dysbiosis). And for the same reasons, it is no coincidence that women suffer so many yeast infections after taking any antibiotics.

## THE BENEFITS OF FRIENDLY BACTERIA IN THE INTESTINAL TRACT

A properly functioning intestinal tract is one of your body's first lines of defense against invaders. In a healthy colon, there are, on average, well over 100 billion beneficial bacteria per milliliter of fecal matter that consume harmful bacteria and other invaders. In the typical digestive tract, because of poor diet and neglect of the colon, the beneficial bacteria count may be as low as four or five per milliliter (not 4 billion, just plain old four). Many researchers now believe that declining levels of friendly bacteria in the intestinal tract may actually mark the onset of chronic degenerative disease.

A healthy intestinal tract balanced with friendly bacteria can:

- Lower cholesterol
- Assist in the digestion of carbohydrates

- Help prevent constipation

- Inhibit cancer

- Protect against food poisoning

- Protect against stomach ulcers

- Protect against lactose intolerance and casein intolerance

- Protect against many harmful bacteria, viruses, and fungi

- Protect against *Candida* overgrowth and vaginal yeast infections

- Prevent and correct constipation and diarrhea, ileitis and colitis, irritable bowel syndrome, and a whole range of other digestive tract dysfunctions

- Improve the health and appearance of the skin

- Enhance nutrition by improving absorption and internally generating B vitamins and vitamin K

- Enhance immunity by killing off invading pathogens and producing immune-boosting biochemicals such as transfer factor and lactoferrin—beneficial bacteria are actually responsible for 60 to 70 percent of your immune system's activity

## GENERAL RECOMMENDATIONS

There can be no true health or recovery from disease unless you have colonies of over 100 trillion beneficial microorganisms flourishing throughout your intestinal tract, aiding in digestion and absorption, producing significant amounts of vitamins and enzymes, and working to crowd out all harmful bacteria. A good probiotic formula containing supplemental friendly bacteria is mandatory to raise your baseline of health. It is absolutely essential for long-term intestinal health and long-term parasite control. When choosing a probiotic supplement, look for the following characteristics:

- Not all strains of beneficial bacteria are created equal. For each type of bacteria, there are recognized super strains. Choose a formula that uses only recognized super strains of beneficial bacteria. They will be identified as such on the label or in the company literature.

- There are many beneficial bacteria that may be contained in a good probiotic, but two are preeminent. *Lactobacillus acidophilus* resides primarily in the small intestine and produces a number of powerful antimicrobial compounds in the gut (including acidolin, acidolphilin, lactocidin, and bacteriocin). These compounds can inhibit the growth and toxin-producing capabilities of some twenty-three pathogens (including *Campylobacter*, listeria, and staphylococci), as well as reduce tumor growth and effectively neutralize or inhibit carcinogenic substances. There are three recognized super strains of acidophilus: DDS, NAS, and BT1386. (It's also important to note that *L. acidophilus* is the primary beneficial bacteria in the vaginal tract. When the presence of the acidophilus is compromised, this allows the bad guys such as *Gardnerella vaginalis*, *E. coli*, or *Chlamydia* to take over. This is particularly important to women to help prevent a whole range of vaginal infections.)

Many researchers believe that declining levels of *Bifidobacteria* in the large intestine actually mark the eventual onset of chronic degenerative disease. *Bifidobacteria* benefit the body in a number of ways. They consume old fecal matter. They also have the ability to remove cancer-forming elements or the enzymes that lead to their formation. This can help protect against the formation of liver, colon, and mammary gland tumors. And in addition to all of that, *Bifidobacteria* are substantial producers of a range of important B vitamins.

- More is not always better. Too many beneficial bacteria in one formula may find the bacteria competing with each other before they can establish themselves in separate areas of the intestinal tract. On the other hand, there are several other bacteria that are extremely beneficial in any probiotic formula. *L. salivarius* helps digest foods in the intestinal tract and makes vital nutrients more assimilable. It also works to eat away encrusted fecal matter throughout the entire colon, helps repair the intestinal tract by providing needed enzymes and essential nutrients, and adheres to the intestinal wall, thereby forming a living matrix that helps protect the mucosal lining.

    *L. rhamnosus* is a powerful immune stimulator. It can increase the natural killing activity of spleen cells, which may help to prevent tumor formation. It boosts the ability of the body to destroy foreign invaders and other harmful matter by three times normal activity and has been shown to increase circulating antibody levels by six to eight times. *L. plantarum* has the ability to eliminate thousands of species of pathogenic bacteria. It also has extremely high adherence potential for epithelial tissue and seems to favor colonizing the same areas of the intestinal tract that *E. coli* prefers—in effect, serving to crowd *E. coli* out of the body. At one time, *L. plantarum* was a major part of our diets (found in sourdough bread, sauerkraut, etc.), but it is now virtually nowhere to be found. Other important friendly bacteria you might find in a good formula include *Streptococcus thermophilus*, *L. bulgaricus*, *B. longum*, and *L. casei*.

- Much has been written about the properties of the soil-based bacteria such as *Bacillus subtilis*, *L. sporogenes*, and *B. laterosporus*. For many people, they can produce a powerful boost to the immune system, but in certain circumstances they may become toxic. It's hard to argue with the great results that many people have had using formulations that contain these cultures. On the other hand, it's possible to get all of the same results using only the cultures that I've mentioned above.

- A good probiotic formulation will usually contain fructo-oligosaccharides (FOS), a sugar that helps promote the growth of beneficial bacteria. For some of these bacteria, FOS can increase their effectiveness by a factor of 1,000 times or more. The key in using FOS is to make sure you use a variety that has been designed to specifically promote the growth of only the beneficial bacteria, not the bad guys.

- Make sure the formula you choose was developed using full-culture processing so that the beneficial bacteria and its powerful supernatant are kept together. The supernatant, which is the medium the culture was grown in, contains a multitude of beneficial byproducts of the growth process, including vitamins, enzymes, antioxidants, and immune stimulators.

- Then there's the question of how many live microorganisms are in your formula when you actually use it. Pick up any probiotic formula, look at the label, and you'll see something like this: "Contains 13 billion live organisms per capsule at time of manufacture." And that's the problem: the words "at time of manufacture." The die-off rate can be astounding. Most formulas will quickly experience a surprisingly large die-off—for example, from 13 billion down to a paltry 13 million—within just sixty days of manufacture, unless they are protected from heat and moisture which accelerate the process. Conscientious manufacturers recommend that both you and the store from which you bought your formula keep probiotics refrigerated. Look for a formula that has been refrigerated from the moment it was manufactured to the day you buy it. An alternative is to look for formulations that use tableting and encapsulation techniques that seal the bacteria from moisture.

- Some manufacturers claim that you need to use enterically coated capsules to protect the bacteria from stomach acid, which kills the bacteria, but this makes no sense. If stomach acid killed beneficial bacteria, then no one who ate fermented foods over the centuries would have received any benefit from the bacteria they contained, since all of the bacteria in those foods would have been destroyed by stomach acid. Nonsense! Bottom line: beneficial bacteria do not need to be enterically coated; they survive stomach acid quite nicely, particularly if consumed without food.

- Start slowly. When you first start using a probiotic supplement, there is a good chance that you will precipitate a die-off of bad bacteria in your intestinal tract. This can lead to excessive gas and stomach rumblings and cramping for 10–21 days. If you experience any problem with your initial dosage, back it down. Start again with one capsule (or even half a capsule) for several days. Build up slowly to the recommended dosage for your particular supplement.

- Eating yogurt (unless you make your own) does not really help. First, the bacteria used to make most yogurt (*L. bulgaricus* and *S. thermophilus*) are not the key beneficial bacteria, although they are indeed helpful. (Some brands throw in a small amount of acidophilus after the fact—just so they can put it on the label.) Even more important, though, much of the yogurt that you buy in the store is now pasteurized after it is made. Pasteurization before the yogurt culture is introduced is essential to the making of yogurt, but pasteurization after the culture has been allowed to grow is done merely to increase shelf life and totally destroys all the benefits inherent in the yogurt.

  Also, a diet high in complex carbohydrates such as fruits, whole grains, and vegetables promotes the growth of *Bifidobacteria* in the large intestine. Heavy meat consumption does just the opposite. And drinking chlorinated water or eating meats and dairy produced with antibiotics totally defeats any program you're on.

So, we've now covered how to clean out our intestines and how to rebuild the population of friendly bacteria that lives there. Next, we will look at the dangers that may be lurking in your mouth.

# CHAPTER 5

# *Your Mouth Is Killing You*

- **Toxic Mouth**
- **Dental Plaque and Proteolytic Enzymes**
- **"Gifts" from Your Dentist**

## TOXIC MOUTH

At any given time, there are more than 500 species of bacteria in your mouth. It is these bacteria that form the sticky, colorless film on your teeth known as plaque, the "gateway" to many health problems. When mineral salts in saliva combine with plaque, hard deposits known as tartar or calculus, which can't be removed by brushing alone, are formed on your teeth. Plaque can build up at your gum line, where even more bacteria can accumulate in the space between your gums and teeth. Toxins produced by the bacteria in plaque irritate your gums and cause them to become inflamed and bleed (a condition called gingivitis). This causes your gums to separate from your teeth, forming spaces between your teeth and gums (pockets) that become infected.

The toxins produced by the bacteria and the infection in these pockets can also stimulate a chronic inflammatory response in which your body turns on itself, and the tissues and bone that support the teeth are broken down and destroyed. As the disease progresses, the pockets deepen, the inflammation and infection increase, and more gum tissue and bone are destroyed. This is called periodontitis.

In periodontitis, the connection between the teeth, gums, and jawbone is broken down—in fact, your jawbone and the ligaments that hold your teeth to your jawbone are literally eaten away. If you think this is something you don't need to worry about, think again! Often, this destructive process has very mild symptoms (at first), so many people are unaware that they suffer from it. About 75 percent of Americans have gum disease and don't know it! The bottom line is that periodontitis results in loosening of the gums from the teeth, and eventually loosening of the teeth from the jawbone—not to mention bad breath and an increasing risk of life-threatening, chronic illnesses such as heart disease.[1]

## Avocado/Soy Unsaponifiables (ASU) to the Rescue

It is now understood that one biochemical in particular is responsible for the erosion of oral structures, the eating away at your jawbone and the ligaments that hold your teeth to your jaw. This oral toxin is called interleukin-1beta

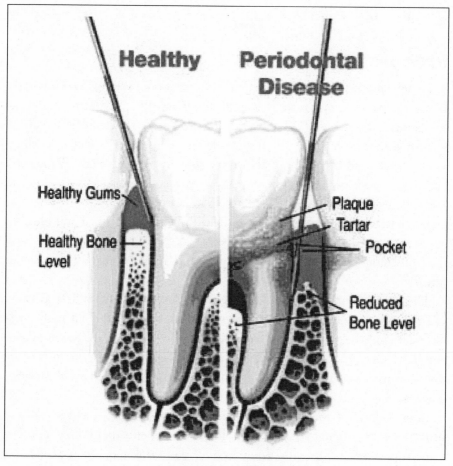

The structure of the tooth.

(IL-1beta) and it is a common mediator of the inflammation process. Your body's counter measure to IL-1beta is a family of biochemicals called transforming growth factor-beta (TGF-beta). It has been identified as one of the factors capable of counteracting IL-1beta's destructive effects and plays a key role in tissue regeneration. Unfortunately, one of the effects of IL-1beta is that it inhibits the production of TGF-beta, the very substance that can counteract it and repair the damage.

A French study conducted by the Laboratory of Connective Tissue Biochemistry and the Maxillary-Facial Surgery Department, University Hospital Center, in Caen, France, found that that a phytosterol/sterolin extract concentrated from the oils found in avocado and soybean fibers (known as avocado/soy unsaponifiables, or ASU) can stop the erosive damage caused by IL-1beta in periodontal diseases. In other words, ASU helps protect against periodontal disease.[2] Another French study conducted by the Faculty of Dental Surgery, University Rene Descartes, in Paris, found that ASU also protects the fibers that hold your teeth in place—the destruction of which is a hallmark of periodontal disease.[3] Bottom line: supplementation with ASU helps protect against and reverse periodontal disease.

## DENTAL PLAQUE AND PROTEOLYTIC ENZYMES

Plaque is formed by a selective attachment and growth of oral microorganisms on a protein-based film that tightly adheres to the surface of teeth. Getting rid of plaque is important because it plays a central role as the catalyst in periodontal disease. The use of systemic proteolytic enzymes for eliminating dental plaque is certainly controversial. There have been several studies that have produced mixed results, and in fact, there are some proteolytic enzymes produced in the body (there are thousands of different kinds) and present in saliva that actually promote the growth of plaque. That said, I have personally experimented with and seen remarkable results using some proteolytic enzyme formulas in which heavy plaque disappeared in a matter of days.

How could this happen? Saliva plays a major role in the health of the oral cavity and the entire body. Saliva is made up primarily of water but also contains minerals and digestive enzymes such as amylase. It seems that some supplemental proteolytic enzymes are able to make their way from your blood to the saliva in your mouth, where they dissolve the protein-based film that bonds the plaque to your teeth, thus allowing the bacteria that cause dental caries to be washed away by your saliva. In fact, it turns out that this very concept is being examined by the National Institute of Dental Health and Craniofacial Research and by Boston University Medical School in an ongoing study titled "Salivary Proteins in Dental Integuments." While the results of the study are not yet available since the projected end date is not until May 2010 (start date was January 1983), the premise of the study offers support for what I've indeed seen with some proteolytic enzyme formulas.

## "GIFTS" FROM YOUR DENTIST

Dentists have accomplished many great things in this country in terms of promoting oral health, but on three key issues, they stand on the wrong side of history and of health: fluoride, mercury fillings, and root canals.

### Fluoride

We'll talk more about the toxic effects of fluoride in your water in a later chapter, but for now it is important to understand that it has no place in water, your toothpaste, or in fluoride treatments from your dentist. The only

---

## THE TOXIC COMBINATION OF FLUORIDE AND ALUMINUM

It has been known for some thirty years that aluminum, once it enters our bodies, has the tendency to accumulate in our brains, where it kills off neurons and leads to memory loss. And thanks to the significant amounts of aluminum found in food emulsifiers, antiperspirant deodorants, hair sprays, baking powder, many toothpastes, much of our drinking water, and most of our cookware, we are exposed to quite a lot of aluminum over the course of our lives. There has been much speculation, therefore, that aluminum may be one of the prime factors in the onset of Alzheimer's disease. The connection between aluminum and Alzheimer's became even stronger when, in 1995, *Neurotoxicology* reported that the widespread use of aluminum salts to purify water could account for the large numbers of people suffering from Alzheimer's.[5]

New research has revealed that fluoride in drinking water makes the aluminum that we ingest more bioavailable. In the presence of fluoride, more aluminum crosses the blood-brain barrier and is deposited in the brain.[6] The combination of aluminum and fluoride causes the same pathological changes in brain tissue that are found in Alzheimer's patients.

relevant question when talking about fluoride and your teeth is: does it actually prevent tooth decay? Let's take a look.

One claim of dental researchers is that just introducing fluoride into a previously unfluoridated city's drinking water supply can reduce its inhabitants' rate of tooth decay by 40 to 70 percent. Sounds impressive, until you find that during similar time frames, dental health improved in nearby communities with unfluoridated water at virtually the same rate, indicating that the improvement resulted from enhanced dental hygiene, not fluoridation. Another claim made in a 1990 National Institute of Dental Research epidemiological study declared that "water fluoridation has played a dominant role in the decline in caries and must continue to be a major prevention methodology." But others who examined the study results found that the difference in numbers of decayed or missing teeth or filled surfaces was minimal—about one-half of a single tooth surface out of 128 total tooth surfaces (less than 0.5 percent difference).[4]

I have actually heard some dentists argue that your tooth enamel is made of fluoride, which is why adding fluoride to your toothpaste and drinking water helps. They are misinformed. Tooth enamel is actually composed of calcium phosphate. The more accurate explanation for how fluoride theoretically helps is that the fluoride bonds with the calcium phosphate, making it harder and more resistant to decay. So, is the theory true? Does fluoride work? There's no question that since fluoridation began, the incidence of dental caries has decreased significantly in the United States. But as we've seen, it's gone down throughout the country, even in areas that don't fluoridate their water. In fact, there is no good statistical evidence that fluoride (either in your water or in your toothpaste) makes one iota of difference in terms of dental health. All of the improvement in dental health that we have seen in the United States can easily be attributed to better dental hygiene (brushing and flossing), not fluoridation.

Finally, fluoride levels in your blood can double within five minutes of brushing your teeth with a fluoride toothpaste, just from the amount absorbed through the cheeks and gums. The amount absorbed in a dentist's office from a fluoride treatment is several orders of magnitude higher.

## Mercury Fillings

The American Dental Association has resolutely maintained for years that "when mercury is combined with the metals used in dental amalgam, its toxic properties are made harmless." If this were true, it would be miraculously fortuitous. Amalgam, which consists of mercury, silver, tin, copper, and a trace amount of zinc, has been used by dentists for hundreds of years—as far back, actually, as the seventh century in China. In the United States, mercury-based fillings made their appearance in the early 1800s.

From the beginning, there were a number of dentists who were concerned by the presence of mercury, since by that time it was fairly well known that mercury was poisonous. In fact, these concerns were so strong that by the mid-1940s several dental societies, including the American Society of Dental Surgeons, had joined to stop the use of amalgam fillings. But amalgam was just too easy to work with, and whatever ill effects people experienced were too far down the road to matter. So, in 1859, the American Dental Association (ADA) was founded primarily to promote the use of mercury amalgam as a safe and desirable tooth filling material. There were no tests done. Amalgam was promoted because it was easy to work with. The reason the mercury was used was because it serves to "dissolve" the other metals and make a homogenous whole.

It would be miraculous indeed if you could use one of the most toxic substances known with no ill effect. How was this defended? Well, the early position was that the mercury reacts with the other metals to form a "biologically inactive substance" so that none of it ever makes its way into your body. This was an interesting *theory* that, of course, turned out to not be true. Numerous studies conducted in the 1970s and 1980s proved conclusively that the mercury from fillings (primarily from mercury vapor created when we chew) makes its way into the body, ending up in our lungs, heart, stomach, kidneys, endocrine glands, gastrointestinal tract, jaw tissue, and our brains. In effect, the denser the tissue, the greater the concentration of mercury.

There have been over 12,000 papers published to date elucidating the dangers of amalgam fillings, but the most compelling of those studies detailed the use of radioactively tagged amalgam fillings in a controlled experiment. In less than thirty days, substantial levels of the tagged mercury was found throughout the body and brain, especially in the liver and kidneys. Studies have shown that within a month of receiving amalgam fillings, kidney function is reduced by well over 50 percent.[7]

Once it became irrefutable that mercury from the fillings was ending up in our bodies, it then became mandatory for the ADA to find a new theory/

defense. Again, not based on clinical studies but rather on convenience, it became the position of the ADA that, yes, perhaps some mercury does make its way into the body, but at levels that are so low it has no effect on our health. And once again, it would be miraculous indeed if that were true. Unfortunately, it is not—like so many other toxic substances, the real problem with mercury is that it is a cumulative poison and the body holds onto a significant percentage of the mercury that enters it.

Mercury is one of the most toxic metals known—even more toxic than lead. And while there is no conclusive evidence that the mercury from fillings causes any particular health problems, there are a number of studies that imply such a relationship. There is strong evidence that mercury lowers T-cell (white blood cell) counts. A number of studies have shown removing amalgam fillings can cause T-cell counts to rise anywhere from 50 to 300 percent. This, alone, implicates amalgam fillings in cancer, autoimmune diseases, allergies, *Candida* overgrowth, and multiple sclerosis (MS). In fact, there have been several studies that have shown that white blood cell abnormalities, such as found in leukemia, tend to normalize when amalgam fillings are removed. Mercury levels in MS patients are, on average, 7.5 times higher than normal.

It has also been shown that mercury interferes with the ability of the blood to carry oxygen—actually cutting its oxygen-carrying capabilities by half. This would account for many instances of chronic fatigue syndrome. Mercury also has an affinity for our brains and is implicated in brain tumors and dementia. The famous "mad hatters" of England were actually hat makers who worked with mercury and eventually went insane. Finally, mercury has an affinity for fetal tissue—reaching higher levels in the fetus than in the mother herself—which accounts for mercury's implication in birth defects.

What about other sources of mercury entering the body? Well, seafood is, of course, a source, as are some other foods we eat. But the amount of mercury entering our bodies from amalgam fillings represents anywhere from 50 to 90 percent of the total amount. Each amalgam filling in your mouth pumps, on average, some 3,000,000,000,000,000 mercury atoms into your body every day.

So why in the world does the ADA continue to support the use of amalgam fillings? One simple answer is: in for a penny, in for a pound. What would the legal ramifications be if the ADA suddenly announced that it, and all the dentists connected with it, had been wrong for well over 100 years and had been slowly poisoning all Americans? Can you spell "class action lawsuit"?

In June 2008, as part of the settlement of a lawsuit, the FDA posted an announcement warning that mercury-based amalgam fillings "may" pose a safety risk for pregnant women and young children (www.fda.gov/cdrh/consumer/amalgams.html). The wall begins to crumble.

## Root Canals

Unfortunately, the sins of the dentist don't stop with fluoride and mercury. They also perform root canals. If a tooth's pulp, which contains nerves and blood vessels, becomes infected or damaged because of decay or injury, your options are often limited. Effectively, your dentist will offer you two choices: either have the tooth pulled or have the nerve removed (a root canal treatment). A root canal consists of removing the infected or diseased pulp from the tooth and sterilizing and refilling the canals with a sealer to prevent recontamination of the root system. The traditional sealer of choice has been gutta percha, although new options are becoming available that overcome the major problem associated with gutta percha—microscopic shrinkage as it dries, leaving empty space in the root that may fill with bacteria.

Nevertheless, the one problem that no sealer can overcome is that no filling can reach into the miles of tubules in the tooth. A tooth is not a solid, inanimate structure. Each tooth is a living structure sustained by some three miles of microscopic tubules running through the hard dentin material. In a healthy tooth, those tubules, which make up a full 90 percent of the actual tooth, can be thought of as the tooth's "arteries and veins."

Once a tooth has had its root filled in a root canal procedure, it no longer has any nourishment circulating through its tubules, but the tubules themselves remain, unfilled. And therein lies the problem: it is physically impossible to fully sterilize the miles of microscopic tubules in a tooth. Some bacteria (including strains of *Streptococcus*, *Staphylococcus*, as well as spirochetes) survive and thrive in these empty tubules. And once sealed in your tooth, no part of your immune system can reach them and destroy them because you have stopped all blood supply to the tooth's interior. For the same reason, no antibiotics that you might take can reach the bacteria. Nevertheless, because the tooth itself is porous, those bacteria and/or their toxins can migrate out into surrounding tissue, where they can "hitchhike" to other locations in the body via the bloodstream. The new location may be any organ, gland, or tissue, and the new colony will be the next focus of infection in a body plagued by recurrent or chronic infections.

Every single root canal leaks, without exception. Bacteria and/or toxins leach out from every tooth treated with root canal. Anyone who has had a root canal has had their immune system compromised to some degree by having to fight a continual low-grade infection that it can never eliminate because it can't reach the source of infection in the tooth. About 25 percent of all people seem to have immune systems that are strong enough to resist the continual infection coming from the tooth, thereby preventing it from taking hold anywhere else in the body for many years. But the other 75 percent can look forward to a whole range of chronic and debilitating diseases, including arthritis, heart disease, chronic infection, chronic fatigue, and eye problems.

The bottom line is that root canals, at this point in time, are to be avoided. With better dental care and by following the dietary principles outlined in this book, you should never have to face the need for a root canal. Incidentally, if you already have a root canal and need to have it removed, it is not enough to simply have it pulled. It is almost a surety that the bacteria have migrated to the bone and tissues adjacent to the tooth's root. You will need to find a dentist experienced in the procedure for removing a root canal tooth, which includes removing the periodontal ligament (which is always infected with toxins produced by *Streptococcus* bacteria living in the dentin tubules) and the first millimeter of bone that lines the socket (which is also usually infected).

## GENERAL RECOMMENDATIONS

- Consider supplementing with avocado/soy unsaponifiables to protect against periodontal disease.

- Consider using proteolytic enzymes to dissolve dental plaque and wash it away. (If the enzyme formula you try doesn't work, try another until you find one that does.)

- Fluoride—If there's any way to keep it out of your city water supply, fight to do that. If it's already there, you have to make sure you remove it at your house so that it doesn't make it into your drinking water, bath, or shower. Also, you'll probably want to avoid fluoride toothpastes, and you'll definitely want to avoid fluoride "treatments" from your dentist.

- Aluminum—Make sure it's not in the water you drink, and you might want to think twice about the antiperspirant you use. Also, look at the cookware you use. Aluminum cookware is, of course, a problem. (Heavy metal detoxification can help here.) Aluminum core cookware is better, but what metal or coating is the food touching? Stainless steel is good, except for the fact that it's a major source of nickel, which is a problem. (Again, regular heavy metal detoxes can help here too.) And teflon cookware contains minute traces of perfluorooctanoic acid (PFOA), a suspected carcinogen. Other types of cookware such as glass may be safer, but may be less satisfactory when it comes to cooking.

- Mercury fillings—Unless you have some chronic health condition, you may not want to go through the expense of having your fillings replaced. However, you would be well advised to start some of the cleansing programs we describe—particularly the colon cleanse and some form of heavy metal cleansing, such as chelation therapy (or the use of a good heavy metal chelating formula). If you need any new fillings, don't use amalgam.

  If you are going to have your fillings removed, go to a dentist who specializes in the removal of amalgam fillings. There's a whole procedure involved to minimize the amounts of powdered mercury that escapes down your throat and mercury vapor up into your nasal passages as a result of the high-speed drill used to remove the amalgam. But keep in mind that no matter how careful the dentist is, significant amounts of mercury will indeed enter your system during the removal process. Always follow up removal with a heavy metal detoxification.

- Root canals—Don't. And if you have one, you may want to consider having it pulled. Look to titanium implants instead. Titanium itself presents some toxicity problems, but it's nothing compared to what leaches out of a root canal.

Several times in this chapter I have referred to heavy metal detoxification. In the next chapter, we'll cover detoxification in detail, with a discussion of how to clean out your liver, gallbladder, kidneys, and blood.

# CHAPTER 6

## Cleansing Your Liver, Kidneys, and Blood

- **The Body's Primary Filter**
- **Eliminating Kidney Stones**
- **Cleansing the Blood**
- **Balancing pH**
- **The Healing Crisis**

recent study was eye-opening: it found that even if you try to live a pure organic lifestyle, some toxins are inescapable—even if you're raised on organic food, living in a "clean" environment, and even located hundreds of miles away from any obvious sources of pollution, you're still going to be toxic. On average, each person in the study tested positive for an average twenty-five known toxins.[1] The study even identified children who were contaminated with toxins that had been banned before they were born! The bottom line is that if you are alive today, you must detoxify regularly. But beyond colon cleansing, what should you do?

Colon cleansing is quite the rage now, with colon-cleansing products on store shelves and on the Internet. Many of these products are worthless (really nothing more than expensive fiber formulas), but a sizeable number are actually quite good. That said, almost every one of these products misses the point. Colon cleansing is not the end of detoxing—it's only the beginning. Colon cleansing, as we've already discussed, is required to clean out the elimination channels so that toxins released from the other forms of detoxification have a clear path out of the body. But the major work of detoxification, the improvements in health that most people are looking for, come from those other detoxes, not from colon cleansing. What "other" detoxes are we talking about?

- The liver/gallbladder cleanse to flush stones, sludge, toxic waste and chemicals, and cholesterol from the liver and gallbladder and to improve liver performance and help regenerate damaged liver tissue.

- The kidney flush to get rid of kidney sludge and stones (as well as gallstones and pancreatic sludge), clear infection and inflammation from the kidneys, and help stimulate renal tissue.

- The blood cleanse to optimize blood activity, eliminate any viral or bacterial contamination, and help the body eliminate any malignant cells.

- Chelation therapy to remove heavy metals from the body, thereby eliminating a major factor in the onset of cardiovascular problems, cancer, and the overall degradation of health.

- Balancing pH to improve oxygen availability and the functioning of the immune system.

- Fasting to clear out old damaged cells and tissue and encourage the growth of new healthy tissue.

With that in mind, let's look at each of these detox programs one at a time.

## THE BODY'S PRIMARY FILTER

Our liver is the primary filter of our body. Good health is impossible without proper function of the liver. Unfortunately, over time, we so abuse and overtax it that illness is the inevitable result.

Next to the skin, the liver is the largest organ in the body. In many ways, it is the most important organ and the last to be considered when it comes to health. In addition to being large, the liver is also a complicated organ involved in at least 200 separate functions. Generally speaking, the liver performs a vital role in regulating, synthesizing, storing, secreting, transforming, and breaking down many different substances in the body. Specifically, these functions include:

- Regulation of fat stores.
- Cleansing the blood and discharging waste products.
- Neutralizing and destroying poisons.
- Protein metabolism, including manufacturing of new body proteins.
- Metabolizing alcohol.

- Managing chemicals and drugs in the blood.
- Aiding the digestive process by the production of bile.
- Helping the body resist infections by producing immune factors and by removing bacteria from the bloodstream.
- Storing vitamins, minerals, and sugars.
- Production of quick energy when needed.
- Controlling the production and excretion of cholesterol.
- Maintaining hormone balance.
- Regenerating its own damaged tissue.

The liver is so important to our well-being that many healers maintain that most diseases cannot develop in the body (that, in fact, no form of cell degeneration can occur) if the liver is functioning in an efficient, healthy manner. Conversely, an unhealthy liver is very likely at the root of most serious health problems. As part of a program to rebuild and repair the liver, we must

- Remove all the excess fat from the liver.
- Get bile flowing freely again.
- Eliminate toxic waste that our livers have filtered out.
- Dissolve and pass out the accumulated gallstones and incipient gallstones that are stored in our livers.
- Regenerate the damaged and destroyed cells of the liver.

## What Harms the Liver?

- Too much protein in the diet. Protein metabolism is especially taxing on the liver since it is the liver that must metabolize complex proteins into simple compounds. The greater the consumption of protein, the greater the stress on the liver.
- Too many simple carbohydrates in the diet. The body converts excess simple carbohydrates into triglycerides, which are then stored in the liver as fat. The more fat stored in the liver, the harder it is for the liver to perform its full range of normal functions.
- Overeating. Too much enzyme-deficient food stresses the liver.

- Drug residues. Virtually all of the drugs that we take (medicinal and recreational) are processed, purified, and refined in the liver—in preparation for elimination from the body.

- Vitamin isolates. Many vitamins in their isolated form are toxic to the body and must be conjugated by the liver to render them harmless and make them available to the cells. Every time you supplement with such vitamins, you stress the liver.

- Alcohol causes inflammation of the liver's tissue. Once the liver is inflamed, it can no longer filter, which causes it to plug up with fat and become even more inflamed. If we consume enough alcohol, we overwhelm the liver's ability to regenerate itself, and the net result is cirrhosis (or hardening) of the liver.

- Toxins, heavy metals, and pesticides. Everything we breathe, eat, and absorb through our skin is purified and refined in the liver.

- Lack of exercise forces the liver to do the elimination work that should be done by the lungs and the skin.

- And, of course, there's always liver disease such as chronic hepatitis C.

## Symptoms of Liver Dysfunction

- Digestive problems
- Constipation
- Low energy output
- Allergies and hay fever
- Arthritis
- Diabetes
- Hypertension
- Obesity
- Infertility

## A Word about the Gallbladder

Alas, the poor gallbladder. Guilty by being found at the scene of the crime, it is the frequent target of the surgeon's knife because of gallstones and other problems. Over half a million gallbladders are removed each year in the United States, making it one of the most frequently performed operations. Women are four times more likely than men to get gallstones.

The gallbladder is not responsible for the production of gallstones—the liver is the culprit, or rather what we do to the liver. The gallbladder is merely a holding area for bile to be used in the digestion of fats and oils. But if our diets are too high in the wrong kind of oils, if we have allergies to dairy and eggs, low levels of stomach acid, too little fiber in our diets, stress, if the liver is not functioning properly, and so on, then the bile produced in the liver (a mixture of cholesterol, minerals, bile salts, pigment, and lecithin) is of a type and consistency that tends to quickly harden into "stones" before it can be passed out of the gallbladder.

Removing the gallbladder does not remove the problem—it merely removes the organ in which symptoms first manifest. Yes, it's true that after gallbladder removal you're *unlikely* to suffer from further gallstones. But on the other hand, you've now traded one problem for two new ones:

1. Since you never corrected the underlying problem of imbalances in the liver, these problems will just continue to get worse—eventually compromising the liver itself.

2. By removing the gallbladder, you also remove its regulating effect on bile. That means that bile is continually dumping into your intestinal tract when it is not needed, and it is available in only minimal amounts when it is needed. The net result is chronic digestive problems and probable long-term nutritional deficiencies.

Far better than removing the gallbladder is a seasonal liver/gallbladder flush combined with a periodic liver-rebuilding program.

## What Can Be Done to Help the Liver and Gallbladder?

Fortunately, your liver has an astounding ability to regenerate itself—if you give it a chance. Giving it a chance means two things:

• The Don'ts—Improper dietary choices particularly affect liver health. You need to eliminate (or at least cut back on) the liver stressors in your diet. Too much protein in the diet is especially taxing on the liver. Too many simple carbohydrates in the diet are converted into triglycerides and stored in the liver. And overeating enzyme-deficient food stresses the liver. The sicker you are, the cleaner your diet needs to be. If you're suffering from serious liver problems, a raw juice diet may be required to give your liver time to regenerate.

• The Do's—Several times a year, you need to do an herbal detoxification/ flush to rebuild your liver. A low-level cleanse using betaine hydrochloride and pancreatic enzymes is also helpful, as is drinking fresh beet/apple juice regularly. You need to regularly include nutritional support for the liver. Look for formulas that contain milk thistle, dandelion root, the perennial herb *Picrorrhiza kurroa*, and artichoke or beet leaf. *Picrorrhiza* has been shown to protect liver cells from the many degenerative changes that would normally be caused by a variety of liver toxins. It appears to be particularly useful in treating both alcoholic liver damage and chronic viral hepatitis.

### Liver/Gallbladder Flush

By cleansing the liver, we're talking about inducing the liver to purge all of the fats, old cholesterol deposits, incipient gallstones, poisons, drug residues, and toxic waste stored therein. Probably nothing else you do (including a colon cleanse) will make a greater difference in your overall health. However, it is vital that you do a colon cleanse before doing the liver cleanse. When the liver dumps, it dumps through the bile duct and into the colon. If the colon is plugged, the waste backs up into the bloodstream and can make you feel extremely ill. This is the reason that the "miracle doctors" always start with a colon detox (see Chapter 3). It's the prerequisite for all the other cleanses in the body—and, of course, it can also produce dramatic healing in its own right. For most people, and particularly for those who have never done a liver cleanse before, it is also vital that you soften any stones that you may have by using a *Chanca piedra*/hydrangea root/gravel root herbal tincture before you do the liver detox. (We'll talk more about this formula when we explore the kidney flush.)

The five-day cleanse is a variation of the liver/gallbladder flush recommended by Dr. Richard Schulze and is the one most people should opt for. It's actually both more gentle and more complete than the one-day purge. For complete step-by-step details on how to do the detox, go to the Detox Center at www.jonbarron.org, but I'll summarize it below. The liver/gallbladder flush has five main components that work together and you need to do all five.

1. **Morning Flush Drink**—This is the heart of the program. In a blender, mix 8 ounces of any fresh-squeezed citrus juice (fresh apple juice or grape juice with all the sediment will work too), 1 lemon, 1 clove of garlic (increase by 1 clove each day), 1 tablespoon of olive oil (increase by 1 tablespoon each day), and a piece of ginger (about one-inch long) along with 8 ounces of pure water. The way the program works is that you starve your

body of fats all day. This allows bile to build up in your liver and gallbladder. Then, in the morning, you have the morning flush drink, which contains your only fat of the day (1–5 tablespoons of olive oil, depending on which day of the flush you're on). This causes the liver and gallbladder to literally "wring themselves out" in an attempt to deal with the oil—squeezing out accumulated fat, cholesterol, softened gallstones, and toxins in the process. The purging action gets progressively stronger each day of the flush. On the last day, when you consume five tablespoons of olive oil (a half cup of oil in one shot) that really squeezes the liver and gallbladder.

2. **Liver Tea**—The tea helps with the flushing process itself, but it also helps minimize any discomfort or nausea. The key herb in the tea is dandelion root, one of the strongest herbal lipotropics known (it flushes fat deposits from the liver). Other herbs that you will find in a good liver tea include ginger, clove, cinnamon, burdock root, and horsetail. Incidentally, some of the other herbs used in the tea (such as uva ursi, parsley root, and juniper berries) are also extremely beneficial to the kidneys.

3. **Liver Tincture**—The tincture is crucial in that it contains herbs that help the liver to rebuild and regenerate itself. A secondary benefit is that it will significantly reduce the liver's release of low-density lipoprotein (LDL) cholesterol, the bad kind. The key herbs include milk thistle, dandelion root, the herb *Picrorrhiza kurroa* (sometimes called kutkin or Indian milk thistle), and artichoke or beet leaf. Some tinctures also include antiparasitic herbs such as wormwood and black walnut. Along with the garlic that you are taking with the morning liver flush drink, this will drive virtually any parasite from your body.

4. **Potassium Broth**—The potassium broth is exactly what its name says: a clear soup broth that's high in potassium. Its main purpose is to make sure that potassium levels stay high to minimize any chance of your heart rate speeding up while you're fasting and losing electrolytes. It's also outrageously high in garlic to help cleanse the liver and further drive parasites from your body. Key ingredients include potato skins, fresh beets, onions, and fifty cloves of garlic.

5. **The Diet**—It is extremely beneficial to incorporate a two-day raw food and three-day juice fast into your five-day cleanse. Even better, though, is to incorporate a five-day raw juice and chlorella fast. In any case, avoid all fats so as to maximize the "wringing effect" of the morning flush drink.

## AN ALTERNATIVE CLEANSE

For those who don't want to do the full liver flush, there is a slow and easy version that will give you 70 to 80 percent of the benefit without the difficulty. As part of your daily diet, just eat one cup of freshly grated beets mixed with olive oil and lemon juice for thirty days straight. Daily use of a liver detox tea is also required. Using one bottle of liver tincture is recommended.

### What Can You Expect?

If you are so inclined (and you should be), you should examine what you deposit in the toilet during the liver/gallbladder flush. Check for "stones." The bile from the liver gives some stones their typical green color, but also look for black, red, and brown stones, as well as stones with blood inside them. During the course of the cleanse, it's not uncommon for some people to pass some 2,000 of these stones. Be glad, because the more you pass, the healthier you become. You may also find untold numbers of tiny white cholesterol "crystals" mixed in with the waste. (Note: Oftentimes, the olive oil is converted into little "soap beads" in the intestinal tract, and many people confuse these little beads with actual stones.)

If you don't notice anything, though, it doesn't mean the flush is not working. Many people don't have gallstones. But they do have toxins in the liver, and those are being purged. In the end, though, it's not what you see, it's how you feel. Wait for a few days after the cleanse and then evaluate. Did you lose weight? Do you feel lighter and cleaner? Did your senses come alive? Does food taste better? Are colors brighter? Is your breathing a little easier, less congested with mucus? These are the tangible results you're looking for.

## ELIMINATING KIDNEY STONES

Thanks largely to the increasing incidence of diabetes around the world, kidney disease and kidney failure are also exploding. Later in the book, we will discuss diabetes and how to minimize and reverse much of the damage it causes to organs such as the kidneys, but there is one major problem to address now—kidney stones. Actually, kidney stones are just the final manifestation of a more insidious problem called kidney gravel: these are stones so small that, unlike a full-blown stone, you don't feel them pass through the ureter. However, they are large enough to block your kidneys' nephrons and the tubules in the collecting duct system, critical parts of the filtration system. Regularly dissolving these incipient stones and flushing them from the kidneys is essential for good health.

How extensive is the problem? Virtually every person has some degree of sludge buildup and some loss of kidney function over time. The only question is how much. Does it reach the point where it causes painful kidney stones to form or the point where it chokes off a critical mass of kidney tissue, ultimately leading to kidney failure? Each year, nearly 100,000 Americans are newly diagnosed with kidney failure, more than 100,000 currently have end-stage renal disease due to diabetes, and an astounding 7.7 million have physiological evidence of chronic kidney disease.[2]

It should be noted that kidney stones or sludge, pancreatic sludge, and gallstones are not related. Having one does not necessarily mean you will have the other. However, a well-designed formula used for eliminating kidney stones and sludge will also help remove gallstones and pancreatic sludge. A good kidney flush formula will contain herbs such as *Chanca piedra*, hydrangea, and gravel root that help to break up stones and sludge. But the formula needs to do more than just break up stones and sludge, it also needs to work as a:

- Diuretic (water removing)
- Antiseptic (infection killing)
- Anti-nephrotoxic and anti-hepatotoxic
- Soother to urinary tract tissue
- Anti-inflammatory
- Stimulator to renal tissue

To accomplish all of this, you need to look for a formula that contains herbs such as marshmallow root, juniper berry, corn silk, *Uva ursi*, parsley root, carrot tops, dandelion leaf, horsetail, orange peel, peppermint, and goldenrod—in addition to the *Chanca peidra*, hydrangea root, and gravel root mentioned above. And be sure to drink fresh-squeezed apple juice, as the malic acid in it also helps to soften the stones.

## CLEANSING THE BLOOD

Blood is one of the most complex organs in the human body. Just under-standing the cascade of clotting mechanisms in the blood requires up to a full year in medical school. But in simple terms, blood has three primary functions:

- It transports things into, around, and out of the body. That includes gases such as oxygen and carbon dioxide as well as nutrients and cellular waste.

- It protects the body from bacteria, viruses, and malignant cells by virtue of the white blood cells that function as part of the immune system.

- It balances the body, including balancing electrolytes, hydration, blood sugar, and so on.

Blood cleansing is required to repair the damage we do to our blood through improper diet and exposure to environmental toxins, not to men-tion exposure to various pathogens. When used regularly, a good blood-cleansing formula works to purify and optimize your blood, cleanse your liver, kill viruses, balance blood sugar, and, of course, drive "malignant spir-its" from your body. It should be noted that human blood is antiseptic— under normal circumstances. In other words, it does not tolerate the presence of pathogens. It is for this reason that many doctors say that blood cleans-ing is nonsense since bacteria and viruses can't exist in human blood. Unfor-tunately, that's a bit naïve. As we know, human existence rarely adheres to "normal" circumstances. The fact is that viruses and bacteria frequently sur-vive in human blood, everything from AIDS to HPV to bacteria implicated in arthritis and Crohn's disease. If you want to be healthy, they must be cleansed.

There are several ways to cleanse your blood. One of the most effective is to use systemic proteolytic enzymes between meals and/or before bed (see Chapter 11). Within a matter of minutes, the enzymes enter the bloodstream and begin cleaning the protein-based detritus out of your blood and stimu-lating the immune cells to consume circulating immune complexes (CICs) in your blood. CICs are large protein molecules that are only partially digest-ed in the small intestine but are nevertheless absorbed into the blood. They can cause allergic reactions and other problems in the body. Ridding the blood of CICs can make a significant improvement in your overall health rather quickly.

What we're talking about here, though, is something different—using herbal blood cleansers to remove toxic residues so that your blood and body resist bacteria, viruses, and cancer. The great blood-cleansing herbs are chaparral, red clover (*Trifolium pratense*), burdock root (*Arctium lappa*), poke root (*Phytolacca decandra*), yellow dock root, bloodroot (*Sanguinaria candensis*), Oregon grape root, mistletoe, goldenseal root, cat's claw, sheep sorrel, and cayenne. These are the herbs you will find in the famous blood-cleansing formulas such as the Hoxsey formula, Essiac Tea, the Dr. Christopher and Dr. Schulze formulas, and my own version of the formula. These formulas can "drive" bad things out of your body or prevent them from entering in the first place.

First of all, though, the designation "blood cleanser" is a euphemism. In fact, this formula (along with every herb in it) is considered by herbalists to be anti-cancer. Variations of this formula have been used for hundreds of years by Native American tribes. The fact that we can't talk openly about the anti-cancer property of herbs and herbal formulas is probably the most political topic in alternative health today. Not surprisingly, many of the individual herbs in these formulas are on the U.S. Food and Drug Administration (FDA) cautionary list, and virtually all of them are on the equivalent Canadian list. You will also find numbers of these herbs on the precautionary lists of European countries such as Switzerland and Germany, and even Australia, for that matter.

Although many people use blood-cleansing formulas as part of their semi-annual liver and gallbladder flush, they should be considered in their own right as important formulas to be used in maintaining optimal health and optimizing the immune system. If well designed using high-quality herbs, they can have powerful and extremely fast acting anti-pathogenic properties.

## Chelation Therapy—Another Part of Blood Cleansing

In 2004, over 427,000 bypasses and 1,295,000 angioplasties were performed in U.S. hospitals,[3] at a cost of over $40,000 each. It works out to approximately $63 billion a year spent on questionable coronary procedures. Questionable because at least 5 percent of the patients die from the procedure; even more people die not long after surgery from complications such as stroke. New studies show that the vast majority of these procedures have no benefit.[4] But it's a small risk and a small price to pay since there's no alternative, right?

Well, not exactly. There's an alternative that's so effective that, in some countries the national health-care systems will not pay for bypass surgery unless this alternative has been tried first. This treatment is called chelation therapy, and it could save hundreds of thousands of lives a year. It costs just a fraction of what a coronary bypass or angioplasty costs, and according to many in the alternative health community, this is the reason the medical establishment is so dismissive of chelation therapy—it would cost them billions of dollars a year. In any case, up to this point, all of the studies that the medical community trots out to invalidate chelation therapy are seriously flawed, either in concept, patient selection, symptom evaluation, or in some cases arriving at conclusions that actually contradict the data being evaluated. On the other hand, the numerous studies that are indicative of chelation therapy's benefits are routinely ignored.

Chelation therapy has two pronounced effects on the body. It chelates (from the Greek word *chele*, meaning "to claw" or "to bind") onto heavy metals such as aluminum, lead, and mercury (particularly those located in the cardiovascular system) and pulls them out of your body. By removing heavy metals from the body, chelation therapy significantly reduces the production of free radicals in the bloodstream and the consequent scarring of the arterial walls.

The net result for most people is a dramatic improvement in the health and condition of their cardiovascular system. If you're in an advanced state of coronary disease, you should seriously consider tracking down a doctor who specializes in chelation therapy.

However, chelation therapy is not for everyone. It involves going to a doctor's office for a series of approximately 30 four-hour intravenous "drip" sessions of ethylenediamine tetra-acetic acid (EDTA). In addition, although it costs a fraction of what bypass surgery costs, it is not inexpensive—usually running a little over $2,000 for the complete set of sessions. On the other hand, if you are not in an advanced disease state, there is the easier alternative of oral chelation.

### Oral Chelation

Oral chelation is not as quick as standard chelation therapy. Nevertheless, given a little time, it can do an extremely effective job at cleaning out the blood. Most formulas are based on EDTA. EDTA works great when administered directly into the bloodstream through standard chelation therapy, but its usefulness when taken orally is open to question. There are some studies that indicate that there may be less than 5 percent absorption when taken orally.

There is an alternative, however. A tincture of cilantro and chlorella has turned out to be remarkably effective as an oral chelator. Why cilantro and chlorella? Because cilantro changes the electrical charge on intracellular deposits of heavy metals to a neutral state, which relaxes their tight bond to body tissues, freeing them up to be flushed from the body.[5] Studies have shown that levels of mercury, lead, and aluminum in the urine increase significantly after consuming large amounts of cilantro.[6] It's worth noting that cilantro can cross the blood-brain barrier and, therefore, appears to be particularly effective at removing heavy metals from the central nervous system.

Once the heavy metals are free, the next step is to actually facilitate their removal from the body. Chlorella possesses the capacity to absorb heavy metals. This property has been exploited as a means for treating industrial effluent that contains heavy metals before it is discharged and to recover the bio-available fraction of the metal in the process. In studies undertaken in Germany, high doses of chlorella have been found to be very effective in eliminating heavy metals from the body—from the brain, intestinal wall, muscles, ligaments, connective tissue, and bone.[7]

Together, these herbs create a powerful oral chelation formula. Phase I clinical trials on this formula, completed in 2005, proved that it can naturally remove an average of 87 percent of lead, 91 percent of mercury, and 74 percent of aluminum from the body within six weeks.[8] Once cleaned out with an initial six-week cleanse, a two-week cleanse every three to four months should be enough to keep you relatively metal free—unless you eat a lot of high-mercury fish or have more than a few amalgam fillings, in which case a cleanse every two months is advisable.

Incidentally, you do not want to use a chelation formula every day because your body actually needs small amounts of some heavy metals. Also, chelation will remove small amounts of beneficial metals such as calcium and magnesium—these are easily replaced, though, when you take a break.

## BALANCING PH

Our bodies function in a very narrow range of acid/alkaline balance (pH). Our blood in particular is very sensitive to these changes. Ideally, blood pH should be slightly alkaline at about 7.45. If it varies by even as little as a few tenths of a point, severe illness and death may result. Unfortunately, most of the food we eat is highly acid-forming in the body (meat, dairy, sodas, alcohol, cooked grains). In the end, it becomes too much for our bodies to handle. If we don't correct the problem by "alkalinizing" the body, disease, sickness, and death are the inevitable result. In effect, alkalinizing the body means that you are removing, or detoxing, the acid imbalance that you have created.

Your body has a number of different pH levels that it has to maintain. Your saliva is slightly alkaline, the stomach is strongly acidic during digestion, the intestines are strongly alkaline, and your urine is slightly acidic (to control bacteria). But the most crucial pH level is your blood. Again, if your blood pH deviates even few tenths of a point from its normal pH of 7.45, severe illness or even death is likely. Considering the importance of pH to the body, it's well worth discussing a little further how it affects the body and how we can help maintain the proper pH levels in our own bodies.

The importance of pH really boils down to two things:

1. Enzymes. Enzymes control every metabolic function in our bodies, and they are integral to our immune system. They function optimally at a specific pH and will become inactive if the pH deviates beyond very narrow limits or a particular enzyme.

## WHAT IS PH?

Representing hydrogen ion concentration, pH is the measurement of the acid/alkaline balance of anything.

- On the pH scale, water is neutral and rates a 7.0.

- Acids (such as hydrochloric acid and citric acid) are rated as numbers less than 7.0. The further away from 7.0 the number is, the stronger the acid. Cow's milk at 6.5 is slightly acidic, soft drinks at 3.0 are strongly acidic, and stomach acid at 1.5 is highly acidic.

- Alkaline substances include everything that rates above 7.0 on the pH scale. Again, the further away from 7.0, the more alkaline the substance. Blood at 7.45 is slightly alkaline; pancreatic juice in your intestines is strongly alkaline at 8.8; and baking soda at 12.0 is highly alkaline.

2. Oxygen. Every cell in our body requires oxygen for life and to maintain optimum health. To put it simply, the more acid the blood, the less oxygen is available for use by the cells. Without going into a discussion of the chemistry involved, just understand that it's the same mechanism involved when acid rain "kills" a lake. The fish literally suffocate to death because the acid in the lake "binds up" all of the available oxygen. It's not that the oxygen has gone anywhere, it's just no longer available. Conversely, if you raise the pH of the lake, oxygen is now available and the lake comes back to life. Incidentally, it's worth noting that cancer is related to an acid environment (lack of oxygen)—the higher the pH (the more oxygen present in the cells of the body), the harder it is for cancer to thrive.

The bottom line is that a balanced pH is vital. An extended pH imbalance of any kind threatens our well-being—threatens, in fact, our very lives. Managing the pH balance of all of our bodily fluids, tissues, and organs is so important that our bodies have developed a system to monitor and balance acid-alkaline levels in every cell and biosystem.

## What Affects pH in Our Bodies

To better understand the system our bodies have developed for maintaining pH balance, we need to take a look at what affects pH (usually making us more acidic) and how our bodies respond to that change.

- Acid-Forming Foods: When they are metabolized, carbohydrates, proteins, and fats produce various acids in our bodies. That means that all meats, fish, poultry, eggs, dairy, cooked grains, and refined sugars are acid forming in the body. Probably at the top of the list of acid-forming foods in the human diet are colas. Not only are they high in refined sugar, which is highly acid forming in and of itself, but most cola contains a large amount of phosphoric acid, not to mention carbon dioxide (an end-product of the acid neutralization process).

- Alkaline-Forming Foods: For the most part, only fresh fruits and vegetables and superfoods such as chlorella, spirulina, barley grass, and wheatgrass are alkaline forming and help your body maintain a proper pH. It should be noted that even though citrus fruits are highly acidic, your body treats them as alkaline so that they are, in fact, highly effective alkalinizers.

When proteins are metabolized in the body, they produce sulfuric acid and phosphoric acid; carbohydrates and fats produce acetic acid and lactic acid. Since these acids are poisonous to the body, they must be eliminated. Unfortunately, they can't be eliminated as acids through the kidneys or large intestine as they would damage these organs. The way the body handles them is to neutralize them by converting them into acid salts by combining them with the minerals sodium, calcium, potassium, and magnesium. Of these, calcium is the most important.

Now, here's the key: your body uses a priority system if there are not enough available minerals to neutralize all of the acids present. Blood is at the top of the heap—your body will steal minerals from anywhere and everywhere before it will let your blood become too acidic. Remember, even a slight deviation in blood pH results in death.

Saliva is at the bottom of the heap. Saliva is the first place your body steals minerals from to balance the blood. That's why pH testing of saliva provides an early warning system for when you are becoming too acidic. At optimum health, your saliva will have a pH of 7.45, the same as your blood. At a pH of 6.5–7.0, you'll find yourself frequently succumbing to colds and sickness. At 5.5 and lower, you can pretty much count on the fact that major disease has already taken hold. Virtually, all cancer patients test strongly acidic on a saliva pH test.

Unfortunately, your saliva doesn't contain a big reserve of minerals, so you soon run out. After extracting what it can from urine and soft tissues (creating a rich environment for the spread of cancer), your body turns to its great mineral bank—your bones. So, if your diet is too acid-forming (too much meat, dairy, simple carbohydrates, phosphoric acid, and sugars), your body will fairly quickly begin to leach calcium from your bones to balance the low pH and avoid death. In effect, your body says osteoporosis is preferable to death.

## How to Balance pH

- Change your diet so that you consume lower levels of acid-forming foods and increase levels of alkaline-forming ones. That is, cut back on meat, dairy, sugar, alcohol, and refined grains; consume more fresh vegetables, fruits, and superfoods such as chlorella, wheat grass, barley grass, and spirulina. Follow the guidelines laid out in Chapter 7.

- In addition, there are several special alkalinizing agents available. Your health food store should have alkalinizing teas or drops available. Coral calcium can help. And there are machines that will "micronize" your water—that is, take your tap water and divide it in two. One stream is acidic and can be used for washing and cleaning; the other stream is alkaline and is used for drinking. Unfortunately, these machines are rather expensive—about $1,000.

Another alternative is to simply magnetize your water. Applying a magnetic field to a pitcher of water for a short period of time can help raise the pH of the water a half point or more, depending on its mineral content. It also offers the added advantage of lessening the surface tension of the water, which makes the water more usable by the cells of your body.

## THE HEALING CRISIS

On occasion when detoxing, particularly during your first few detoxes, you may experience some symptoms, often referred to as a healing crisis (Herxheimer's reaction). It is characterized by a temporary increase in symptoms during the cleansing or detoxification process. Reactions, when they occur, are almost always mild, but on rare occasions can be severe.

There are three primary triggers for a detox reaction:

1. Any large-scale die-off of bacteria can release a significant amount of toxins present within the actual bacteria. The stronger those toxins are and the more bacteria present to release them, the stronger the cleansing reaction. Colon cleansing, the use of probiotics, digestive enzymes, immune enhancers, and pathogen destroyers can all trigger bacterial die-off.

2. Any detox that causes the organs of the body (particularly the liver, which is a storehouse of drug and poison residues) to purge their stored poisons and toxins can trigger a cleansing reaction, as can the use of an herbal blood cleanser.

3. Any program, such as fasting or the use of weight-loss herbs, that causes a rapid breakdown of fat cells (which are a storehouse for toxins) can be accompanied by a detox reaction.

The bottom line is that the body must go through an elimination process to achieve good health. There will be ups and downs. Symptoms, if

# THE HEALING POWER OF FASTING

Although not system specific, as are the other programs we've mentioned so far, when it comes to detoxing, fasting nevertheless can play a major role. The principles of fasting are simple. First, when you deprive your body of food, your body begins to consume itself to survive. Being geared to self-survival, your body chooses to consume damaged cells and toxic cells first, saving the healthiest for later. Second, it takes a tremendous amount of energy and puts a tremendous strain on your body's organs to process food. (Check your heart rate after eating a large meal and observe how exhausted you feel.) When you fast, your body diverts that energy to repair and rebuilding.

No matter what medical doctors may say, the process of fasting works. In fact, a simple thought confirming the necessity for periodic fasting is the fact that human beings are the only animals that eat when they're sick. Think about that for a moment. Have you ever observed how dogs or cats, for example, stop eating while they're recovering? They intuitively understand the healing power of fasting.

Numerous books on fasting are available to help guide you through the process. There are four levels of fasting worth considering:

- The pure water fast. This is the most powerful fast, but also produces the most toxic side effects. I do not recommend it unless you have a great deal of experience in fasting or are working directly with a qualified healer.

- The master cleanse, which adds maple syrup and lemon juice to the pure water fast, helps even out some of the blood sugar swings experienced on the pure water fast. In other words, it's a bit easier.

- Juice fasting. Fasting on fresh juices helps smooth out many of the discomforts of fasting by keeping blood sugar levels balanced.

- Chlorella fasting. Even gentler is supplementing your juice fast with chlorella throughout the day. As a bonus, the chlorella adds to the impact of the detox by escorting many toxins (including heavy metals) out of your body. (If you're allergic to chlorella, you can use any of the other green superfoods.)

When fasting, make sure you drink large amounts of water to flush the toxins and organic compounds from your body. In Chapter 3, we discussed the herbal colon-activator formula that provides both cleansing and healing to the entire gastrointestinal system—it's highly recommended that you use such a formula while fasting to accelerate removal of toxins from the colon. If not, you will have to take a colonic or an enema every day. Also, using a water-soluble fiber, such as psyllium seed husks, while fasting will help "escort" toxins out of the body.

they appear, are usually mild, but in some cases can be severe. Understand that the symptoms you experience are indicative of the cleansing, purifying process that is underway. Go as slowly as your body needs to so that your elimination is gradual and comfortable. Also, keep in mind that this is not an endurance contest. If symptoms become too severe, stop the detoxification and regroup. You can always restart the detox again at a later date.

## Easing Your Way through the Healing Crisis

- Drink plenty of fresh water, juices, and herbal teas to flush the body of toxins.

- Use a colon stimulation formula to make sure that you are eliminating waste promptly. Symptoms frequently disappear immediately after a good bowel movement.

- Use psyllium seed husks, ground flaxseed, or oat bran daily to absorb toxins and to help speed their transit through the system.

- On occasion, a good enema or colon irrigation can provide relief.

- Sometimes, rest is the best therapy.

- And, on rare occasions, a reduction of the dosage or temporary cessation may be required.

## One Person's Experience

The follow story comes from a letter I received from a competitive cyclist who went through a healing crisis while detoxing. His reactions were on the severe side to be sure, but it's instructive to see how the crisis ended.

The thirty-day colon cleanse went without a hitch. I lost 10–15 pounds, maybe more. This is excellent news for a competitive cyclist because weight loss without losing muscle mass is a win-win situation.

After I was done with the colon cleanse, I began the liver/gallbladder detox. The first day I had some cravings for food and that night I dreamed I was at a banquet stuffing my face. I thought, "Oh no, I'm supposed to be fasting," and then woke up and realized I hadn't broken my fast. I had interesting dreams almost every night of the five days.

On the second day, I had a headache in the morning and, when I got home around 4 P.M., the headache still persisted. I tried to make the potassium broth, but the smallest tasks seemed monumental, and I lay down in bed and started to burp a little. I couldn't sleep, the headache got worse, and I began to feel as if I was going to be ill. Eventually, I had my first bout of vomiting and "dry heaves." The only way I can describe the next hour or so is that it was like how "going cold turkey" from heroin is portrayed in the movies. I had several sessions of vomiting, hot and cold sweats, and one of the worst headaches of my life.

The first session of vomiting was the carrot juice I had consumed or so it looked like it. The second time was what may have been ancient maraschino cherries or tapeworms(?)—chunks of red, but not blood. Round three brought up some mucus-like substance and some yellowish, bile-like fluid. The "heaves" were so bad that I was thinking I might have to stop the detox. The final bout was the worst and brought up yellow bile(?) with red "blood" specks in it, seemingly from the deepest recesses possible (or that I had ever experienced).

Exhausted and not wanting to be too far from the toilet, I sat back in a reclining chair and fell asleep. I woke up in an hour and immediately noticed that my sinuses were clearer, my headache was gone, and I felt like a million bucks. A chiropractor friend confirmed that it was probably the effects of toxins being released by my liver into my system and that I may have gotten rid of some bad stuff.

## GENERAL RECOMMENDATIONS

### Liver

- Liver/gallbladder flush. A liver/gallbladder flush twice a year (more often if you are ill) to eliminate any accumulation of liver fat, toxins, and incipient gallstones is mandatory.

- Liver-rebuilding tonic. In addition to flushing, you need to regularly partake of a liver-rebuilding formula. Herbs such as milk thistle, which are usually found in these formulas, stimulate the liver to rebuild itself. *Picrorrhiza kurroa*, another herb frequently used, is probably an even stronger liver protector and rebuilder. And herbs such as dandelion root, barberry, artichoke, and beet leaf are lipotropics that help clean fat out of the liver.

- Regular consumption of fresh apple/beet juice is profoundly beneficial to the liver. Start with small servings and build slowly to avoid uncomfortable detox reactions.

Note: Never do a liver cleanse without first cleaning out the colon to provide an outlet for the toxins released by the liver. And again, it is also highly recommended that you do a kidney flush program that incorporates herbs such as *Chanca piedra* and gravel root to soften any gallstones before doing the liver detox.

### Kidneys

If you have access to a full kidney cleanse formula, then by all means use it. If it's in a liquid form, mix it with a quart of diluted apple juice and drink a pint a day for four days. Do this every two to three months to keep your kidneys free flowing. And remember, a good kidney formula not only helps cleanse and rebuild the kidneys, it is also tonic for the gallbladder and pancreas.

### Blood

- Cleansing. Go on an herbal cleansing of the blood two to four times a year (even more often if you are ill).

- Oral chelation. Use a cilantro/chlorella tincture: start with a six-week detox, then twice a year after that do a two-week detox. As an alternative, you can use a good EDTA-based oral formula.

- Alkalinize or die. Cut way back on acid-producing foods such as meat, dairy, sugar, soda, refined grains, etc., and add alkalinizing foods such as chlorella and fresh vegetables to your diet. Drink water that has been magnetized, use micronized water, or add alkalinizing drops to your water to raise pH.

- One final thought on pH: it makes sense to test the pH of your saliva on a regular basis as a touchstone for your overall health. You can pick up pH paper specifically designed for this purpose at most health food stores. Make sure you test in the morning before brushing or eating as these things can temporarily alter the pH in your mouth. Just spit out a couple of times into the sink, then onto the pH paper. Ideally, your pH should be about 7.45. If it tests below 7.0, you should get aggressive in terms of alkalinizing your body.

We've now concluded our discussion on detoxification. In the next chapter, we will explore how to improve your diet and nutrition.

# PART THREE
## *Diet and Supplements*

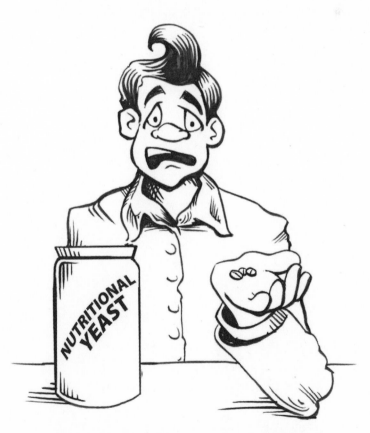

**Do these come in chocolate truffle?!?**

# CHAPTER 7

## Diet—The Slow Killer

- **The Four Problem Areas**
- **Everything You Always Wanted to Know about Fats**
- **The Importance of Carbohydrates**
- **Protein: What about Meat and Dairy?**
- **Frankenfoods: Genetic Engineering, Irradiation, and Microwaves**

Probably no topic has been more discussed (and is more confusing) than what constitutes the optimum diet. Almost every day, we are presented with another book promoting a new type of diet—the caveman diet, the blood-type diet, the Ornish Plan, the high-carbohydrate diet, the Pritikin Diet, the Atkins Diet, the Zone, the South Beach Diet, and on and on. It is not my goal in this chapter to detail an optimum diet plan for you. Even if that were my intent, it couldn't be done in a single chapter. Instead, what I want to do is arm you with enough information so that you can selectively evaluate any plan you might be interested in and intelligently choose those parts that might work for you. So, with that in mind, let's step back and take an objective view of the situation.

Let me begin by categorically stating that medical doctors don't study health and nutrition in medical school. The average time spent is one class of one hour a week for eight to ten weeks. That's it. If you read two good books on the topic, you know more than 99 percent of all the doctors in the world. Just because a doctor, or the *Journal of the American Medical Association*, makes a pronouncement on health and nutrition does not necessarily make it true, no matter how peer reviewed it may be. And as for government agencies, they are under intense lobbying pressure, as evidenced by "modifications" to the food pyramid in the United States to promote industry (such as the dairy industry) over health or the passage of the European Food Supplements Directive, which was designed to promote the use of prescription drugs by restricting access to herbs and supplements across an entire continent.

When it comes to the "authorities" in health and nutrition, just think of some of the nonsense you've been "fed" over your lifetime. Remember, it was these same authorities who at one time told you that margarine was good and that butter was bad, that diet had nothing to do with cancer, and that allowed soda pop to be sold at schools. In fact, just think of hospital food— and keep in mind that doctors are in charge of the overall programs in hospitals. If hospital food represents the medical community's definition of healthy, healing food, then we need to rely on a different group of experts.

## THE FOUR PROBLEM AREAS

Eliminating bad fats from your diet makes all the sense in the world. Cutting refined carbohydrates and minimizing high-glycemic grains and starchy vegetables is also a healthy thing to do. Eating enough of the right kinds of proteins is important, as is eating high-quality food grown to produce the maximum nutritional value. It all makes sense, but this simple advice has become lost. Quite simply, we are once again being seduced by our love of broad-stroke generalizations. Let's go into a little detail and see what the real story is.

Once you've cleaned out and repaired your food processing and waste removal systems, you're ready to begin the process of rebuilding your body. Keep in mind that your body is rebuilding itself all the time. The actual life cycle of a blood cell, for example, is approximately four months. That means you replace your entire blood supply every 120 days. The question is: what will determine the quality of that blood? What are you going to be building that new blood from—fast-food burgers and fries? Understand, it's not only your blood, but every cell and organ in your body that's being replaced. For the most part, you get an entirely new body every seven years. It doesn't take a genius to realize that the better your nutrition, the better the "quality" of your new body.

Unfortunately, it's not quite that simple. Any attempt to optimize the nutrition we take into our bodies must address four key problem areas:

1. Plastic fats

2. Refined carbohydrates

3. Bad proteins

4. Frankenfoods

## EVERYTHING YOU ALWAYS WANTED TO KNOW ABOUT FATS

It wasn't that long ago that fat was the number one culprit in our diets. Every doctor and food commercial on TV promoted low-fat, lean foods. And we responded: fat consumption in Western society dropped significantly over the last twenty years. But surprisingly, obesity soared at exactly the same time, to the point that the U.S. is now among the fattest countries in history (with the rest of the world working hard to catch up).

What was wrong with the fat theory? Aren't fat calories bad for you, and don't they contribute to obesity? The answer is no—at least not when stated in such simplistic terms. As it turns out, there are good fats and bad fats, and I'm not talking about unsaturated and saturated fats. Again, why anyone would listen to the medical establishment when it comes to diet and nutrition is still mind-boggling to me. Listening to a doctor about nutrition just because they went to medical school is like listening to a plumber about your clogged arteries just because they specialize in cleaning out clogged pipes.

The current dogma promoted by the medical community when it comes to fat is:

- Fat is bad.

- Saturated fat is bad.

- Trans-fat is bad. (A complete reversal on their part, incidentally, over the last ten years.)

- If you have to eat fat, polyunsaturated vegetable oils are the way to go. These are the bottled oils you buy in the store (corn oil, canola oil, and safflower oil). Omega-3 fatty acids are probably good for you, but the alternative health community is moving much too fast in adding these fats to all kinds of food.

But it turns out that the truth is quite different. With that in mind, let's explore the reality behind the facts.

## Is Fat Unhealthy?

Is fat bad for you? Hardly; in fact, it's essential for good health! Fats are the ultimate energy storage system. Your body stores fat for long-term energy use. Think of bears that live off their fat for months at a time while they hibernate in winter. On the other hand, if you're eating every day, your body doesn't really need to store fat for future use, so what is necessary for survival for bears can be a quick ticket to the cemetery for humans. Nevertheless, even though excess fat of the wrong kind may be deadly, certain fats are essential for life and health and are required in sufficient quantities.

To understand the real story behind fats, it's worth approaching the issue from two angles: common sense and biochemistry. But first, since, as they say, you can't tell the players without a scorecard, here are the players:

### SATURATED FATS

Meat (grain fed), dairy, chocolate, coconut oil, and palm oil

### ESSENTIAL FATTY ACIDS (POLYUNSATURATED FATS)

*Omega-6 fatty acids*

Linoleic acid: Safflower, sunflower, corn, hemp, soybean, walnut, pumpkin, canola, and sesame oils

Arachidonic acid: Via synthesis from linoleic acid and consumption of grain-fed meat

Gamma-linolenic acid (GLA): Black currant seeds and evening primrose oil

Dihomo-gamma-linolenic acid (DGLA): Brown algae

*Omega-3 fatty acids*

Alpha-linolenic acid (ALA): Flaxseed, canola oil, hempseeds, greens, walnuts and soy, range-fed meat, cage-free eggs

Eicosapentaenoic acid (EPA) and docosahexaenoic acid (DHA): Fish, marine animals, algae, and from the breakdown of ALA

### MONOUNSATURATED FATS

*Omega-9 fatty acids*

Olives and avocados

Hydrogenated and partially hydrogenated oils are artificial creations, and the primary source of trans-fatty acids. Once promoted as a healthy alternative to saturated fats by the medical establishment, they are now recognized as one of the primary killers in our diets. It's also important to understand that most substances that contain fats or oils actually have more than one kind. Canola oil, for example, contains omega-3s, -6s, and -9s. Meat contains not only saturated fat, but also omega-6s and -3s. The table shows the predominant fat that each food provides.

## Is Saturated Fat Bad?

Not all saturated fat is bad; in fact, a certain amount is essential, and some saturated fats are extremely health promoting. Prolonged experience with the Atkins Diet has shown that natural saturated fat does not necessarily raise cholesterol levels and clog arteries (although the diet itself quite likely promotes osteoporosis and colon cancer). The simple truth is that the whole issue of saturated versus unsaturated fats is mostly false.

Certain saturated fats are extremely healthy and even essential to good health, such as coconut oil. For a number of years, coconut oil has been vilified by the medical health authorities due to its saturated fat content, but not all saturated fats are alike. Coconut oil is unique in its structural makeup. It is not only the highest source of saturated fats (92 percent), but included in that number are the medium-chain triglycerides (MCTs), which are extremely beneficial to the body. In addition, approximately 50 percent of these MCTs are made up of lauric acid, the most important fatty acid in building and maintaining the body's immune system. The only other source of lauric acid found in such high concentrations is mother's milk.

## Trans-Fats—Decidedly Unhealthy

Is trans-fat bad? Absolutely! In fact, in earlier editions of this book I called products made with trans-fats (partially hydrogenated oils) the number one killer in our diet. But this is one area that has seen a dramatic change in the last ten years. Whereas at one time medical authorities promoted these products as "healthy" alternatives to saturated fat products such as butter, these same authorities gradually became aware (about thirty years after the alternative health community) that trans-fats were, in fact, decidedly unhealthy. They are major contributors to cancer, heart disease, and diabetes. Over the last couple of years, government agencies have jumped on board and started pressuring food companies and restaurants to ban trans-fats from our diets. And even if late, they are correct. These oils are absolutely unnecessary and have no place in your diet or in any of the foods you eat—if you wish to be healthy.

## Polyunsaturated Vegetable Oils—Proceed With Caution

Unfortunately, the same government authorities and health experts who are now warning us away from trans-fats are pushing us toward polyunsaturated vegetable oils. But are these good for us? Not necessarily. Because of the quantity and quality of polyunsaturated fats in foods, they have replaced trans-fatty acids as the number one killer in our diets—a statement that probably comes as a surprise to most of you.

First, let's talk about why essential fatty acids (EFAs), a group to which polyunsaturated oils belong, are so important. Among other things, they are the main components of all cellular membranes—inside and out—where they protect against viruses, bacteria, and allergens. They are the key building blocks of all fats and oils, both in our foods and in our bodies. They play a key role in the construction and maintenance of nerve cells and the hormone-like substances called prostaglandins, and they help decrease cholesterol and triglyceride levels in the blood. The bottom line is that essential fatty acids are vital to our health, the primary healing agents in the body. According to some estimates, as many as 90 percent of all people are deficient in at least one of them.

In point of fact, all fats are actually fatty acids, consisting of one part fat (which is not water soluble) and one part acid (which is). Omega-3 and omega-6 fats are not only good for you, they are, in fact, essential—your body can't produce them, which means you must get them in your diet. However, due to the extreme sensitivity of omega-3s to light and oxygen, they have been removed from virtually all processed foods so that the foods have a longer shelf life. The sad fact is that our lack of these key EFAs has been linked to many of today's diseases and afflictions, including hair loss, lack of energy, skin problems, heart and circulatory problems, and immune disorders (including arthritis).

Now let's talk about the problem associated with EFAs. For most of human existence, we have eaten foods containing omega-6 fatty acids (linoleic acid and arachidonic acid) and omega-3 fatty acids (DHA, EPA, and alpha-linolenic acid) in a ratio of about 1:1 to 2:1. Over the last fifty years, however, that ratio has changed to 20:1 or 30:1, even in some cases as high as 50:1. Our diets now include huge amounts of highly refined oils that are extracted from plants and used for cooking or in prepared foods (at the insistence of medical authorities). These oils—corn, safflower, cottonseed, peanut, and soybean—are all high in omega-6s. As a consequence, we have dramatically decreased our intake of omega-3s as found previously in whole grains, beans and seeds, and seafood—and now get our omega-3s primarily as the secondary fatty acid in our highly refined bottled oils and meat, which accounts for the increasing distortion of the fatty acid balance toward omega-6s.

In other words, for most of us, we face the cruel paradox that the higher our intake of omega-3s, the worse the omega-6/omega-3 fat ratio gets in our bodies. This crops up in areas of our diet that we don't even think about. For example, grass-fed beef contains omega-6 and omega-3 fatty acids in close to the healthy 2:1 ratio. But grain-fattened beef, which most people eat, contains fat in an imbalanced ratio that parallels the ratios found in the grains used to fatten them—20:1, 30:1, and even 50:1 in favor of omega-6.

There are numerous studies that show how deadly this is. For example, a Korean study found that the ratios of serum omega-6 to omega-3 fatty acids were highly indicative of prostate cancer risk. The researchers concluded that omega-6 polyunsaturated fatty acids have a tumor-promoting effect while omega-3 acids have a protective effect.[1]

## Taking Omega-3 Fatty Acids

Right now, omega-3 fatty acids are "hot." Over the next couple of years, they are set to become the number one additive in functional foods. And obviously, based on what we've already talked about, that's a good thing, right? Sort of . . . well, almost . . . but not necessarily!

Omega-3 fatty acid comes in six forms, but three are of primary interest to us:

- Alpha-linolenic acid (ALA) is the complex form of omega-3 that's found in most plants, such as flax. It's not actually useful to the body until it's broken down into its two constituents, EPA and DHA.

- Eicosapentaenoic acid (EPA) provides profound anti-inflammatory activity, enhances the immune system, and provides numerous cardiovascular benefits, including thinning the blood and lowering blood pressure.

- Docosahexaenoic acid (DHA) is a major fatty acid in sperm and brain phospholipids, and especially in the retina. Dietary DHA can reduce the level of blood triglycerides in humans, which may reduce the risk of heart disease. It also appears to play a major role in preventing and relieving Alzheimer's disease and depression.

The primary sources of ALA supplementation are vegetarian, most notably flaxseed. The primary sources of EPA and DHA are fatty fish such as salmon and krill (cold water, shrimp-like invertebrates). Most of the alpha-linolenic acid we consume must be converted into DHA and EPA. Unfortunately, this process, which is governed by a particular enzyme (delta-6 desaturase), is significantly inhibited (up to 50 percent or more) by an over-abundance of linoleic acid, which comes from excessive omega-6 fatty acid consumption. The enzyme is "used up" in the desaturation process involved in getting rid of excess omega-6 fats and no longer available for converting ALA. The delta-6 enzyme is also inhibited by the trans-fatty acids and by high levels of insulin, a problem today when obesity and diabetes are soaring. And the process of delta-6 desaturation slows with aging.

Each of these factors can lead to an accumulation of ALA, which is counterproductive, but alleviating that build-up is relatively easy:

- Stop using all plastic fats—all hydrogenated vegetable oils and all super-refined vegetable oils. The high temperatures that these oils are exposed to dramatically changes their structure. Highly refined and cold-pressed oils are not the same, and they behave very differently in the body.

- Stop cooking with oils high in omega-6 fats, such as safflower, sunflower, and corn oils, and instead shift to walnut, olive, coconut, and avocado oils, as well as organic butter (in moderation). And if you need to use oil for high-temperature frying or sautéing, use small amounts of avocado oil or rice bran oil.

- Shift your diet away from high-glycemic, refined carbohydrates and move to a more Mediterranean style diet to help lower insulin levels.

- Finally, an effective method of counteracting slowed desaturation of linoleic acid is to provide the delta-6 desaturated metabolite, gamma-linolenic acid (GLA), directly through supplements. Desaturation of linoleic and especially alpha-linolenic acid increases dramatically in the elderly with GLA supplementation. One other advantage to GLA supplementation is that much of the GLA is converted to DGLA, which competes with and prevents the negative inflammatory effects that arachidonic acid otherwise causes in the body. Key sources of GLA are evening primrose oil, black currant oil, and borage oil.

An obvious question comes up when talking about ALA: why bother if you can just take fish oil or krill oil supplements and not have to worry about conversion? The answer is that each source has its own benefits. Fish oil is good because it is already broken down into the useable EPA and DHA. Krill oil contains phospholipids specially integrated with omega-3 essential fatty acids. This unique structure provides important cell membrane building blocks in the right ratios for use by the body. And as for flaxseed oil, although it needs to be broken down, it also happens to be outrageously high in lignans, phytochemicals shown to have significant anti-cancer properties. Flax picked up a bad rap several years ago based on a bogus study that said it may promote prostate cancer.[2] But no one in the study was supplementing with flax oil—the subjects' high ALA readings came as a result of other oils and fats they were eating, particularly from meat. In other words, the increased incidence of cancer associated with ALA was far more likely the result of a wildly skewed omega-6/omega-3 ratio. So, the "warnings" concerning flax damn a valuable component of a healthy lifestyle based on faulty information and let the true killers—highly refined, high omega-6 oils—go free.

## Rancidity

All oils are sensitive to heat, light, and exposure to oxygen. Over time, depending on the level of exposure and the particular oil, they can turn rancid—noticeable as off-taste and odor. Oils turn rancid through two chemical processes: hydrolysis and oxidation. Both affect the taste and odor of the oil and can degrade its nutritional value. But our primary concern when it comes to health is oxidation. As we will explore in detail in Chapter 10, oxidation means free radical production, which can present major health problems. Rancidification can produce large numbers of highly reactive free radicals and is to be avoided. To delay the development of rancid oil, it is best to store all oils in the refrigerator or a cool, dry place. Most highly refined oils that you buy in the supermarket can easily keep for a year or longer—in some cases, almost indefinitely—but there are other health trade-offs involved in using highly processed, refined oil. Extra-virgin olive oil, on the other hand, will also keep about a year after opening without the trade-offs. Other unrefined vegetable oils that you buy in the health food store will keep about six months. Rancidity is only a problem for unsaturated fats and oils; saturated fats such as coconut oil do not turn rancid.

# THE PROBLEMS WITH PROCESSING OILS

An important factor to remember, particularly as omega-3 fatty acids are being introduced into functional foods en masse, is their sensitivity to heat, light, and processing. In other words, their value may be somewhat negated (and even turned upside down) in many of these foods if the manufacturers don't know what they're doing. This brings us to a key issue regarding fats and oils: processing. Over the years, I have talked frequently of the dangers of highly refined oils—plastic fats, if you will—but what exactly does that mean? What follows is a generic description of the process involved in getting oils out of seeds (or in this case, coconut copra) and onto your grocer's shelves.

The first step in the process is for the copra (which is about 64 percent oil content) to be cleaned up. Dirt and other foreign materials are removed by hand. Metallic objects are removed by magnets. The cleaned copra next passes through a series of grinders and flakers, which take the pieces down to about an eighth of an inch in size. The material is then placed in driers, where the moisture is taken down to 2–3 percent. Oil is then extracted from the dried copra by means of a mechanical press. The extracted expeller oil, containing fine solids, is conveyed to the filtration section for purification, then pumped into storage tanks.

But there is still oil in the pressed copra cake. "Waste not, want not." So, the cake goes to a solvent extraction plant, where it undergoes continuous washing with hexane for more efficient extraction of the oil from the cake. This chemically extracted oil is pumped to the filtration section for blending with the expeller oil and further purification. Unfortunately, trace amounts of hexane remain in the oil. Is this a problem? Yes, because hexane is a petroleum-based solvent that can seriously impact health. Side effects from exposure to hexane include dizziness, drowsiness, dullness, headache, nausea, weakness, unconsciousness, and abdominal pain. Also, hexane tends to concentrate in the meal that is left, which is sold as animal feed and can cause anemia in livestock. A number of hexane compounds are carcinogens, according to the Environmental Protection Agency and are classed as hazardous substances. Hexane also poses a serious environmental threat as it is a hydrocarbon polluter and produces ozone and air pollution.

## Refining

Once extracted, the oil "needs" to be refined, which involves the treatment of the crude oil with a lye solution to reduce the free fatty acid (FFA) content to 0.05 percent. This is done primarily to prevent spoilage—to help the oil last an eternity on the grocer's shelf. However, free fatty acids are not necessarily bad: conjugated linoleic acid (found in meat and dairy products), for example, is a naturally occurring free fatty acid that has been shown to improve nutrient usage, promote muscle tone, significantly reduce body fat, and have anti-tumor properties. But why in the world would we want something like that in our vegetable oil?

In addition, other impurities in the oil, such as gums, phosphatides, pigments, and other oxidation products, which would "impair" the taste, odor, shelf life, and other "desired" properties of the oil are likewise removed. This degumming and neutralization process is accomplished by means of phosphoric acid and more lye.

The now "neutral" oil is mixed with bleaching earth (a type of clay) and activated carbon to give the oil a lighter color. Final purification is accomplished using filters, presses, and polishing filters. At which point, the oil is pumped into storage tanks.

## Deodorizing

All edible oils and fats contain certain compounds that give the particular oil its identifiable taste and smell. In all commercial oils, these compounds are removed to make the oil as neutral tasting as possible (after all, who wants to eat anything that has any flavor?). This process is called deodorization, and because of the high temperatures involved, it is extremely damaging to the oil.

Refined bleached oil from refining is first transferred to a de-aerator operating under a vacuum for removal of any air in the oil. The oil then passes through a series of heaters, where the temperature is raised high enough for efficient steam distillation and deodorization—upwards of 200°C (450°F). At these temperatures, the fundamental structure of many oils is changed into a different form of fatty acid through a process called isomerization. These new forms are not beneficial to the human body. The high heat also causes a small amount of trans-fatty acids to be formed. Finally, steam is blown through the oil to vaporize those components of the oil that actually give it any lingering odor or taste. The fully deodorized, tasteless, and refined oil then passes through a cooler and polishing filter basket for removal of any fine suspension before being finally pumped to the storage tank.

What's left is an oil that is virtually colorless, odorless, and tasteless, which can last for years in a bottle with no danger of spoilage. On the other hand, it has no connection with the beneficial oil that was originally contained in the seed or nut. It is now a "plastic fat," fundamentally changed in structure, that offers no benefits to the human body—a plastic fat that is actually quite harmful. In addition, all of the beneficial phytochemicals (such as the lignans, which are an integral part of the oil complex and play a key anti-cancer role) have been removed.

## THE IMPORTANCE OF CARBOHYDRATES

If you believe much of what's circulating in the news today, carbohydrates are killers—responsible for everything from obesity to diabetes. Nonsense! Not all carbohydrates are bad. In fact, our bodies need carbohydrates. Most of our organs and tissues, including the muscles and our brain, run on carbohydrates. As Joel Fuhrman states in his book, *Eat to Live*, "It is impossible to glean all the nutrients needed for *optimal* health if your diet does not contain lots of carbohydrate-rich food. Fresh fruits, beans and legumes, whole grains, and root vegetables are all examples of foods whose calories come mainly from carbohydrate. It is the nutrient-per-calorie ratio of these foods that determines their food value."

The concept of *nutrient density* that Dr. Fuhrman mentions is key to truly making sense of dietary issues. The U.S. Department of Agriculture (USDA) maintains a National Nutritional Database (www.nal.usda.gov/fnic/cgi-bin/nut_search.pl). Compare sirloin steak to romaine lettuce, for example, and you will be greatly surprised: romaine lettuce not only has far more nutrients than sirloin, but it also more than holds its own when it comes to protein per calorie as compared to sirloin. Surprise! On a per-calorie basis, romaine lettuce contains 100 times the calcium, over 20 times the magnesium, and infinitely more antioxidants, phytochemicals, and fiber than sirloin. Which food do you think is more beneficial to your body?

And it's not just leafy greens that are nutrient dense—fruits of all kinds are packed with vitamins, minerals, antioxidants, phytochemicals, and fiber. And even whole grains have more nutrient density than meat and dairy. Now, to be sure, many grains are high-glycemic and trigger an insulin response and contribute significantly to allergies and autoimmune disorders, but not all grains do so. (The glycemic index was developed by diabetes researchers as a measure of the insulin impact of particular foods. Foods with a higher rating on the glycemic index cause a higher insulin response.)

Understand that your body can only use glucose (or its stored form, glycogen) as energy; everything must get broken down to these forms first. These are your body's primary and preferred energy sources and are sometimes referred to as blood sugar. If there is too much glucose in your blood (hyperglycemic), your pancreas produces insulin to shuttle the sugar out of your blood and into your cells; if there is too little sugar (hypoglycemic), your body produces glucose from the stored glycogen, which gets rid of the insulin so you can build up more sugar in your blood. Hyper- and hypoglycemia are the extreme conditions of high and low blood sugar, respectively.

The bottom line is that you need carbohydrates for energy. They power every part of your body and energize it to work, run, jump, think, breathe, and more. As long as you're using your body, you need glucose. When you are hungry, you find it hard to think and work because you're running out of glucose, and your brain needs more fuel.

## Types of Carbohydrates

The key to how carbohydrates are used in the body is how quickly they break down in the digestive tract. This is largely determined by their fundamental structure.

- Simple, or short-chain, carbohydrates don't need to be broken down at all. They are instantly available to the body as sugars. To say that all sugars are bad, as is often now stated, is an oversimplification. There are times that your body truly needs an instant influx of energy foods. And many sugars such as mannose play a key role in our immune systems. However, there is no question that, in general, a sustained high-level intake of sugars spikes insulin levels and eventually contributes significantly to major health problems, such as obesity, high cholesterol, high triglycerides, and diabetes.

- Complex, or long-chain, carbohydrates cannot be utilized by the body until they are broken down. Complex carbohydrates consist of hundreds or thousands of sugar units linked together in single molecules. Theoretically, since they are not instantly available to the body, they should raise glucose levels more slowly and be healthier than simple sugars. But that is not always the case: some long-chain carbohydrates, such as potatoes, bananas, all refined grains (and many whole grains too), and maltodextrin (which is frequently added to processed foods) break down very quickly and are virtually indistinguishable from straight sugar in their effects on the body.

There are two things that prevent complex carbohydrates from doing this. First, fiber cannot be digested by humans, and it has no calories because the body cannot absorb it. The more fiber present in a food, the more slowly the carbohydrates bound to that fiber break down. That's why high-fiber fruits and vegetables, such as broccoli, prunes, and berries, tend to be very low on the glycemic index. In general, these foods, although they are pure carbohydrates, can be eaten abundantly on any low-carbo-hydrate dietary program. Incidentally, not all fibers are the same, a distinction usually lost in translation. Some fibers (glucomannans) slow sugar absorption, whereas other fibers (beta-glucans) lower the risk of heart disease, and some merely provide bulk (wheat bran).

Second, if the simple sugars in a complex carbohydrate are not assembled in a straight line but rather include many branches, it slows the breakdown of the carbohydrate dramatically because the enzyme amylase does not work on branches. Examples of branched carbohydrates include the gums such as guar and xanthan.

Whichever form of carbohydrate you eat, if digested, it appears in the circulatory system as glucose, on its way to the cells where it is used for energy. The key is how long that process takes. If it is spread out over several hours, there is no spike in blood sugar and insulin levels, the body does not store fat, and you get sustained energy over a prolonged period of time.

## The Negative Impact of Refined Carbohydrates

So, given this background, and understanding that there are both good and bad carbohydrates, let's cut to the chase. When people say "carbohydrates are bad," what they really should be saying is "refined carbohydrates are bad." Refined carbohydrates include all refined and processed foods, such as:

- Everything made with white flour: most snack foods, most baked goods (specifically, breads and rolls), and most pasta

- White rice

- Cold cereals and most hot cereals

- All sugar foods, including cakes, candies, many bottled juice drinks, and soda. Soda, particularly colas, may be the single worst "food" ever invented. Soda contains approximately one teaspoon of sugar per ounce of soda. (Artificial sweeteners are even worse.) That works out to about 12 teaspoons per can, or 32 teaspoons per "big gulp" drink. Many sodas, particularly colas, are also high in phosphoric acid, which leaches calcium out of your body at an astounding rate, eventually leading to osteoporosis.

When grain is made into refined white flour (primarily to prolong shelf life), more than thirty essential nutrients are largely removed. All fiber, wheat germ, and essential fatty acids are removed; only the starch is left. Of the natural nutrients removed, only synthesized vitamins $B_1$, $B_2$, and $B_3$, and iron are put back in to create one of the first (dating back to the early 1940s) "functional foods"—enriched flour. This truly is a creative definition of the word *enriched* considering that "un-enriched" whole-wheat flour contains 44 percent more vitamin E, 52 percent more pantothenic acid, 65 percent more folic acid, 76 percent more biotin, and 84 percent more vitamin $B_6$, not to mention more magnesium, calcium, zinc, chromium, manganese, selenium, vanadium, and copper.

As for fiber, enriched white bread has just 25 percent as much as real whole wheat. And keep in mind that much of the bread now marketed as "whole wheat" is in truth white bread with burnt sugar added for coloring. Several years ago, one company even added sawdust (calling it "cellulose" on the label) to replace the lost bran and advertised it as "high-fiber" bread. How can this be? Quite simply, it is legal to describe flour as "whole wheat" on the label even when the bran and germ have been removed. Buyer beware! You need to look at the ingredient list to see if the bread is 100 percent whole wheat or mostly white flour with just a little bit of whole wheat added just so it can be featured on the label.

Refined carbohydrates negatively affect the body in a number of ways:

- They are acid-forming in the body (see Chapter 6).

- They are converted to triglycerides in the body and stored as fat.

- They all rank high on the glycemic index (with no redeeming nutritional value, unlike whole fruits and vegetables that are also high on the glycemic index).

# THE GLYCEMIC INDEX

The glycemic index, and identifying high-glycemic foods, is one of the hot areas of nutritional science right now. Not to make light of it, it is an extremely important dietary consideration, but with two huge "howevers." Diabetics have been using the glycemic index for years to help in controlling their insulin levels. Quite simply, foods that adversely affect blood sugar by elevating insulin levels are considered "high-glycemic" foods, and foods that do not elevate insulin levels are "low glycemic."

High-glycemic foods can cause your body to store fat, make you feel fatigued, cause your brain to go "fuzzy," and lead to heart problems such as elevated LDL ("bad") cholesterol levels and high blood pressure. Obviously, these are conditions to be avoided. Keep in mind that high-glycemic unprocessed fruits and vegetables have compensating benefits. Raisins, for example, are high glycemic, but also one of the highest antioxidant foods known. With that caveat in mind, high-glycemic foods that cause elevated insulin levels and concomitant problems include:

• Bananas

• Raisins

• Carrots

• Potatoes

• Corn

• Breads, cereals, pastas, and rice of all kinds

• Virtually all snack foods

• Sugars of all kinds and sodas

There are two "howevers" to the glycemic index:

1. Chewing. If you chew your food well enough, it slows down the entire eating process, which spreads out the glycemic response. It also allows the amylase in the saliva to effectively start breaking down the carbohydrates, which takes a huge burden off your pancreas. And it allows time for your stomach to signal your brain that you're full (it normally takes twenty minutes for your brain to catch up with your stomach), so you end up eating less.

So, how much do you need to chew your food? There's an old saying: "You should drink your solids and chew your liquids." What that means is that you should chew the dry food you eat until it turns to liquid in your mouth (about forty chews per mouthful), and that you should swish liquids back and forth in your mouth (chew them, as it were) an equal number of times. This helps mix enzymes into the food or liquid and begin the digestive process.

2. Fiber. The presence of fiber in a meal slows down the absorption of carbohydrates in the intestinal tract. Beyond that, there are also several natural fibers that can be taken as supplements with meals that block carbohydrate receptor sites in the intestinal tract, thereby further slowing the absorption of high-glycemic carbohydrates and the resulting glycemic response. These include high-fiber foods such as nopal cactus, konjac mannan (glucomannan), and fenugreek (*Trigonella foenum-graecum*). We will cover these particular fibers in more detail in Chapter 20 when we focus on diabetes.

## Sweeteners

There's no denying that, as a species, humans have a sweet tooth. Trying to suppress it doesn't work, so, in some way, we have to accommodate it. Most sweeteners (sugar, maple syrup, honey, rice syrup, blackstrap molasses) have similar effects on the body when used at equivalent levels of sweetness. The more natural alternatives do have the advantage of containing supporting nutrients, which have been removed from refined sweeteners such as table sugar. So, if you use the alternatives (and you should), you still need to limit the amount.

The sugar alcohols (mannitol, maltitol, xylitol, and sorbitol) provide another "natural" way to go. Think of sugar alcohols as sweet-tasting alcohols that are incompletely absorbed in the small intestines so that they produce virtually no glycemic response and are low in calories. This makes them popular sweeteners among diabetics and people on low-carbohydrate diets. On the down side, they are expensive and may cause intestinal distress. Erythritol is the best of the bunch—it is 70 percent as sweet as table sugar, yet it is virtually non-caloric, does not affect blood sugar, does not cause tooth decay, and tends not to cause the same gastric side effects as the other alcohol sugars.

Which brings us to the artificial sweeteners, aspartame and sucralose. Quite simply, don't go there. Aspartame has been associated with everything from tumors to tremors to blindness. And sucralose is based on a false premise: that because it's a totally artificial molecule, your body can't recognize it and passes it out unused. We're talking about all the sweetness of sugar, clean taste, and no downside—what more could you ask for? Unfortunately, the truth is that about 15 percent of the sucralose you consume does not pass out of the body, and side effects are already being reported, including a significant reduction in the weight of the thymus after just twenty-eight days of use. This has profound implications for the long-term viability of your immune system.

Finally, let's talk about lo han and stevia. Lo han is a non-caloric, low-glycemic sweetener made from the lo han fruit (lo han kuo). It has all kinds of positive attributes and one huge negative—its taste, which is very pronounced. Stevia has a glycemic index rating of zero and is virtually non-caloric. It has a definite aftertaste, but compared to lo han is remarkably clean tasting. It has one major downside: the U.S. Food and Drug Administration (FDA) will not approve its use as a sweetener—it can only be used in supplements. Why? Stevia has undergone numerous toxicity tests, not one of which has shown any harmful effects. It has stood the test of time, having been used for centuries in South America with no indication of harmful side effects. And thousands of tons of stevia have been consumed in Japan (where stevia is the alternative sweetener of choice) since the mid-1970s, again with no evidence of side effects. Today, stevia is cultivated and used in foods throughout East Asia, including China (for over twenty years), Korea, Taiwan, Thailand, and Malaysia. It can also be found in use in Brazil, Paraguay, Uruguay, and Israel. But throughout the United States, Canada, and Europe, the health authorities would rather you use aspartame and sucaralose. It definitely makes you wonder what the agenda is here, because it certainly isn't health or safety.

### High-Fructose Corn Syrup (HFCS)

No discussion of sweeteners would be complete without talking about high-fructose corn syrup (HFCS). HFCS is made by using enzymes to convert cornstarch to fructose and then blending it with glucose to produce the desired sweetness. A 90 percent fructose version is most commonly used in baked goods, and a 55 percent version is used in soft drinks. Manufacturers love high-fructose corn syrup because it is cheaper than table sugar and easier to transport and work with (because it's a liquid).

Unfortunately, the human body is not designed to handle high levels of isolated fructose. Since the dawn of man, humans have consumed fructose—mostly in fresh fruit, where the fructose is actually bound to the fruit fiber, thus slowing its absorption in the body—limiting intake to about 16–20 g per day. The heavy use of HFCS, though, has resulted in significant increases in consumption of fructose *isolate*, leading to typical daily consumption reaching an average of 85–100 g of fructose.

The problem is that fructose is absorbed differently than other sugars, and fructose isolate even more so. It causes major health problems:

- Exposure of the liver to such large quantities of fructose leads to rapid stimulation of the breakdown of fats and the concomitant rapid accumulation of triglycerides. This contributes to reduced insulin sensitivity, insulin resistance, and glucose intolerance.

- Unlike glucose, fructose doesn't stimulate insulin production, which means it isn't utilized for energy, but rather is stored in the liver as triglycerides.

- Again, unlike glucose, HFCS doesn't increase leptin production or suppress production of ghrelin, hormones that play a primary role in appetite control. The net effect is that the more HFCS you eat, the more you want. In effect, HFCS is addictive and encourages weight gain and obesity.

- It appears that HFCS distorts the body's magnesium balance, thereby accelerating bone loss.

Yes, it's true that medical authorities and publicity-seeking politicians finally took on trans-fats, but that was a relatively easy target. Let's see if they will take on high-fructose corn syrup, which in my opinion has replaced trans-fats as the number one dietary killer.

## PROTEIN: WHAT ABOUT MEAT AND DAIRY?

Let's begin by cutting through all the nonsense and take a look at what kinds of food our bodies were designed to handle, then figure out what that means for us today. And the best way to do that is by first identifying the key characteristics of our "eating and digestive" systems, then seeing which animals we match up with and what they eat. The key indicators that we're going to look at are the teeth, the stomach, and the length of the digestive tract. The human eating machine looks like this:

- Teeth: All of our teeth are nearly of the same height. Our canines project only a small amount, and our molars are broad-topped.

- Stomach: The human stomach is slightly elongated, approximating the shape of a kidney bean.

- Digestive tract: The average adult has a digestive tract (measured from mouth to anus) about 30–33 feet long. This means that the ratio of the length of a person's digestive tract as compared to their height (also measured from mouth to anus) is approximately 10–12 times the length of their body.

**Carnivores (Meat Eaters): Lions, Tigers, Etc.**—The first thing you notice about carnivores is that their teeth are nothing like those found in humans. They have huge canines for striking and seizing prey, pointed incisors for removing meat from bones, and molars and premolars with cusps for shredding muscle fiber. In carnivores, the teeth of the upper jaw slide past the outside of the lower jaw so that prey is caught in a vice-like grip. In general, carnivores don't chew much; mostly, they just tear chunks off and swallow them whole.

An examination of the carnivore intestinal tract reveals a short (relative to the length of their body) bowel for fast transit of waste out of the body. The actual length of the carnivore bowel is approximately 3–5 times the length of the body—again measured from mouth to anus—a ratio less than half that found in humans. Fast transit of waste for carnivores is essential for two reasons. The faster the transit, the less opportunity for parasites to take hold. Also, meat tends to putrefy in the intestinal tract, so fast transit limits exposure to the byproducts of putrefaction.

Most of the digestive process occurs in the carnivore's stomach (which is a round, sack-shaped structure with a high concentration of acid salts for digesting animal muscle and bone). Food usually remains for days at a time in a carnivore's stomach while it is digested (to a large extent) by enzymes present in the raw meat itself (a process called autolytic digestion). In addition, carnivores are adapted to process huge amounts of food at a time (up to 25 percent of their body weight or more), then eat nothing for days at a time. This doesn't sound very much like the human digestive process (except on all-you-can-eat nights at the Trough and Brew Restaurant).

**Herbivores (Plant Eaters): Cows, Deer, Etc.**—Herbivores have sharp chisel-shaped incisors for cutting, no upper incisors in some cases, and small incisor-like canines. Their molars and premolars are flattened with ridges. Their teeth and upper jaw meet the lower jaw so that lateral movement of the lower jaw produces the grinding actions to break down plant materials. In herbivores, the incisors are dominant, the canines usually depressed, and the molars broad-topped.

Herbivores also tend to have extended, compound stomachs. As for the herbivore bowel, at 20–28 times the length of the body (from mouth to anus), it usually runs almost eight times longer than a carnivore's, since plant matter (unlike meat) is not prone to putrefaction, thus rendering quick elimination moot. Again, not much like us.

**Omnivores (Roots, Berries, Meat, Nuts): Bears, Wild Pigs, Etc.**—No animal is really adapted to eat all things, but if any animal comes close, it would be the bear. Typical foods consumed by bears include ants, bees, seeds, roots, nuts, berries, insect larvae such as grubs, and even flowers. Some meat, of course, is eaten by bears, including rodents, fish, deer, pigs, and lambs. Grizzlies and Alaskan brown bears are well-known salmon eaters. Polar bears feed almost exclusively on seals, but then, what vegetation is there for them to eat in the frozen wastes of the Arctic? And, of course, anyone who has read *Winnie the Pooh* knows that many bears love honey.

Other than the ants, grubs, and rodents, the bear diet sounds a lot like the typical Western diet. For this reason, many people conclude that the natural human diet is that of an omnivore. But remember, we're stepping back and taking a look physiologically where we fit in, and on those counts, we don't match the omnivores. The biggest difference is in the teeth. Omnivores have the sharp canines of the carnivore and the pronounced incisors of the herbivore. They also have molars that are both pointed and broad-topped. That's not even close to a human set of teeth.

**Frugivores (Fruit and Nut Eaters): Gorillas, Orangutans, Chimpanzees, Etc.**—In the frugivore, all the teeth are nearly of the same height. The canines are a little projected and the molars are broad-topped. (Sound familiar?) Unlike the carnivore jaw, which is vertically mobile for biting or tearing, the jaw of the typical frugivore is laterally mobile to allow for chewing.

As for the bowel of the frugivore, it runs about 10–12 times the length of the body from mouth to anus, the same as found in the human body. The stomach of the frugivore is typically long and extended (a complex structure), containing a tenth of the acidic salts and pepsin found in a carnivore's stomach. Again, the same as in humans.

So, here we have our match, but what does it mean? Are we restricted to fruits and nuts? No. In fact, the frugivores we most closely resemble, the wild chimpanzees, periodically eat live insects and raw meat. Among the great apes (the gorilla, the orangutan, the bonobo, and the chimpanzee) and ourselves, only humans and chimpanzees hunt and eat meat on a frequent basis.[3] Gorillas have never been observed hunting or feeding on any animals other than invertebrates such as termites and ants. Nevertheless, chimpanzees are largely fruit eaters, and meat comprises only about 3 percent of their diet—far less than is found in the typical Western diet.

So far, the discussion of our natural diet is based on observation and hypothesis. Is there any science to back it up? In fact, there is: in 1979, Dr. Alan Walker, an anthropologist from Johns Hopkins University, in Maryland, published research based on a careful examination of fossil teeth and fossilized human remains with electron microscopes. As Dr. Walker and his associates reported, "Preliminary studies of fossil teeth have led to the startling suggestion that our early human ancestors (*Australopithecus*) were not predominantly meat-eaters or even eaters of seeds, shoots, leaves, or grasses, nor were they omnivorous. Instead, they appear to have subsisted chiefly on a diet of fruit."[4]

## Should We Eat Meat?

Is a vegetarian diet automatically healthier? Not necessarily. Some people actually do better when they include small amounts of meat in their diet—although, to be sure, a balanced vegetarian diet appears to offer some protection against cancer and heart disease. Other factors in our diet, however, affect our health to a much greater degree than whether or not we eat meat.

The bottom line is that, ethical questions aside, eating small amounts of meat, chicken, or fish probably comes down mostly to a personal choice. If you choose to, you can include meat in your diet without any significant health problems—with the following provisos:

- Keep the amount small—3 ounces of meat a day or less. Heavy consumption of meat significantly compromises beneficial bacteria in the colon, resulting in a 1,000 percent increase in the levels of harmful bacteria and a concomitant 90 percent drop in the levels of the beneficial bacteria. High consumption of meat also tends to push the body's pH levels into the acidic range, which presents major health risks, including cancer and osteoporosis. Epidemiological studies at Harvard Medical School showed that "men who eat red meat as a main dish five or more times a week have four times the risk of colon cancer than men who eat red meat less than once a month." They are also more than twice as likely to get prostate cancer. A recent study found that women who had more than one-and-a-half servings of red meat a day doubled their risk of hormone receptor–positive breast cancer.[5]

- If you're going to eat meat, buy only organic meat to avoid exposure to the whole range of chemicals, growth hormones, and parasites present in today's mass-produced beef and chicken, or the high levels of toxic metals present in most fish. Just as an example, over 90 percent of today's chickens are fed arsenic compounds, which have been government-approved additives in poultry feed for decades and are used to kill parasites and to promote growth. And while we're on the subject of chickens, according to a government study, over 90 percent of all chickens are infected with leukosis (chicken cancer). As for those chickens with too much cancerous tissue to be sold, well . . . they're destroyed, ground up, and fed back to the chickens that we ultimately buy and eat! If organic isn't available locally, pressure your supermarket to carry it as an option.

## What About Dairy?

The average American typically eats close to 600 pounds of dairy products a year, which makes it the single largest component of his or her diet. Unfortunately, this may not be as healthy as the milk ads on TV would lead you to believe. Even if the cow's milk you get is free of chemicals, growth hormones, allergenic proteins, blood, pus, antibiotics, bacteria, and the viruses typically found in milk, you still have major problems.

Cow's milk is not designed for people. For one thing, it has twenty times the casein of human milk. Human milk is designed to take an infant from 8 pounds to 40 pounds in 18 months, while cow's milk is designed to take a calf from 90 pounds to 1,000 pounds in about 24 months. Incidentally, the high level of casein is just one of several reasons that humans do not digest milk proteins very well, leading to numerous allergic reactions and high levels of mucus in our sinuses and bowels. As a side note, until 1947, the forerunners of Elmer's® glue were based on cow's milk casein—thus, Elmer's picture (Elsie the Cow's husband) on the label.

In addition, the cow's milk you buy in the store and the cow's milk that comes from a cow are not really very similar. First, homogenized milk is not natural and presents serious health risks. The theory behind homogenization sounds simple: break up the fat particles in milk so they stay suspended in the milk and don't rise to the top, forming the layer of cream that used to be the trademark of all bottles of milk. Unfortunately, once you make the fat particles that small, you've also made them so small that they are easily absorbed into the body and clog your arteries.

Second, there's the problem of the growth hormone used in dairy cows (in the United States) to increase milk production. This growth hormone, called bovine-somatotropin (BST) and recombinant bovine growth hormone (rBGH), was developed by Monsanto. It was supposed to be identical to the actual growth hormone found in cows. In fact, as part of its 55,000-page application to the FDA, Monsanto submitted a chart identifying the 191 amino acids contained in BST showing that they absolutely matched the amino acid chain found in natural growth hormone. However, it seems that the application is inaccurate. The problem occurs at amino acid 144, which was supposed to be lysine in both the natural growth hormone and in Monsanto's BST—it isn't. In 1994, Bernard Violand, a Monsanto scientist, published evidence that amino acid 144 in Monsanto's growth hormone is, in fact, epsilon-N-acetyl-lysine, a freak substance.[6] Whoops! But then you probably think that once this problem came to light, totally nullifying the Monsanto application, that BST was recalled. Sadly, no, not in the United States.

The FDA gave its approval for the sale of Monsanto's BST in 1993, but in Canada and the European Union, BST remains unapproved because of strong circumstantial evidence that it may promote cancer in cows and humans. Understand, this change in one amino acid is not insignificant: the replacement of one amino acid can drastically change the configuration of a protein, and configuration determines the properties and effects of a protein. Although the chemically detectable difference between true BGH and Monsanto's BST is slight, the effects of the two hormones on the human body may be quite different indeed.

It should also be noted that the body digests milk differently once gastric juices begin to flow at around 18–20 months old. Before gastric juices flow, milk is alkaline and non-mucus-forming in the body, but once gastric juices enter the picture, they turn the milk acidic, forming mucus, causing sinus problems, allergies, colds, etc. That's why every animal except man weans its young off of milk. Think about that for a moment.

Another factor to consider is that milk proteins are large and tend not to break down completely. Cow's milk proteins damage the human immune system. Cow's milk contains many proteins that are poorly digested and harmful to the immune system, such as casein, alpha-lactalbumin, and beta-lactaglobulin. Repeated exposure to these proteins may eventually lead to disease. Your body views these large proteins as foreign invaders, which stimulates an allergic response. This takes the form of both excess mucus running out your nose and encasing your stools, and increases in circulating

## CALCIUM AND MILK

Milk is often pitched as a great source of calcium. It is not. Yes, it has a high calcium content, but the human body is able to utilize very little of it. In fact, because of the way the body deals with milk, consumption of milk actually leaches calcium from the bones. It is a myth that we need milk for calcium. There are many far superior sources of calcium, such as sesame seeds, broccoli, Chinese cabbage, and collard greens. It's worth noting that there's more calcium in three-quarters of a cup of collard greens than in a cup of cow's milk.

The problem with milk is that because of its high sulfur and phosphorus content, your body needs to buffer it with even more internal calcium than you get from the milk itself. Besides, even if the absorption issue was not enough by itself, the 10 to 1 ratio of calcium to magnesium found in milk is too high and devastating to the human body. If you have any doubt about this, just consider the fact that Americans are among the highest consumers of dairy in the world and yet we have one of the highest incidences of osteoporosis in the civilized world!

immune complexes (CICs), which ultimately end up lodged in your body's soft tissue, promoting swelling and water retention. Quite simply, cow's milk is one of the primary allergy-producing foods you can eat. In fact, the FDA now requires that products containing dairy carry a food allergen warning! And of course, this is all above and beyond the issue of lactose intolerance, which affects those who lack sufficient lactase to break down the milk sugar lactose and thus suffer major intestinal distress.

## Health Conditions Associated with Milk Consumption

There are many problems associated with consuming dairy. Many of these are probably conditions you are already noticing in your own body, particularly those that relate to allergies, diabetes, and autoimmune disorders.

- Heart disease. Research has shown that, of all dietary factors studied, milk carbohydrates played the biggest role in the development of heart disease in men over 35, and nonfat milk played the biggest role in the development of coronary heart disease in men over 45.[8] Interestingly, this problem seems only to occur with homogenized milk.

- Cancer. Genetically engineered bovine growth hormone (BGH) causes an increase in insulin-like growth factor (IGF-1) in the milk of treated cows. It also survives pasteurization and human intestinal digestion and can be directly absorbed into the human bloodstream, particularly in infants. IGF-1 is known to transform human breast cells to cancerous forms, causing breast and colon cancer. BGH is banned in Europe and Canada. A 1989 study in *Nutrition and Cancer* linked the risk of developing non-Hodgkin's lymphoma to the consumption of cow's milk and butter.[9] High levels of the cow's milk protein beta-lactoglobulin have been found in the blood of lung cancer patients, suggesting a link with this cancer as well. Ovarian cancer rates parallel dairy-eating patterns around the world. The culprit seems to be galactose, the simple sugar broken down from the milk sugar lactose.

- Allergies and asthma. Poorly digested bovine antigens (substances that provoke an immune reaction) like casein become "allergens" in allergic individuals. Dairy products are the leading cause of food allergy, often revealed by diarrhea, constipation, and fatigue. Also, many cases of asthma are reported to be relieved and even eliminated by cutting out dairy. The exclusion of dairy, however, must be complete to see any benefit.

- Arthritis. Antigens in cow's milk may also contribute to rheumatoid arthritis and osteoarthritis. When antibody-antigen complexes (resulting from an immune response) are deposited in the joints, the result is pain, swelling, redness, and stiffness. These complexes increase in arthritic people who eat dairy products, and the pain fades rapidly after patients eliminate dairy products from their diets.

- Diabetes. Consumption of cow's milk has been associated with insulin-dependent diabetes. The milk protein bovine serum albumin (BSA) may lead to an autoimmune reaction aimed at the pancreas. Beta-caseine, a protein found in cow's milk, can trick the immune system into attacking and destroying the insulin-producing beta cells of the pancreas.

- Colds, flu, and sinus problems. Doctors who recommend dairy-free diets often report a marked reduction in colds, flu, sinusitis, and ear infections. In addition, dairy is a tremendous mucus producer, which puts a tremendous a burden on the respiratory, digestive, and immune systems. Removing dairy from the diet has been shown to shrink enlarged tonsils and adenoids, indicating relief for the immune system.

- Colic and ear infections in children. One out of every five infants in the United States suffers bouts of colic. Another common problem among infants receiving dairy, either directly or indirectly, is chronic ear infections. You don't typically see this painful condition among infants and children who aren't getting cow's milk into their systems.

- Childhood anemia. Cow's milk has been shown to cause loss of iron and hemoglobin in infants by triggering blood loss from the intestinal tract. This is one reason the American Academy of Pediatrics recommends that infants not drink cow's milk. Also, some research shows that iron absorption is blocked by up to 60 percent when dairy products are consumed in the same meal.[10]

- Vitamin D toxicity. Records show that dairies do not carefully regulate how much vitamin D is added to milk. (Milk has been "fortified" with vitamin D since deficiencies were found to cause rickets, even though the vitamin is easily obtained through minimal exposure to sunlight.) A study reported in the *New England Journal of Medicine* showed that of forty-two milk samples, only 12 percent were within the expected range of vitamin D content.[11] Testing of ten infant formula samples revealed seven with

## DISEASE-LADEN MILK

Milk has played a major role in the development of the "super bacteria" that have recently emerged to plague our health. In 1990, the U.S. Department of Agriculture allowed the dairy industry to increase the antibiotic residue standard for milk (one part per hundred million) by a whopping 10,000 percent to one part per million. The problem is that at this level of constant intake, the antibiotics destroy the probiotic colonies normally found in the intestinal tract of the cows, which then allows harmful bacteria to flourish and develop resistance to a whole range of antibiotics. There are fifty-two kinds of antibiotics and fifty-nine bioactive hormones found in milk.

One consequence of the mass-production dairy farm is an increase in cow breast infections. To cure the infections, farmers use large doses of antibiotics, which can also get into our intestinal tract, killing good bacteria colonies in human digestive systems and making us resistant to a whole range of antibiotics. Joseph Beasley, M.D., and Jerry Swift wrote in *The Kellogg Report* that even "moderate use of antibiotics in animal feed can result in the development of antibiotic resistance in animal bacteria—and the subsequent transfer of that resistance to human bacteria."[7]

It is important to note that the U.S. Food and Drug Administration (FDA) states that milk must be dumped if antibiotics exceed the one part per

more than twice the vitamin D content reported on the label; one sample had more than four times the label amount. The net result is that heavy consumption of milk, especially by small children, may result in vitamin D toxicity.

### The Bottom Line on Dairy

Milk is great food—if your goal is to grow up and become a 1,200-pound cow. Clearly, commercial milk is not a health food. Is drinking milk a better option than getting your calories from donuts and soda? Of course, but that doesn't make it a healthy food. If you must drink milk, drink raw, unpasteurized, organic milk, if possible. Absolutely avoid milk that has added growth hormones and antibiotics, and, if possible, avoid homogenized milk.

An even better choice, though, is goat's milk, if you can tolerate the taste. It is much closer to human milk in composition. You also have the option of million now allowed. It must also be dumped if it has too many somatic cells, white cells (pus) that can indicate mastitis, an udder infection. But is it? Due to budget restrictions, the FDA can only do so much to enforce these laws, and most of us just have to hope that farmers are doing their job in proper testing. Some would say this is not the case. In 1990, an FDA survey found excessive levels of antibiotics and sulfa drugs in 51 percent of seventy milk samples taken in fourteen cities. The *Wall Street Journal* reported months later that the FDA had actually found drugs in 80 percent of the samples.

Which leads us to the next issue—store-bought milk is often disease laden. Some estimate that 9 million cows in America are not healthy; half the herds in America have cows infected with bovine leukemia virus and Crohn's disease. It doesn't take a huge mental leap to make a connection between the high consumption of milk in the United States and the fact that 40 million Americans now suffer from irritable bowel syndrome. Why are cows so diseased? Largely it is because of their tortured environments. A typical cow in nature produces an average of 10 pounds of milk per day, but mass-production dairy cows injected with growth hormones and antibiotics can produce upwards of 50 pounds of milk per day. The average California cow, for example, produces a mind-boggling 19,825 pounds of milk each year! That's got to hurt.

a number of grain-, nut-, and rice-based milk alternatives—in moderation because they tend to be high glycemic. I do not recommend soy milk.

## Protein Alternatives

Fermented soy is a "reasonable" part of the diet when used in "reasonable" amounts. Soy becomes a problem food when used as the main protein or as a large-scale dairy replacement in the diet. Too much of a good thing is bad. And too much of any single dietary component is bad: no matter how healthy a food is, if you overindulge in it, disease will result, not health.

In large amounts, the high levels of phytoestrogens in soy become problematic. Also, soybeans have the highest levels of phytic acid of any grain or legume. Phytic acid is a substance that can block the uptake of essential minerals (calcium, magnesium, copper, iron, and especially zinc) in the intestinal tract. Phytic acid is neutralized in fermented soy, such as tempeh and miso, but not in soy milk or tofu. Soy also contains goitrogens, which are substances that depress thyroid function. These are not a problem in small amounts, but a significant problem when consumed in larger amounts.

Soy is especially not appropriate for children, particularly as a major component of their diets. I'm not a big fan of soy milk for children of any age, but especially for infants. The phytoestrogens are really more than their bodies were designed to handle. Fermented soy products, however, can provide lifelong breast cancer protection when served in moderation to girls between the ages of five and nine.

While I don't endorse soy or whey as protein mainstays, eggs (organic from free-range chickens) are a great source of useable protein, but they top the charts when it comes to food allergies. Eggs are one of the most common food allergens in infants, young children, and adults. The most allergenic proteins in egg whites are ovalbumin, ovomucoid, ovotransferrin, and lysozyme. As for egg yolks, they contain three highly allergenic proteins: apovitellenins I and VI and phosvitin.

What's left as a protein alternative? Actually, quite a lot in addition to any small amounts of beef, chicken, or fish you might consume. Sprouts and sprouted (or soaked) seeds and nuts are certainly options, but the big five I recommend when it comes to protein supplements are:

- Rice protein
- Spirulina
- Yellow pea protein
- Chlorella
- Hemp protein

They are all highly bioavailable proteins, easily beating meat and coming in just behind eggs and whey. But they offer one huge advantage: they are hypoallergenic.

## FRANKENFOODS: GENETIC ENGINEERING, IRRADIATION, AND MICROWAVES

### Genetic Engineering

Genetic engineering is already widespread. Today, around 70 percent of all the processed food that you buy in America—including soft drinks, ketchup, potato chips, cookies, ice cream, and corn flakes—contains genetically engineered ingredients. It's important to understand that genetic engineering

# THE BLOOD TYPE DIET

Right now, the Blood Type Diet and its variations are all the rage. They are based on an entirely different approach to determining the optimum diet than I have outlined. The basic idea behind these diets is that blood types evolved from the lifestyles and diets of different groups of humans over the millennia; therefore, you need to eat the diet natural to the group from which you are descended. The cornerstone of the diet is the premise that certain proteins/glycoproteins in food, called lectins, ape the glycoproteins on red blood cells, thus triggering immune reactions from the matching blood type. Is the premise valid?

Probably not so much. Yes, there is no question that different foods definitely have high allergy potential for many people, but the problem appears to be less with the lectins than with the ability of the digestive tract to fully break down the proteins in food. This is evidenced by the fact that the simple addition of supplemental digestive enzymes with meals and proteolytic enzymes between meals can often help reduce food allergies dramatically. In fact, there is little evidence that lectins, other than a handful of exceptions such as ricin (which will affect any-one of any blood type), present a problem for the human body of any blood type.

But that aside, doesn't the Blood Type Diet work for some people? Absolutely! Simple math works in its favor. If you tell an O, an A, or an AB not to eat dairy because they don't have the right blood type, then you've just told the vast majority of people in the world not to eat dairy. Considering all of the problems associated with commercial dairy we've already discussed, a lot of people are going to feel significantly better on the diet, regardless of blood type. (Chalk that up in the win column for the diet.) On the other hand, you've also just told a lot of Asians (they have the highest percentage of blood type B in the world) that they'll thrive on dairy. Probably not such a good thing since about 90 percent of all Asians suffer from lactose intolerance. (And that would need to be chalked up in the loss column.) Bottom line: if the diet works for you, then use it, but understand that your good results are probably based more on casino odds than science.

has been going on for thousands of years. All of the different varieties of vegetable seeds, rose bushes, fruits, and vegetables that you buy in the supermarket are the result of genetic engineering in the form of cross-pollination. And it's not just plants—many breeds of cattle, dogs, and cats are the result of crossbreeding, all designed to enhance certain traits and suppress others.

Some people claim that cross-pollination and selective breeding are not genetic engineering, claiming that this term is strictly reserved for modern gene-splicing techniques. In fact, genetic engineers themselves employ cross-pollination and selective breeding in their arsenal of techniques, but they now call it "molecular breeding." So, what's different today? We've gone beyond the limits of nature. With cross-pollination, the limits on what nature allows are much narrower. You can't crossbreed a tomato with a flounder, for example—nature doesn't allow it. Now, however, through the miracle of gene splicing, you can force nature to accept it. In fact, tomatoes have already been grown with flounder genes inserted to keep the tomatoes from freezing. (Great for the farmer, I suppose, but what about the person who makes an Italian dish with these tomatoes and then puts the leftovers in the freezer expecting them to keep for several months, only to find that they never froze and went bad?)

Is this necessarily bad? No, not necessarily. Keep in mind that just because nature allows something doesn't make it good. Nature allowed African bees and honeybees to crossbreed and produce the so-called killer bees. On the other hand, some of the results of gene splicing have been positive. Cotton plants that resist boll weevils without pesticides, for example, are probably not so bad—theoretically. It produces clean cotton and saves the environment from millions of gallons of pesticides each year. On the other hand, there are questions emerging as to how sustainable these high yields are and whether or not insects develop resistance to the genetic modifications.[12] Unfortunately, whether you like it or not, genetic modification is here to stay. Insect- and herbicide-resistant transgenic cotton is now planted on some 75 percent of the total area in the United States and South Africa and over 50 percent in China.[13]

There are, however, major concerns. Strains of genetically engineered corn have had unintended consequences, such as poisoning butterflies. But the biggest concern is the uncontrollability of the process. Already, scientists are pressing into some very dangerous areas, such as exploring the possibility of using genetically engineered plants to "grow" medicine. The problem is that if this is done, it is almost guaranteed that, at some point, these "medicine" crops will escape and contaminate all related crops. And what's medicine for one person is poison to another. Already, it is virtually impossible to find any soy (organic or otherwise) that has not been tainted by genetically modified soy. It is simply impossible to prevent the pollen from being carried on the wind or spread by insects and "infecting" clean fields. As Jeff Goldblum's character kept repeating in the film *Jurassic Park* when told there was no chance that the dinosaurs could escape or breed by themselves, "Life will find a way." And once the dinosaurs escape the park, you can't bring them back. Gene pool pollution is forever!

In the end, I think the problems with genetic engineering are barely understood at the moment but will emerge with much greater clarity as the years go by. To be on the safe side, avoid genetically modified foods as much as you can. As the saying goes, "Better safe than sorry."

## Irradiation

Let me begin by stating that you don't need to worry about "radioactive" foods. That's not an issue. The latest techniques in food irradiation have significantly reduced the amount of "radiation" that food is exposed to and also make use of non-radioactive forms of radiant energy, such as electrons. But even when "hard" irradiation from gamma rays was used, the food never became "radioactive." The health issue has never been about food being "radioactive." Radioactivity is a red herring.

The theory behind irradiation is very simple. Expose food to extremely high doses of radiant energy and you kill all living organisms (bacteria, parasites, fungi, etc.) in that food, thus eliminating a major cause of disease and spoilage. Everyone wins. The consumer is "safer" because of the elimination of potentially dangerous contaminants, and the food processor is happier (and wealthier) because he or she no longer loses any product to spoilage.

The problem is that the fundamental purpose of irradiation is to break chemical bonds in the living tissue of insects, bacteria, molds, and so on, for the specific purpose of killing them. Unfortunately, if the process is strong enough to destroy those pests, it is also strong enough to fundamentally change chemical bonds in the molecules of the food itself and produce radiotoxins and aflatoxins—no matter the dosage or the source.

What are radiotoxins and aflatoxins? Again, they have nothing to do with radioactivity. The word *radiotoxins* was first coined by Russian researchers experimenting with food irradiation to describe the molecules created in the food exposed to irradiation. Since that word was considered frightening to American consumers, the FDA came up with a couple of "softer" terms. They now call the known molecules, such as formaldehyde and benzene (both carcinogens), that are created by irradiation "known radiolytic products." As for those chemical molecules created by irradiation that have never before been seen on the planet, the FDA came up with the equally delightful "unique radiolytic products."

In addition to destroying all bacteria and parasites and producing radiolytic byproducts, irradiation has the added "benefit" of destroying nutrients—as much as 70 percent of vitamins A, $B_1$, and $B_2$ in irradiated milk and about 30 percent of the vitamin C. Irradiation also has the ability to accelerate the growth of aspergillus mold, which produces the most potent natural carcinogens known to man, called aflatoxins.

But this all seems so theoretical. If irradiation were truly dangerous, wouldn't there have to be hard evidence available somewhere that proves it? And there is:

- In the FDA's final report approving food irradiation, it stated that when up to 35 percent of the laboratory animal's diet was irradiated, feeding studies had to be terminated because of premature mortality or morbidity.[14]

- At the University of Illinois, the Department of Medicine fed irradiated food to mice, and 17 percent of the animals had to be killed or died due to respiratory problems so severe they couldn't even move around their cages.[15]

- Researchers at the Medical College of Virginia fed rats with irradiated beef. All the male rats died of hemorrhagic syndrome within thirty-four days.[16]

In approving food irradiation, the FDA started with 441 studies, including the three I just mentioned. It accepted 226 for further review, but then narrowed it criteria and selected only sixty-nine for in-depth review. Of these, the FDA itself reported that thirty-two showed adverse effects and thirty-seven studies showed safety problems. Then, without explanation, it eliminated all but five studies (including every negative study) and said it would base its decision on those five studies alone. Maybe it's just me, but

I'm not sure this kind of "science-based" assessment gives me a warm, comfy feeling when it comes to irradiated foods.

So, what foods do you have to worry about? Well, just about everything. Foods already approved for irradiation include fruits, vegetables, wheat, flour, herbs, spices, nuts, seeds, peas, pork, chicken, and beef—and most of it is unlabeled. The FDA requires a label stating that a food has been irradiated only if it was irradiated as a "whole food" and then sold unchanged. But if you process it in any way, if you add any other ingredients to it, it no longer requires a label stating that it, or any of its ingredients, was irradiated. To put it simply, an irradiated orange would require a label, but irradiated orange juice would not. This is very disturbing.

## Microwaves

The problem with microwaved food is similar to the problem with irradiated food. Although the actual processes are different, the results are similar—they are both disruptive to the fundamental structure of the food itself. Microwave ovens cook by creating friction in molecules, causing them to spin rapidly first in one direction and then another, switching directions millions of times a second. The friction caused by all this molecular agitation heats the food, but it also changes the food. With what result?

- Consumption of microwaved food appears to cause hemoglobin (red blood cell) levels to drop.[17]

- It causes white blood cell counts to drop, thereby damaging your immune system.[18]

- It destroys important phytochemicals. One study, for example, showed that microwaved broccoli lost 97 percent of its flavonoids, 74 percent of its sinapic acid, and 87 percent of its caffeoyl-quinic derivatives—these are all known cancer protectors. By comparison, steamed broccoli loses a mere 11 percent, 0 percent, and 8 percent of the same antioxidants.[19]

## GENERAL RECOMMENDATIONS

### Fats

It only makes sense to eliminate all hydrogenated oils and trans-fatty acids. When possible, buy and use organic, unrefined, cold-processed vegetable oils. Use avocado oil for cooking: it has a very high smoke point and will not burn or smoke until it reaches 255°C (491°F), which is ideal for searing meats and stir-frying. Another good cooking oil is rice bran oil. Also, unrefined virgin coconut oil is very healthy for any use other than high-temperature cooking. For low-temperature cooking and salads, olive oil and walnut oil are best. Surprisingly, butter in small amounts is fine, provided that you can get butter that doesn't contain antibiotics and hormones.

## Carbohydrates

- Minimize sugar consumption.

- Minimize the consumption of high-glycemic starches such as potatoes.

- Mimimize the consumption of refined grains, including anything made with white flour. If you're going to eat grains, make them whole grains.

- Minimize the consumption of grains in general, unless they are slow cooked at temperatures below 118°F.

- When it comes to grains, don't just think wheat (the least healthy grain). Look to grains such as amaranth, quinoa, and barley.

- And consider eating your grains in their healthier forms—as sprouts and as juices from the grain grasses, such as wheatgrass and barley grass juice.

- Minimize the consumption of bottled and canned juices, which are effectively little more than sugar water.

- Avoid like the plague anything that contains high-fructose corn syrup.

- Start incorporating supplements that contain carbohydrate/insulin modifiers (such as *Gymnema sylvestre*, nopal cactus, and fenugreek extract) into your diet.

## Meat and Dairy

Cut back on the quantity of meat, pork, chicken, and dairy in your diet, and make sure that what you do consume is organic. Fish, of course, is okay, if you can be sure it's free of heavy metals and toxins and hormonal "modifications." Incidentally, pesticide levels are far more concentrated in the animal flesh and dairy we eat than in the fruits and vegetables sprayed with those pesticides. The animals consume these pesticides day after day in their feed, steadily concentrating all of the pesticides they eat through their entire lives in their flesh. The higher up the food chain you go, the more concentrated the pesticides become. A cow eats hundreds of pounds of clover to make a few gallons of milk, thus concentrating the pesticide in that milk. Then again, it takes 10 pounds of milk to make 1 pound of cheese and 21 pounds of milk to make 1 pound of butter—concentrating the pesticides even more in the foods you eat.

In March 2008, *BMC Neurology* published the results of a study confirming that exposure to pesticides increases the likelihood of developing Parkinson's disease and that risk increases with long-term, repeated exposure (www.biomedcentral.com/1471-2377/8/6). Be warned.

## Overall Eating Plan

Any diet that promotes extremes (whether it's high protein, low carb, or low fat) will not serve you well in the long term. In addition to being unsustainable for most people, extreme diets have consequences: for example, the Atkins Diet may help you lose weight and lower cholesterol and blood pressure in the short term, but it's also likely to contribute significantly to colon cancer and osteoporosis in the long term. Low-fat diets, on the other hand, may promote heart health, but they deny your body the essential fatty acids and lignans it needs to prevent cancer. In the end, a version of the so-called Mediterranean diet is likely to work best:

- Lots of nutrient-dense fresh vegetables and greens.

- Lots of fresh whole fruit.

- Lots of fresh-squeezed juices (more vegetable than fruit).

- Eat organic when possible. Avoid genetically modified and irradiated when possible.

- Moderate consumption of sprouted (or soaked) seeds, nuts, and beans.

- Eliminate as much processed and cooked food from your diet as possible. Instead of canned or frozen, eat fresh.

- Low consumption of grains (whole grains, if you do eat them, and sprouted grains and grain grasses are fine). Eliminate as much refined flours, grains, and sugars as possible. Instead of white bread, eat whole wheat. Even better, instead of whole-wheat bread, eat lettuce wrap sandwiches. Instead of cake and ice cream for dessert, eat fresh fruit.

- Replace low-value foods such as potatoes and iceberg lettuce with high-value foods such as sweet potatoes and almost any of the richly colored vegetables such as romaine lettuce, spinach, Brussels sprouts, broccoli, and beets.

- As much as possible, eliminate all snack foods and fast foods. Replace with prunes (an extremely powerful antioxidant), raisins, and all of the berries.

- Reduce your intake of meat, pork, chicken, and dairy.

- Moderate consumption of low-mercury fish (if at all). As a rule of thumb, avoid bottom feeders such as shellfish (pollution concentrates at the bottom) and firm-textured fish that are higher up the food chain such as shark, tuna, and swordfish. The safest fish are ocean-caught high-oil fish such as salmon. Avoid farm-raised fish—although generally low in mercury, they consistently test high in PCBs and dioxin.

- Supplement with superfoods such as spirulina, chlorella, pre-sprouted barley, wheatgrass, barley grass, and white chia seed.

So, what does that leave you? Actually, thousands of choices. Virtually, everything that we've talked about eliminating is easily replaced with a healthier version. If you can't find the organic meats and dairy you want, or the whole-grain foods you're looking for, talk to your local supermarket manager. In most cases, they will get it if you ask. Even Wal-Mart announced that it intends to become the largest seller of organic foods in the world.

Of course, if you are in an advanced state of illness, you better clean up your act totally and eat no meat and no cooked food. In fact, ideally, you should go on a raw juice fast—at least until you get well. Once you're well, and have maintained that state for several months, you can bring back some minor indulgences. The worse you eat, the more often you will need to cleanse and detox and make use of supplements.

## My Diet

What do I personally eat? At one time, I was totally vegetarian, primarily for ethical reasons. (Anyone who has any awareness of how cattle, poultry, and pigs are treated on modern "super-farms" must think twice about consuming products produced by this system. It is incredibly cruel.) Unfortunately, after years of speaking engagements around the world, I got tired of eating iceberg lettuce with second-rate Italian dressing for lunch, and white rice and dead vegetables for dinner. I broke down and started eating small amounts of chicken and fish. My diet now consists of:

- Fresh juices, superfoods, and freshly ground flaxseed for breakfast.

- Large fresh salads, with a variety of greens and vegetables, with the occasional small piece of organic chicken or clean fish such as wild salmon for lunch. I'm talking about *substantial* salads, piled with healthy items such as avocado, sprouts, zucchini, palm hearts, and artichoke hearts. Also, sometimes I'll substitute a plate of lightly steamed or baked vegetables for the salad.

- Dinner is light: a small bowl of soup or sometimes fresh fruit and vegetables or a bowl of slow-cooked, whole-grain cereal so that the enzymes are still active (never heated above 118°F).

However, I still have an occasional slice of pizza, maybe once a month. Also, more often than I should, I still indulge my "sweet tooth" and have dessert every now and then, particularly when having dinner with friends. Hey, living longer is only part of the deal—you've got to enjoy your time here too.

So, now we've covered the basics on food—proteins, fats, and carbohydrates—except for one more important ingredient—water. Let's take a closer look at water: how much we need for optimum health and how to judge the quality of our water.

# CHAPTER 8

## Dying of Thirst

- **How Much Water Do We Need?**
- **The Questionable Quality of Our Drinking Water**
- **Worry about the Water You Bathe In**
- **Increasing Bioavailability with Magnetics**

Clean water for drinking, bathing, and growing food is one of the most precious commodities on the planet. You constantly read in the news about how we're running out of oil and energy—how these resources can only last another 20–30 years. While that's probably not true, it's still longer than we have for clean water. Already in many parts of the world, lack of clean water is the biggest problem facing huge numbers of people.

According to a recent United Nations investigation, half of the world's 500 biggest rivers are seriously depleted or polluted. All of the twenty longest rivers are disrupted by big dams. One-fifth of all freshwater fish species either face extinction or are already extinct. The Nile and Pakistan's Indus are greatly reduced by the time they reach the sea; some major rivers, such as the Colorado and China's Yellow River, now rarely reach the ocean at all. Other rivers, such as the Jordan and the Rio Grande, are dry for much of their length. And thanks to global warming (whether caused by humans or a natural phenomenon), the problem is only likely to accelerate as worldwide drought becomes the norm.

Why is water so important? Quite simply, it's essential for life. And the sad fact is that most people just don't get enough. And I'm not talking about Third World countries ravaged by drought—the vast majority of people living in the industrialized world (even where water is abundant) are dehydrated.

## HOW MUCH WATER DO WE NEED?

In advanced societies, thinking that tea, coffee, alcohol, soda, or other forms of manufactured beverages are desirable substitutes for the purely natural water needs of the daily "stressed" body is a common, but potentially deadly, mistake.[1] Water is the solvent in our bodies, and as such, it regulates all the functions of our bodies, including the action of all the solids dissolved in the water. Up to 60 percent of the human body is water; the brain is composed of 70 percent water; 83 percent of our blood is water; and our lungs are nearly 90 percent water. In fact, every function of the body is monitored and pegged to the efficient flow of water. Think for a moment of just a few of the functions that water regulates:

- The movement of blood
- The transport of nutrients into our cells
- The movement of waste out of our cells
- The flow of lymph fluid
- The movement of nerve impulses through our nerves
- The movement of hormones throughout our bodies
- The functioning of our brains

If we become dehydrated, all of these functions (and a thousand more) are impaired. Unfortunately, that's exactly what happens for the vast majority of us. Over time, as we become increasingly dehydrated, our thirst mechanism gradually fails, which leads to even more dehydration. Even when our thirst mechanism is functioning properly, it's not a reliable indicator of dehydration since "thirst" is one of the last symptoms of dehydration to manifest. Symptoms of chronic dehydration include allergies, asthma, chronic pains, constipation, acidosis, dry skin, and the shrinking of internal organs and thinning of skin associated with aging—to name just a few.

Understand, we can function quite well and for quite a long time without sufficient water. The body quickly adapts and starts extracting more water from your stools, for example. In fact, there are some health experts who claim that your body does quite well without drinking any additional water—just by making use of water found in the food you eat. But these experts confuse adaptation with health. Adaptation leads to compromise, which leads to diminished health over time.

At the very minimum, we lose (and must replace) approximately 2.5 quarts (liters) of water a day. But that's the minimum. Ideally, in addition to any water in our food, we need to consume 64 to 96 ounces of pure water a day. Pure, fresh (not bottled or canned) fruit and vegetable juices may be substituted for some of this quantity—as may limited quantities of non-diuretic herbal teas (without sugar). In general, however, pure water is the key.

## THE QUESTIONABLE QUALITY OF OUR DRINKING WATER

When you look at the big picture, government authorities have done a remarkable job in providing "clean" water for most developed countries. Water-borne epidemics such as cholera are almost unheard of in the developed world. On the other hand, acknowledging what has been accomplished does not mean that we should close our eyes to the problems that exist.

Keep in mind that the "maximum contamination levels" that water districts so proudly adhere to merely represent a compromise standard designed to be economically feasible for local districts to meet. They in no way come close to the safety standards established by the U.S. Safe Water Drinking Act. Drinking water in Europe and throughout the rest of the world is little different, and in many cases even worse.

On average, drinking water in the United States currently contains over 2,100 toxic chemicals that are known to cause cancer, cell mutation, and nervous disorders. This is not particularly surprising considering that there are close to 100,000 chemicals now in everyday use—with over 1,000 new ones added every year. In fact, according to the Environmental Protection Agency (EPA), United States industries generate some 79 million pounds of toxic waste each year that is *not* disposed of properly.

What is probably more surprising to most people, though, is that 53 million Americans unknowingly drink tap water that is polluted by feces, radiation, or other contaminants, according to the EPA. Also, some 45 million people drink water contaminated with the parasite *Cryptosporidium*, which killed more than 100 people in Milwaukee, Wisconsin, in 1993. And over half of all Americans drink water that has been used at least once before! (You probably shouldn't think about this particular statistic too long if you have any tendency toward a weak stomach.) Each year, at least 400,000 cases of illness in the U.S. can be attributed to contaminated water.

## Contaminants in Water

### Chlorine

Chlorine is the primary disinfectant used to purify drinking water. Let me make it absolutely clear that I am not advocating eliminating chlorine from the purification process. That would make no sense, because chlorination controls many water-borne diseases, including typhoid fever, cholera, and dysentery. However, it should be understood that:

- Chlorine is one of the most toxic substances known. It does everything from drying your skin and destroying your hair to wiping out the beneficial bacteria in your colon.

- The byproducts of chlorination (such as chloroform, trihalomethane, dichloro-acedic acid, and MX), which are found in drinking water, are all proven carcinogens.

- According to the U.S. Council on Environmental Quality, the cancer risk among people drinking chlorinated water is 93 percent higher than among those whose water does not contain chlorine. There is a higher incidence of cancer of the esophagus, rectum, breast, and larynx and a higher incidence of Hodgkin's disease among those drinking chlorinated water. A January 2007 study in the *American Journal of Epidemiology* found that people who drank chlorinated water were at 35 percent greater risk of bladder cancer than those who didn't, and those who spent time in swimming pools, showers, and baths boosted their bladder cancer risk by 57 percent.

- Chlorine has been strongly implicated as a major factor in the onset of atherosclerosis and its resulting heart attacks and strokes.

- As we discussed earlier, chlorine in your drinking water devastates beneficial bacteria in the intestinal tract, leading to a state of dysbiosis and a severely compromised immune system.

- By the same mechanisms that chlorine narrows blood vessels that feed the heart, it also narrows the blood vessels that feed the brain. Consequently, chlorine has been implicated as a major factor in the onset of senility.

There's no question that the use of chlorine in drinking water has helped stop the spread of many virulent water-borne diseases. On the other hand, there's also no question that chlorine in our drinking water presents serious long-term health implications. The bottom line on chlorine is that it needs to remain part of the water purification process for now, but you need to remove it from your water once it reaches your house before you drink it or bathe in it.

## Monochloramine

Several years ago, in an effort to reduce the carcinogens in drinking water, the EPA began exploring other disinfection options and found several advantages to monochloramine. While it isn't quite as good a disinfectant as free chlorine, it doesn't react with the natural organic molecules, so no trihalomethanes (considered a carcinogen) are formed. Plus, it lasts longer, a sort of a time-release disinfectant. However, recent studies have found that when monochloramine is added to water, the water will then dissolve almost any lead it encounters. While homes are rarely constructed with lead pipes today, there are still several sources of lead along the pathway from the water district to the kitchen faucet. The water mains are usually made of plastic or cast iron, with a service line running from the main to each home. In a lot of older houses, that service line is lead pipe. Another source is brass alloys in water meters, which contain lead. In houses, flow regulators, check valves, water meters, and faucets—even lead-free brass faucets—can contain up to 8 percent lead. Even copper pipes in many modern houses are soldered with lead.

How bad is the problem? In early 2004, officials in Washington, D.C., a city whose water district had recently switched to monochloramine as a disinfectant, discovered abnormally high levels of lead in homes across the city—some levels as high as 48,000 parts per billion (ppb). The EPA stipulates an action limit of 15 ppb of lead for drinking water to be safe. That's 3,200 times the safe limit!

## Fluoride

At the risk of appearing to be a Luddite, let's take a look at the use of fluoride in drinking water. Exactly what is water fluoridation? In fact, all water contains some natural fluoride. Fluoridation, however, is the process of adjusting the level of fluoride in the water supply upwards to theoretically protect against tooth decay. This concentration varies from 0.7 to 1.2 parts per million (ppm). "Organic" fluoride is present naturally in soil, water, plants, and many foods (tea, for example, is an extremely high source of fluoride—even when made with unfluoridated water). However, the "industrial" fluoride used in water fluoridation is not organic fluoride, it is a toxic waste product. American industry loves water fluoridation because instead of paying to dispose of a toxic waste, they now get paid by cities for selling them this same toxic waste to be added to your drinking water as a "health enhancer." It's probably no surprise, then, that the industries producing fluoride byproducts are some of the biggest proponents (and backers) of water fluoridation.

Fluoride is a potent toxin (used as a pesticide for roaches, ants, and rats) that accumulates in the body (about 50 percent a day for adults and 75 percent a day for children). Each exposure stays in your body and adds to the accumulated levels. And that's the key, because we are constantly exposed to high levels of fluoride other than in our water. It is in our toothpaste, which can double the level of fluoride in the blood within five minutes of being used, just from the amount absorbed through the cheeks and gums. It is sprayed on our food—apples and grapes are particularly high in fluoride for this reason. It is present in pharmaceutical drugs ranging from birth control pills to antibiotics. It is in sodas, which are manufactured from fluoridated water. Once you look at the scope of the problem, you realize there is no way in the world to determine what your fluoride intake is—just that it's far higher than is healthy.

Does it work? That's a question of more than some debate. There's no question that since fluoridation began, the incidence of dental caries has decreased significantly in the U.S. But it has gone down throughout the country as a whole, even in states that don't fluoridate their water. In fact, there is no good statistical evidence that fluoride (either in your water or in your toothpaste) makes one iota of difference in terms of dental health. All of the improvement in dental health can easily be attributed to better dental hygiene (brushing and flossing), not fluoridation. Countries such as Canada, Finland, the former East Germany, and Cuba continued to see a drop in tooth decay rates even after they abruptly stopped fluoridation. In fact, as New Zealand's former chief dental-health officer, John Colquhoun, a one-time proponent of fluoridation, said, "When any unfluoridated area is compared with a fluoridated area with a similar income level, the percentage of children who are free of dental decay is consistently higher in the unfluoridated area."[2]

Which brings us to the key question: Is it safe? Well, to be fair, community water fluoridation is supported by the U.S. Public Health Service, the American Dental Association (ADA), the American Medical Association (AMA), the American Heart Association, the American Cancer Society, and the National Academy of Sciences. Nevertheless, it's probably worth noting that the U.S. Public Health Service, at the same time that it supports water fluoridation, pushes for a reduction in our daily fluoride intake. Perhaps someone can explain that curious little inconsistency. As for the ADA, it's on the horns of a dilemma—to admit that promoting the use of fluoride was a mistake would open up the floodgates of litigation. And the AMA, even though it supports fluoridation, has repeatedly published articles in its magazine proving the dangers of fluoride. No one ever said this has to make sense. . . .

On the other hand, the devastating, toxic effects of fluoride are well documented by mainstream organizations. Numerous articles have appeared in the *New England Journal of Medicine* and the *Journal of the American Medical Association* challenging the safety of fluoridation. The Pasteur Institute in France and the Nobel Institute in Sweden have caused fluoride to be banned in their respective countries because the health risks from using fluoride far outweigh any possible benefit. Fluoridation is also banned in most of Western Europe, Finland, Chile, and Japan.

Health problems associated with fluoride include the following:

- Up to a 39 percent increase in various cancers, including an astounding 80 percent increase in rectal cancer. Scientists at the National Institute of Environmental and Health Sciences and the EPA have come out against fluoridation because they have confirmed that it does not reduce tooth decay and there is clear evidence that fluoride causes cancer.

- Destruction of the immune system.

- Inhibition of blood enzymes and blood cell production.

- Genetic changes in sperm and in other cells.

- A dramatic increase in heart-related deaths.

- Brittle bones. One of the claims for fluoride is that it helps build bones, a claim so deliberately misrepresentative of the truth that it borders on the criminal. Yes, it is true that some studies confirm that fluoride builds thicker bones, but it is a gross misrepresentation to cite those studies without also mentioning that fluoride makes bones more brittle.[3] And there are numerous studies that have appeared in the *Journal of the American Medical Association* showing a significant increase in hip fractures in areas with fluoridated water.[4] In addition, a 1991 study published in the *American Journal of Epidemiology* reported that water fluoride was correlated with more than double the hip fracture rates compared to areas with unfluoridated water.[5]

- Chronic fatigue.
- Gastrointestinal disturbances.
- Increase in infant mortality and miscarriages.
- Skin rashes after bathing.
- Dizziness.
- Vision problems, including blindness.
- Mottled teeth.

Also, new research has revealed that fluoride in drinking water makes the aluminum that we ingest more bioavailable. In the presence of fluoride, more aluminum crosses the blood-brain barrier and is deposited in the brain. The combination of aluminum and fluoride causes the same pathological changes in brain tissue that we see in Alzheimer's patients.[6] Now, I'm not saying that aluminum/fluoride is the cause of Alzheimer's—that would be premature. But it might be prudent to limit your exposure until we know more one way or the other.

Does anyone have the right to force such a potentially toxic substance into your drinking water for no proven benefit? (At least with toothpaste, you have a choice to buy a non-fluoride brand.) There are now at least ten studies that prove as fluoride intake goes up, so does tooth decay! There is no reasonable justification for the use of fluoride in water. If you can, keep it out of your community's water supply. If it's already there, make sure you remove it before drinking or bathing in it.

### Biofilm

Biofilm, which is found on the inside of water pipes and on the inside surfaces of office water coolers (where the water bottle sits on top of the cooler) is the accumulated sludge comprised of corrosion products from the pipes themselves and colonies of bacteria, viruses, and algae present in the water. Bacteria in biofilms form large, organized colonies and can exhibit unique properties. Some strains of *E. coli*, for example, are up to 2,400 times more resistant to chlorine when found in biofilms than when found floating free in water. Once established, biofilms are difficult to remove. In addition, biofilm contributes to further pipe corrosion and can deplete the chlorine used to disinfect drinking water. Some authorities consider biofilm to be a "tempest in a teapot," while others consider it to be a major health crisis in the making. Either way, you can be sure you'll hear much more about it over the next few years.

## Pharmaceutical Residues

The prevalence of pharmaceuticals in water is nothing new. What has changed, though, is our ability to detect trace amounts of these contaminants in the water. We are now finding pharmaceuticals such as heart medication, steroids, synthetic hormones, and antidepressants in river systems and groundwater used for drinking supplies where we never detected them before.

During 1999–2000, the U.S. Geological Survey conducted the first nationwide investigation of the presence of pharmaceuticals, hormones, and other organic contaminants in over 100 streams in some thirty states. Ninety-five contaminants were targeted, including antibiotics, prescription and nonprescription drugs, steroids, and hormones. Eighty-two contaminants were found in at least one sample, 80 percent of the streams tested positive for one or more contaminants, and 75 percent had two or more contaminants. And 13 percent contained an astounding twenty or more targeted contaminants.

There is no widespread treatment used by municipal water plants that removes these contaminants. Once these drugs enter the water supply, you end up drinking them unless you remove them yourself at home. Are the levels significant? Probably not significant enough to produce *acute* effects, but more than likely significant enough to produce subtle behavioral and reproductive changes. It's worth noting that a 2005 U.S. Geological Survey found that in some Potomac River tributaries nearly all of the male smallmouth bass caught were abnormal "intersex" fish. So maybe the effects are not so subtle after all!

## Don't Drink Tap Water

With all due respect for the great job performed by water departments in all of the states and cities, you still shouldn't drink tap water. It may not kill you immediately, but it will compromise your health over time. Tap water, well water, and bottled water are all suspect. Instead, drink filtered or distilled water. And if you're on the road and you're thirsty, picking up some bottled water at a convenience store is a better alternative than drinking from the water fountain or buying coffee or soda. But keep in mind, bottled water is fundamentally a crap shoot—you never know what contamination level you're going to get. Even bottled distilled water is suspect. While distillation removes all impurities from water at the time of distillation, contamination can occur during bottling, packaging, storage, and handling. If available, choose bottled water with the "sterile" label, which means that the water has been sterilized after bottling.

## WORRY ABOUT THE WATER YOU BATHE IN

As it turns out, it's not enough just to worry about the water you drink—the water you bathe and shower in is equally, if not more, important. Your skin is more than just a shrink-wrap to cover your body. It is your largest organ, weighing in at around six pounds. Stretched out, it averages about 20 square feet. Your skin is a major organ of transportation in your body. It moves wastes such as sweat and carbon dioxide out of your body, and it moves vital nutrients such as oxygen and moisture into your body. As an organ of transportation, the skin can easily let in harmful substances (pesticides, hormones, etc.) as well as beneficial substances, if you are not careful.

As the most visible organ in your body, it serves as a "canary in the coal mine," constantly indicating the state of your overall health. If your skin is dried up, wrinkled, gray, and generally unhealthy in appearance, it is a strong indicator that all of the other less visible organs in your body (heart, liver, kidneys, etc.) are very likely seriously compromised as well.

Your skin is composed of two basic layers. The external layer is called the epidermis. Before any substance can enter the body, it must first pass through the tough outer layer of the epidermis. This is the skin's major barrier, consisting of tightly-packed dead skin cells and roughly about the thickness of tissue paper (except on the soles of the feet and palms of the hands, where it is generally much thicker). So many dead cells are constantly being lost from this layer that it is totally replaced about every five weeks. By the age of 70 each of us has shed about 40 pounds of dead skin. The inner layer, the dermis, is generally between 1.5–2.0 millimeters thick. Here, a rich field of blood and lymphatic vessels can quickly carry any toxic substance that reaches it throughout the body. In one square inch of skin, there are 625 sweat glands, 90 oil glands, 19 million cells, 19 feet of blood vessels, and 19,000 sensory cells.

Our skin is not the impervious barrier that we were led to believe in during our school science classes. For example, you absorb more chlorine during a 15-minute hot shower than you do drinking 8 glasses of that same water throughout the day. Actually, when you shower, you absorb more chlorine through your lungs as vapor produced by the small droplets of hot water than you do through your skin. So much for that nice safe feeling you had drinking bottled filtered water. . . .

Just for fun, stop by your local swimming pool supply store and pick up a chlorine test kit. Fill a glass with some of your local tap water and test it with the kit. The water will change color according to how much chlorine there is in the water. Now, fill up another glass with water from the tap. This time, soak your hand in the water for 60 seconds before testing. Notice how the water shows no chlorine. In just 60 seconds, you absorbed all of the chlorine in the water into your body through your hand. The absorption factor is that dramatic. (The younger you are, the more absorbent your skin tends to be. And women should take special note that breast tissue is the most absorbent tissue in the body. Soak your breast in the same water, and it will clean out all of the chlorine in just 20 seconds.)

The trick is that if you want to make sure you are not absorbing toxic substances into your body, you have to avoid contact with the skin. That means that in addition to the chlorine in your bathing water and swimming pool, you need to be concerned about a wide range of toxins. If you must handle them at all, then always wear gloves when handling items such as pesticides, household cleaners, hair dyes, solvents, and paints.

## INCREASING BIOAVAILABILITY WITH MAGNETICS

Although all water consists of the same basic hydrogen and oxygen molecules ($H_2O$), water nevertheless varies according to how these molecules bond together to form "water molecule groups." To put it simply, it is in the size of these groupings that water differs. The smaller the groupings, the more bioavailable the water is—that is, the more easily it is able to pass through cell walls and to circulate through your body as a whole.

What holds water molecules together in clusters is surface tension. This is what you see when you wash your car and the water beads up in droplets on the hood. When washing your car, you use detergent to break that surface tension, which makes the water "wetter" and better able to clean. Obviously, you can't use detergent to improve the bioavailability of your drinking water. But you can use magnetics. Applying a magnetic field to your drinking water breaks its surface tension, making it wetter and more usable by your body. In addition, there's a strong secondary benefit—applying a magnetic field to water can raise its pH (acid/base balance), depending on which minerals are present in the water.

## GENERAL RECOMMENDATIONS

You need to treat the water that comes into your house to remove the chlorine, fluoride, chemical residues, heavy metals, bacteria, parasites, and other contaminants in your water. And you need to remove all of these toxins not only at the tap where you drink, but also where you bathe and shower. How do you do it? You have four choices:

1. Get a high-end filtering system for the entire house that treats the water where it enters your house. It needs to remove all contaminants (bacteria, heavy metals, fluoride, etc.), not just chlorine. This is obviously the most expensive way to answer the problem ($1,500–$2,500, on average), but if you actually get a good system that removes all of the toxins, it's the best way to go.

2. A good water distiller will provide the "cleanest" water you can get, but you need to be sure it incorporates a charcoal filter, since toxins like chlorine vaporize and recondense along with the water you're trying to clean. There's one other question to consider: distilled water, by definition, has no mineral content. For years, there has been much debate as to whether that's good or bad. "Distillerites" claim that demineralized water is more natural, like rain water and glacier water, and that minerals in drinking water end up in your joints. The argument against distillers is that most animals drink water that has had contact with the ground and acquired a high mineral content. Prime examples are the high-mineral water of the Hunzas and the coral calcium water of the islands off of Okinawa, two

areas renowned for the age and health of their inhabitants. I don't think it matters, provided that if you drink distilled water, you add ionic trace minerals to it before you drink it. You also need to understand that because it's devoid of minerals, distilled water is bio-electrically dead, which is another reason you want to add trace minerals. And as for the question of mineral-laden water leading to joint deposits, studies have proven that the calcium that deposits in joints comes from inside the body, leached from your own bones because of too much acid in your diet, not from the water you drink.

3. Reverse osmosis units produce a good quality drinking water. The main problem is that they waste a huge amount of water—many gallons of waste for each usable gallon. I'm not really sure that's justifiable nowadays with the looming water shortage we face.

4. A good water filter can do the job, but keep in mind that it will cost you. To find one that will truly remove *all* of the bad stuff while leaving in the beneficial minerals, you will need to pay $250 to $300 at the minimum. It will require several stages and several different kinds of media to remove chlorine, biochemicals, drug residues, fluoride, heavy metals, and ultra-small pathogens such as *Cryptosporidia*. And no, the self-contained filters that mount on your faucet and the ever popular filter/pitcher combinations won't do the trick. They just don't offer enough contact time for water and the filtering medium. They may improve the taste of the water, but they won't protect your health.

  • Drink 8–12 glasses of pure water a day. When possible, use glass to hold your water, not plastic (and especially not the thin plastic used in most sports bottles). Absolutely avoid drinking water that has a strong plastic smell or taste.

  • Apply a magnetic field to your water for 1–20 minutes, depending on how large the glass or bottle is.

  • If you're not using a central home purification system, remember to get a good shower filter to remove the chlorine from the water you shower in. Also, understand that the filter is on the shower, not the bath. The bath water (unless you fill the tub from the shower) will still be toxic. However, there are filters you can buy that hang on the spout and clean the water used to fill the tub.

So, now we've covered the basics on food—proteins, fats, carbohydrates, and clean water—but what about the nutrients inside our food? Are we getting enough? Do we need to supplement? What kinds of supplements should we use? Let's explore all that in the next chapter.

# CHAPTER 9

# Vitamins, Minerals, and Phytochemicals

- **Why We Need to Supplement**
- **Fundamentals of Good Nutrition**
- **Minerals**
- **Vitamins and Phytochemicals**
- **A Short-Sighted Approach**

## WHY WE NEED TO SUPPLEMENT

You often hear doctors say there's no need to supplement if you eat a balanced diet. If only that were true. Fast-food diets consisting of burgers, fries, pizza, and sodas have minimal nutritional value beyond proteins, fats, and carbohydrates. And even if you try and eat a balanced diet, the food we eat today is not the same as the food eaten 50–100 years ago. We have to compensate for the loss of "value" in our food.

- It takes eighty cups of today's supermarket spinach to give you the same iron you'd get from just one cup of spinach grown fifty years ago.

- According to a Rutgers University study, it now takes nineteen ears of corn to equal the nutritional value of just one ear of corn grown in 1940.

- There is less than half the protein in today's wheat as in the wheat our grandparents ate.

- Much of our soil is so depleted that our farm crops depend *entirely* on the chemical fertilizers they are fed in order to grow. That means that most of the food we eat is devoid of virtually all the trace minerals we need for survival.

When you think about it, what we've done is exchanged quality for quantity. You can't keep increasing your yield per acre, at the same time steadily depleting your soil year after year, and not expect to lose something in the process. And what's been lost is the quality of our food.

## Organic versus Non-Organic

As we've just seen, most of the food sold in our supermarkets is nutritionally compromised. Part of the solution lies in locally grown organic foods, which hearken back to the more nutritionally beneficial foods of fifty years ago. (Incidentally, locally grown organic food is not necessarily "greener" than food shipped across country, but it tends to have higher nutritional values as many nutrients tend to degrade quickly after picking.) Consider the following comparisons between organic and conventionally grown food:

- Organic snap beans have thirty times the manganese, twenty-two times the iron, and twenty-three times the copper of the conventionally grown variety.

- Organic cabbage has four times the calcium and potassium of the cabbage you buy in the supermarket.

- Organic lettuce is five times higher in calcium, fifty times higher in iron, and 170 times higher in manganese.

- Organic tomatoes are twelve times higher in magnesium, sixty-eight times higher in manganese, and almost 2,000 times higher in iron.

- And the biggest study of its kind, the recently completed Newcastle University study, conducted throughout Europe over a four-year period, found that organic produce was indeed "cleaner" than non-organic produce and contained up to 40 percent higher levels of antioxidants than non-organic.[1] As Professor Carlo Leifert, the study coordinator, said, the government is wrong about there being no difference between organic and conventional produce. "There is enough evidence now that the level of good things is higher in organics."

It should be noted, however, that the organic label by itself is no guarantee of high nutritional value, just low contamination levels. Nutrition levels depend on how many tons of organic fertilizer are used per acre and whether or not the soil is remineralized, both expensive propositions. The best rule of thumb is to find growers you know and trust (perhaps at your local farmer's market) and stick with them. I'm also very excited about some of the work I've seen recently in hydroponics, in which plants are grown in super-high-density, all-natural, organic-nutrient broths. Under these conditions, one sees nutrition levels that are off the charts and contamination levels that are virtually undetectable. The possibilities over the next five to ten years are incredibly exciting.

## Nutritional Stress

A second factor we have to consider is nutritional stress. We're just exposed to far more environmental and pollution stresses than our bodies were ever designed to handle—more than the human body has ever before been required to handle in the history of the world. Even if you were able to consume an all-organic, optimized diet, it takes far more of the protective phytochemicals that food provides than we can possibly get in our diets, even if the food we ate was of the highest quality. Our bodies were never designed to handle:

- High levels of radiation from dental x-rays and high-altitude airplane flights

- Organophosphate pesticide residues

- Totally artificial fats (hydrogenated oils, trans-fatty acids, homogenized fat, and ultra-refined polyunsaturated vegetable oils)

- High levels of refined sugar (the average American now consumes more than 137 pounds a year)

- A totally fiberless, white flour diet (including breads, pastas, cakes, pastries, tortillas, etc.)

- Constant exposure to disruptive electromagnetic fields

- Chlorine and fluoride in our water

- Continued, unrelenting, high-stress jobs and living situations

The bottom line is that if you live in an industrialized country in the world today, you must supplement to maintain your health—to reduce the risk of cancer, heart disease, and degenerative diseases of all kinds, to retard the aging process, and to protect against toxic injury.

## FUNDAMENTALS OF GOOD NUTRITION

Before we can determine which supplements we need to take, we need to take a quick look at the fundamentals of nutrition—that is, proteins, fats, and carbohydrates as nutrients (see Chapter 7 for more detail). For many people, this is where their nutritional knowledge begins and ends. They count calories and compare ratios of fat calories to total calories. In most hospitals, the sole concern of the certified nutritionists who prepare hospital food is putting together a proper balance of proteins, fats, and carbohydrates. As you will soon learn, this is tantamount to nutritional insanity.

Proteins are essential for the growth and repair of all body tissues. They are made of amino acids, some of which your body can produce by itself, and some of which must be included in your diet. A great deal is made about the need for protein, but the fact is our protein requirements are not really very large and are easy to fill. The official Reference Daily Intake (RDI) for protein is approximately 50 grams (g) per day, but if you're at all active you probably need more. To figure out your protein requirement, it works out to 0.33–0.50 grams per pound of your "ideal" body weight (or about 0.75–1.0 gram per kilo), depending on activity. Keep in mind that 50 g is only about 1.8 ounces. A performance athlete might need to double that, but that's still only 3.6 ounces a day.

Theoretically, milk is a top-rated protein, but in reality it's not. As we've already discussed, it messes up the pH (acid/alkaline balance), which results in incomplete digestion. It also has large proteins, such as casein, alpha-lactalbumin, and beta-lactaglobulin, which are difficult to digest and can cause allergic reactions. Meat and fish are fine, but surprisingly not that efficient—they provide only about 20–25 percent protein. You need about 10–12 ounces of meat to get 2.5 ounces of protein. That's about four times the maximum healthy level of 3 ounces per day of meat. Eggs are the most efficient, bioavailable source of protein around, but are also extremely allergenic. Surprisingly, some of the best sources of protein are vegetarian. Spirulina and chlorella are both high in actual percentage of protein (60–80 percent compared to meats) and are also in a more bioavailable form. Rice protein and yellow pea protein are also great sources, particularly in combination, and they're hypoallergenic. Hemp protein is a good balanced food, but has only about half the available protein of rice and pea.

In addition to protein, we need to talk about fats as nutrients. We've already discussed the importance of supplementing your fat intake with omega-3 fatty acids, but which source is best? Fish oil is good because it is already broken down into the forms of omega-3 fatty acids that your body can use, eicosapentaenoic acid (EPA) and docosahexaenoic acid (DHA). The omega-3s in flax oil come in the form of alpha-linolenic acid, which your body breaks down into EPA and DHA. For most people, this is not a problem, but for those who have an overabundance of omega-6 fatty acids in their diet, it is. On the other hand, flax oil is high in lignans, phytochemicals shown to have significant anti-cancer properties. Krill oil is another alternative. Krill are small, shrimp-like creatures and their oil contains phospholipids specially integrated with omega-3 fatty acids. This unique structure provides important cell membrane building blocks in the ratios used by the body and may be far better utilized than other omega-3 oils. And remember, omega-3 fatty acids that have been cooked, processed, or exposed to air for any length of time are most likely compromised and no longer healthy. Supplementing with 3–4 g of krill or fish oil, or 1–2 tablespoons of flax oil is probably all you need, provided you lower your intake of omega-6 fatty acids.

Carbohydrates are the body's short-term energy foods. Simple carbohydrates, such as sugar and white flour, are utilized by the body in a matter of minutes. Complex carbohydrates take time to break down and are, therefore, utilized over a matter of hours. This allows for a more balanced insulin response in the body. The best carbohydrates are fresh fruits and vegetables (non-starchy)—pure and simple. Buy organic and wash thoroughly. Ultra-long-chain carbohydrates, such as pre-sprouted barley, are another great source. Supplementing is not really the issue. Shifting your sources from high glycemic to low glycemic, though, is.

That covers the basics of nutrition. Now, let's take a look at the more subtle issues—the areas where supplementation truly is an issue.

## MINERALS

Your body is actually made mostly of minerals and water. As it turns out, your overall health is determined far more by minerals than proteins, fats, carbohydrates, or even vitamins. Calcium, for example, is not only used to build strong bones and teeth, but it is present in every cell in the body and is instrumental in the transporting of nutrients in and out of those cells.

But getting your minerals is not necessarily that easy. Want some iron? Why not grind down a nail and eat the shavings? Want some calcium? Why not do what the Three Stooges did and shuck some oysters, throw the meat away, and eat the shells? Sound silly? Well, what do you think is in most of the multivitamin/multimineral pills you buy? The simple fact is that your body can't handle straight minerals. They carry an electric charge that is opposite that of your intestinal wall, so they stick to the wall and can't pass through. Once stuck to the intestinal wall, they are "pushed" along and out of the body. In the end, you absorb only about 3–5 percent of the straight minerals you consume. To get around this, many supplement makers use chelators, substances to mask the electric charge, thereby tricking your body into absorbing the minerals. But keep in mind that only means absorption through the intestinal wall. You still have to convince the cells of your body that these inorganic mineral isolates are useful.

On the other hand, plants pull minerals straight out of the ground and then biologically transform them into the very substance of the plant itself. Not surprisingly, your body likes this form of mineral much better. Want some iron? How about eating some beets. Want some calcium? How about ground sesame seeds, collard greens, or carrot juice.

## Major Minerals

Calcium—We live in a calcium obsessed society. Every health expert tells us to supplement with more and more calcium. For the past few years, coral calcium has been one of the hottest supplements in the alternative health market. But the simple truth is that the vast majority of people get more than enough calcium in their diets. In fact, most people get too much.

The average American consumes 600 pounds of dairy products a year—that's almost two pounds per day—and yet osteoporosis rates in the United States are among the highest in the world. Not long ago, researchers at Yale University analyzed thirty-four published studies from sixteen different countries and found that the countries with the highest rates of osteoporosis (including the United States, Sweden, and Finland) were those in which people consumed the most meat, milk, and other animal-based foods. The study also showed that African-Americans, who consume, on average, more than 1,000 milligrams (mg) of calcium per day, are nine times more likely to experience hip fractures than are South African blacks, whose daily calcium intake is only about 196 mg. On a nation-by-nation basis, people who consume the most calcium have the weakest bones and the highest rates of osteoporosis.

Few people know that our worldwide obsession with calcium started in the 1950s under pressure from the American dairy industry. Before then, historically, people didn't consume much calcium and had very few problems with osteoporosis. What they did consume was magnesium—almost five times as much magnesium as we consume today. The key point is that the health of our bones depends far more on other factors such as magnesium, boron, and vitamin D than it does on calcium. Consumption of too much calcium is just plain damaging to your bones and your health in general.

Magnesium—Without calcium, you cannot live, but without adequate amounts of magnesium to balance that calcium, you will find yourself falling victim to hardening of the arteries, arthritis, diabetes, and senility. Magnesium is the activating mineral for close to 400 different enzyme reactions in the body (that we know about)—more than any other mineral. So, too little magnesium impacts your body negatively in hundreds of ways. And what makes the problem even worse is that magnesium is much harder for your body to absorb and utilize than calcium. This fact alone makes a joke of the standard 2:1 ratio of calcium to magnesium found in most supplements. Based on absorption, the ratio provided by most supplements is much closer to 6:1 or even 8:1 in favor or calcium—a very unhealthy ratio. Magnesium is the most important major mineral needed by your body, and unfortunately, the one that is most often depleted.

## Trace Minerals

Ten years ago, few people knew much about trace minerals, which were almost never included in any commercial vitamin/mineral formula. But today, almost everyone knows that trace minerals are, quite simply, those essential elements needed by your body in very small amounts (less than 100 mg a day) for health and life. Every second of every day, your body relies on soluble major and trace mineral ions to conduct and generate billions of tiny electrical impulses. Without these impulses, not a single muscle, including your heart, would be able to function, your brain would not function, and cells would not be able to use osmosis to absorb nutrients.

Among other things, soluble trace minerals are:

- Ionized conductors of the body's electrical current necessary for body functions.

- Catalysts and activators of other nutrients.

- Building blocks of enzymes, hormones, and other natural agents used by the body to perform specific functions.

- Necessary for balancing body fluids, fluid pressures, and pH.

- Needed to keep certain heavy metals from accumulating in the body. Trace minerals are often administered in hospitals as part of the treatment for such disorders as lead poisoning.

- Essential for digestion and assimilation. High amounts of chlorides, for example, are necessary for the body to make hydrochloric acid. Still other minerals are used in the assimilation process.

Traditionally, eating fresh grains, fruits, and vegetables grown in nutrient-rich soil and drinking mineral-rich water have been the primary supply for the full spectrum of ionically charged minerals. Unfortunately, naturally occurring, nutrient-rich soil is almost nonexistent on commercial farms. Aggressive farming techniques have stripped most trace minerals from the soil. The simple truth is that the use of nitrogen fertilizers to make plants grow is relatively cheap and is therefore the foundation of modern farming methods. Remineralization of the soil, on the other hand, is very expensive and produces no "visible" results. It merely makes the food healthier to eat—not a particularly profitable benefit.

When people consume a diet derived from such depleted crops, the intake of essential trace minerals becomes inadequate, leading to poor health and disease. What are some of these key trace minerals? Actually, there are several dozen of them, including copper, tin, silver, gold, and lithium, but three of the most important are:

- Selenium—essential for preventing cancer

- Boron—essential for preventing osteoporosis

- Chromium—essential for regulating blood sugar levels.

## VITAMINS AND PHYTOCHEMICALS

The dictionary defines a vitamin as "an organic compound naturally occurring in plant and animal tissue and that is essential in small amounts for the control of metabolic processes." A simpler definition is that vitamins are co-enzymes whose primary role is to help your body's enzymes do their job. For example, the enzyme responsible for breaking down alcohol, alcohol dehydrogenase, uses vitamin $B_6$ (pyridoxine) as its cofactor. When vitamins are available in limited amounts, enzyme reactions are inhibited.

Phytochemicals are the hot "new" discoveries in nutritional science. They include things such as sulforaphane from broccoli, resveratrol from grapes, and lycopene from tomatoes. You can think of phytochemicals as vitamins, plant-based hormones, and antioxidants in the process of being discovered. This is not necessarily a quick process. It wasn't until fifty years after it was discovered that vitamin E was declared a vitamin.

## It's Not That Simple

You would think that supplementation of vitamins and minerals would be pretty easy. Figure out where people are likely to be deficient, then make a pill that supplements for those suspected deficiencies—you know, a one-a-day multivitamin kind of thing. Determining the best supplement to take would then be a simple job of reading the label. Unfortunately, it's not that simple. There are actually two problems.

1. Natural and synthetic vitamins are not necessarily the same thing.

2. In nature, nutrients do not exist in isolation but rather in nutrient complexes. And as it turns out, our bodies require the complexes, not the isolates.

Actually, most vitamins in isolated form are toxic to the body, and like all toxins, they have to go to the liver to be detoxified. The liver does this by combining the isolates with a protein in a process called conjugation. The problem with conjugation is that you only get the benefit of as much of the vitamin as the liver can manage to conjugate; and every time you force the liver to conjugate vitamins to detoxify them, you're putting additional stress on the liver.

## Natural versus Synthetic

Vitamins can be classified as totally natural, co-natural, or synthetic. Very few vitamins that you buy are totally natural. Why? Quite simply, cost. Direct extraction of vitamins from foods is prohibitively expensive. For example, acerola cherries, one of the best natural sources of vitamin C, contain only 1 percent vitamin C by weight. Most supplements that list acerola cherries as their vitamin C source contain only a small percentage of vitamin

C from the cherries—the rest is synthesized vitamin C. Co-natural vitamins are derived from vegetable and animal sources through the use of solvent (primarily hexane) extraction, distillation, hydrolysis, or crystallization—but, by definition, they haven't undergone any conversion or chemical alteration during the extraction process.

Synthetic vitamins can be derived from either natural or chemical sources. What makes them synthetic is that they undergo a process of "conversion," either as a result of the extraction process or from pure chemical buildup. Synthetics are, at best, about 50 percent as effective as natural vitamins and in many cases actually suppress the body's ability to absorb the natural portion of the vitamin.

Note: Light passing through a natural vitamin always bends to the right due to its molecular rotation. Synthetic vitamins behave differently—that same ray of light splits into two parts when passing through a synthetic, one part bending to the right (*d* for dexorotary), the other to the left (*l* for levorotary). So, a natural vitamin E fraction, for example, is easily identified by the *d* as in "d-alpha-tocopherol" and the synthetic by the *dl* as in "dl-alpha-tocopherol."

## What You Actually Get in the Store

Many commercial-grade vitamin and mineral concentrates are synthesized by the large pharmaceutical and chemical companies from the same starting material they make their drugs from (coal tar, wood pulp, petroleum products, animal byproducts, waste and fecal matter, ground rocks, stones, shells, and metal).

- At one time, vitamin $B_{12}$ (cobalamine) was extracted from activated sewage sludge. It is now grown from bacteria and then stabilized with cyanide (thus becoming, cyanocobalamine).

- Most vitamin D is made from irradiated oil.

- Much of the vitamin E used in all supplements is produced in commercial laboratories.

- Supplemental calcium, for the most part, is either mined from the earth, ground from old bones, or made by grinding up oyster shells—just like the Three Stooges used to do it.

Another surprise is that the term *organic*, when applied to supplements, does not mean the same thing as it does with food. For supplements, all the word *organic* means is that the molecule contains at least one carbon atom (as in "organic chemistry"). In other words, a supplement can be labeled 100 percent organic and not be natural at all. And many so-called natural vitamins have synthetics added to "increase potency" or to standardize the amount in a capsule or batch. Vitamin manufacturers may also add a synthetic salt form of the vitamin to increase stability. These synthetics are easily identified by the terms *acetate*, *bitartrate*, *chloride*, *gluconate*, *hydrochloride*, *nitrate*, and *succinate*.

## A Holistic Entity

Modern medicine refuses to define the human body as a holistic entity, but rather sees it as a grouping of separate parts and pieces. Not surprisingly, that same paradigm has been applied to nutrition. In other words, modern nutrition is based on the concept that key nutrients can be identified and isolated. Unfortunately, the reality is quite different.

Twenty-five years ago, vitamin C (ascorbic acid) was all the rage. Then, suddenly, after years of people scarfing down ascorbic acid, it was discovered that your body really couldn't absorb ascorbic acid very well, unless the bioflavonoids hesperidin and rutin were present. Suddenly, all vitamin C was sold with bioflavonoids. Then it was discovered that you really could not absorb vitamin C very well (even if the bioflavonoids were present) unless calcium was also present. Again, suddenly, all vitamin C was sold with calcium. Two questions that any thoughtful person might want to ask are: What value were people getting all those years they were consuming just ascorbic acid? As it turns out, not much. And was there any source for vitamin C available for all those years that packed ascorbic acid with its bioflavonoids and calcium? And the answer is: of course! Oranges, grapefruits, acerola cherries, and camu camu. Nature packages the whole deal together!

Several years ago, beta carotene was "discovered," and suddenly, beta carotene supplements appeared everywhere. At first, the press touted the anti-cancer properties of beta carotene. Then it touted other studies proving it didn't prevent cancer, and in fact might even promote it. As it turns out, both negative studies used synthetic beta carotene in their evaluations. And, surprise, almost all of the beta carotene found in generic supplements on the market today is an isolated synthetic made from acetylene gas.

Once again, if we turn to nature, it has already packed all of these healthy nutrients together in a complex but natural source. The seaweed *Dunaliella salina*, for example, contains all of the popular carotenoids including beta-carotene, plus a whole slew of others, such as alpha carotene and zeaxanthin. Carrots contain approximately 400 carotenoids in addition to beta carotene, and many of those carotenoids are far more powerful than beta carotene.

Another example is vitamin E. For decades, most vitamin E has been pure synthetic dl-alpha-tocopherol or, if you're lucky, d-alpha-tocopherol. But even d-alpha-tocopherol comes up short. As it turns out, vitamin E is actually a complex containing at least eight components—four tocopherols and four tocotrienols. The reality is that d-alpha is, at best, only number six when it comes to importance for the human body. All four of the tocotrienols and gamma-tocopherol turn out to be more important than d-alpha.

I could give other examples, such as the B vitamins, where science has continually come up short in identifying the key factors that make them work. The bottom line, though, is that in nature vitamins do not exist in isolation—they exist in complexes. Although it is conceivable that science may someday identify all of the key nutrients contained in nature so we don't keep finding out what components we forgot to include, it is, nevertheless, an impossibility that science will ever identify how all of these nutrients interact with and support each other. The mathematical possibilities are just too immense. There are literally thousands of nutrients (remember the antioxidants and phytochemicals) that our bodies require to remain healthy, and the possibilities for the synergistic interaction of all of these nutrients is astronomical. Keep in mind that there are some 400 carotenoids alone, and every day there are new phytochemicals (not to mention whole new classes of phytochemicals) being identified.

## A SHORT-SIGHTED APPROACH

In the early 1940s, a government program was established to determine the Minimum Daily Requirement (MDR) you would need of each essential nutrient to prevent the onset of disease. Testing was simple: withhold a certain nutrient (let's say vitamin C) until disease (in this case, scurvy) appeared.

At that point, the appropriate nutrient was introduced back into the diet until the disease disappeared. The amount that it took to make the disease go away was the MDR. The Recommended Dietary Allowance (RDA) was then established as a small percentage above the MDR to allow a safety margin. Recently, the RDA was replaced by the designation DV (Daily Value), and even more recently by the Reference Dietary Intake (RDI).

The problem with this whole approach is that it deals only with short-term deficiencies. What are the long-term implications (ten, twenty, or more years down the line) of nutritional deficiency? The answer is now becoming apparent for all but the blind or governmentally challenged to see: an epidemic of cancer, heart disease, diabetes, osteoporosis, etc. And what makes it all even more ludicrous is that as pathetically low as the RDA/DV/RDI is, a U.S. Department of Agriculture National Food Survey of 21,500 people found that *not a single person* consumed 100 percent of the U.S. RDA from the foods they ate.

## GENERAL RECOMMENDATIONS

So, what's the best overall (one-a-day kind of thing) supplement? The best way to look at the question of an overall supplement is to break it into three categories: optimum, acceptable, and "avoid at all costs."

### Optimum

- One good choice is to use concentrated "food-based" vitamin complexes. Such supplements will contain concentrated forms of liver, yeast, and wheat germ, for example.

- Another alternative is a superfood combination that contains things like spirulina, chlorella, flower pollen, nutritional yeast, wheat grass, barley grass, pre-sprouted barley, chia seeds, powdered beets, etc., to provide a full complement of vitamins and minerals. The actual amount of vitamins and minerals you get will be less than in other options, but the bioavailability will be better. However, watch out for fillers. Superfoods are expensive, and many manufacturers "water" their formulas down by adding large amounts of things such as inexpensive fibers and lecithin. These are not bad things, they just aren't nutrient dense and their primary value is that they're relatively inexpensive.

  Also, it's important to make sure that your superfood provides good sources for the B vitamins and for vitamin D. For many years, it was thought that edible seaweeds, fermented soy foods, and spirulina contained high levels of $B_{12}$. Unfortunately, they don't. What they contain are $B_{12}$ analogues (chemical look-alikes) that your body cannot use.[2] You'll need another source of $B_{12}$. As for vitamin D, recent studies have found that more than half of all people have too little vitamin D in their bodies. The big surprise was that a third of those who were deficient were taking vitamin D supplements. Make sure your superfood provides adequate amounts of vitamin D (1,000–2,000 IU)—and get some sunlight on your body.

- Probably the best choice is to use "food-formed" supplements. Instead of being chemically manufactured, food-formed supplements are cultivated using a live biodynamic growing process. By growing nutritional yeast or probiotics in a "super-dense nutrient broth," you end up with a "living" vitamin/mineral compound that is comprised of a highly complex, interlocking system of vitamins, enzymes, minerals, active bioflavonoid groups, microproteins, complex carbohydrates, and countless other naturally occurring food constituents. These supplements are not perfect—they are limited by the wisdom of the grower and what is put into the nutrient broth. For example, if vitamin E is put into the broth as d-alpha-tocopherol, that's all that will end up in the supplement. Highly bioavailable, yes. Complete, no. (Note: Food-formed vitamins are heated after the "brewing" process is complete to inactivate the yeast so it cannot grow inside the human body.) These supplements are easy to identify, as any manufacturer using this process to make their vitamins will proclaim it in large letters on their label and on their website.

## Acceptable

It's possible to find high-quality vitamin/mineral supplements at the health food store that use only co-natural vitamins and no synthetics. The problem with supplements based on co-naturals is that they can never be complete. They will never contain unknown factors such as vitamin $B_{29}$, which will not be identified for another hundred years. What co-naturals are useful for is "spiking up" a supplement based on one of the optimum options above. An example would be a "food-based" supplement augmented with co-natural vitamins E and C.

## Avoid At All Costs

Supplements made in whole, or part, from synthetics are not an option. At their best, they are only 50 percent as effective as a natural vitamin. At their worst, they actually may carry harmful side effects. Key red flags to look for in ingredient lists are dl-alpha-tocopherol, ascorbic acid, and oyster shell calcium.

## Essential Fatty Acids (EFAs)

Since the omega-3 EFAs have been removed from virtually all of the foods we normally eat, supplementation is essential. Here are the best ways to get your EFAs:

- If you're taking a daily dose of freshly ground flaxseed, you will probably be getting all of the alpha-linolenic acid (ALA) you need. Otherwise, you should supplement with 1–2 tablespoons daily of organic, cold-pressed, high-lignan flaxseed oil or 3–4 g of fish or krill oil.

- Borage oil is more potent and less expensive than either evening primrose oil or black currant oil and is an effective choice for gamma-linolenic acid (GLA). The supplemental dosage for an adult is one or two capsules of an extract standardized to 0.5 g gammon acids taken three times a day.

## Trace Minerals

There are now many good sources of trace minerals available. You will see them described as "colloidal minerals" or "ionic minerals" or "sea minerals." Take your pick and use one. Trace mineral deficiency is epidemic in America because of the poor quality of our diets, so supplementation is essential. Note: You will find it almost impossible to get the trace minerals you need in an overall supplement. Trace minerals are hard to absorb unless they are in a "liquid" form that the body can use.

Humic and fulvic acid and zeolite can also provide useful sources of trace minerals, in addition to providing detoxing capabilities. The problem with all three, though, is that they are extremely "source"-dependent, in terms of efficacy and also contamination. Many sources of these three ingredients are contaminated with heavy metals and even radioactive components. If you are planning on using them for supplementation, you will need to find a company that you trust to use only premium sources.

## Phytonutrients

At the moment, the best source for phytonutrients is still real food. Foods you will want in your diet include:

Broccoli, Brussels sprouts, and kale—for the sulforaphane and di-indolyl-methane.

- Garlic and onions—for the allyl sulfides.

- Red grapes (including seeds)—for the proanthocyanidins and the resveratrol.

- Green tea—for the polyphenols.

That covers the basics of supplementation. Now, let's look at the power of antioxidants to quench free radicals.

# CHAPTER 10

## Antioxidants and Free Radicals

- **Free Radicals and Disease**
- **Antioxidants to the Rescue**
- **What is ORAC?**
- **The Ultimate Antioxidant**
- **Antioxidant Foods**

## FREE RADICALS AND DISEASE

A free radical is a cellular killer that wreaks havoc by damaging DNA, altering biochemical compounds, corroding cell membranes, and destroying cells outright. In this sense, a free radical can be thought of as an invader attacking the cells of your body. More technically, a free radical is a molecule that has lost one of its electrons and become highly unbalanced. It seeks to restore its balance by stealing a vital electron from another molecule.

Scientists now know that free radicals play a major role in the aging process as well as in the onset of cancer, heart disease, stroke, arthritis, and possibly allergies and a host of other ailments. The link between free radicals and the "aging diseases" is the most important discovery since doctors learned that some illnesses are caused by germs.

In a very real sense, the free radical process in our bodies is much the same as the process that causes fuel to burn, oil to go rancid, or an apple to turn brown if you slice it open and expose it to air. It is as though our bodies rust from the inside out, causing, among other things, dry, wrinkled skin. But wrinkles are the least of our problems. When the process gets out of control, it can cause tumors, hardening of the arteries, and macular degeneration, to name just a few of the problems.

Think of free radicals as ravenous molecular sharks—sharks so hungry that in little more than a millionth of a second, they can be making a frenzied attack on a healthy neighboring cellular molecule. A single free radical can destroy an enzyme, a protein molecule, a strand of DNA, or an entire cell. Even worse, it can unleash, in a fraction of a second, a torrential chain reaction that produces a million or more additional killer free radicals.

## What Causes Free Radicals?

There are four primary sources of free radicals:

- The environment: Air pollution, cigarette smoke, smog, soot, automobile exhaust, toxic waste, pesticides, herbicides, ultraviolet light, background radiation, drugs, and even certain foods can all generate free radicals in the body.

- Internal production: Our bodies are constantly producing free radicals as a byproduct of normal metabolic functions.

- Stress factors: Aging, trauma, medications, lack of sleep, disease, infection, and "stress" itself all accelerate the body's production of free radicals, often by a factor of eight times or more.

- Chain reactions: When a free radical steals an electron to balance itself out, it creates a new free radical in the molecule from which it stole the electron. In many cases, the new free radical will seek to balance itself out by stealing an electron, and on and on. And remember, even one free radical is capable of destroying an entire cell or a strand of DNA.

## Types of Free Radicals

There are several types of free radicals in the body. Four types are particularly destructive to the body:

- Superoxide radical: This free radical tries to steal its much-needed electron from the mitochondria of the cell. When mitochondria are destroyed, the cell loses its ability to convert food to energy and dies.

- Hydroxyl radical: This free radical attacks enzymes, proteins, and the unsaturated fats in cell membranes.

- Lipid peroxyl radical: This free radical unleashes a chain reaction of chemical events that can so totally compromise the cellular membrane that the cell bursts open, spews its contents, and dies.

- Singlet oxygen: Not technically a free radical, this metabolite can never-theless cause destruction in the body.

## ANTIOXIDANTS TO THE RESCUE

Your body is constantly replacing and repairing cells damaged by free radicals, but with the way we live and abuse ourselves, our bodies are bombarded with more free radicals than they can handle. By supplementing with antioxidants, we help our bodies keep up with the carnage. It's even possible to get ahead of the game and reverse damage.

Antioxidants are compounds that render free radicals harmless and stop the chain reaction formation of new free radicals. There are three sources of antioxidants. Several metabolic enzymes and peptides produced by the body, such as glutathione, are extremely effective free radical scavengers. (Unfortunately, the body's ability to produce these biochemicals fades dramatically as we age.) Many nutrients in foods and plants are also powerful antioxidants; among these are vitamins E and C, beta carotene, and the proanthocyanidins (including grape seed extract and green tea extract). Cutting-edge research is continually uncovering new antioxidants in foods and plants from around the world.

Many scientists now believe that free radicals are the major villain in both aging and disease. The amount of cells destroyed over the years by free radicals is enormous. Free radicals literally "eat away" the major organs of the body. The use of antioxidant supplements at a maintenance level may provide the ultimate defense against premature aging and a compromised immune system. At therapeutic levels, antioxidants may actually play a significant role in reversing many of the effects of aging and disease.

## WHAT IS ORAC?

Years ago, there was a television advertisement for dog food with the jingle, "My dog's better than your dog. My dog's better than yours. My dog's better 'cause he eats Kennel Rations." No, this section is not about dog food, but with a little bit of paraphrasing, you've got a jingle for one of the hottest topics in nutrition today. "My antioxidant's better than your antioxidant. My antioxidant's better than yours. My antioxidant's better 'cause it has a much higher ORAC rating."

Drinks based on noni and mangosteen were all the rage for several years, then along came açaí. Currently mangosteen, wolfberry, goji, and pomegranate are the hot antioxidants. All of these are good antioxidants and I like them all, but how does one cut through the noise and nonsense and find the truly effective antioxidants?

ORAC is a standardized test adopted by the U.S. Department of Agriculture (USDA) to measure the "total antioxidant potency" of foods and nutritional supplements. ORAC stands for Oxygen Radical Absorption Capacity. It provides a precise way (with certain key limitations) of establishing the free radical–destroying power of a particular food or supplement. Currently, all testing for ORAC values is done by Brunswick Laboratories under a grant from the USDA. The ORAC unit has become an accepted industry standard for measuring antioxidants. The test combines a measure of both the time an antioxidant takes to react with a free radical and also its antioxidant capacity in a given test sample. In most cases, it is expressed as "per 100 grams of sample." (This will become very significant a little later in our discussion.)

Sounds simple: the higher the ORAC value, the more potent the antioxidant. Unfortunately, as always, the reality is more complex.

## What ORAC Numbers Don't Tell You

Even if we assume that the tested ORAC figures are accurate, it is important to understand that having a high ORAC value in and of itself does not confer any particular advantage. That's because not all antioxidants that are confirmed as present in a test tube can be absorbed and utilized by the human body. It doesn't matter how high the value is in a test, if it doesn't work in the body, it has no value to you. In addition, different antioxidants target different free radicals. Taking a supplement with an ORAC value of 17,000 that targets one group of free radicals still leaves you vulnerable to the ones not targeted.

Also, keep in mind that different antioxidants work in different areas of the body. The herb *Ginkgo biloba*, for example, works in the brain and cardiovascular system, whereas curcumin is active in the colon and silymarin in the liver. Again, having 5,000 ORAC units working in the brain isn't much consolation if you have liver problems.

ORAC value tells only a very small part of the story. Saying that pycnogenol is twenty times more powerful than vitamin C, for example, is meaningless when it comes to scurvy. In that regard, vitamin C is infinitely more powerful than pycnogenol. Or to say that mangosteen is ten times stronger than noni is also meaningless. When it comes to raising nitric oxide levels, noni is infinitely stronger because mangosteen doesn't do that. On the other hand, mangosteen appears to have much stronger anti-pathogenic activity than noni. So ORAC value by itself presents a very incomplete picture.

Finally, there is a limit to how much you can benefit from an increased intake of antioxidants. The maximum number of ORAC units the body can handle in a given day is about 3,000 to 5,000 units. This is because the antioxidant capacity of the blood is tightly regulated, so there is an upper limit to the benefit that can be derived from antioxidants. Taking in 25,000 ORAC units at one time (as reputedly occurs with some mangosteen drinks, if you believe what you read on some websites) would be no more beneficial than taking in a fifth of that amount (at least in terms of its ORAC value). The excess is simply excreted by the kidneys. Let me rephrase this to make it even clearer. Taking more than 3,000–5,000 ORAC units a day of the same antioxidant is a bit like using a tank to go to the grocery store—it's overkill. And promoting those super high numbers in advertising is a bit like a car dealer trying to convince you to buy that tank for your grocery shopping in the first place. It's less than honest.

## Comparing Apples to Apples

Now, let's go back to the issue I mentioned above—that ORAC values are normally calculated on the basis of 100-gram portions. The reason is that ORAC was originally developed to give data on whole foods, and 100 grams works out to just under a four-ounce portion. It is essential, therefore, to make sure that the comparison cited for ORAC values is based on equivalent volumes (or servings). When sellers of mangosteen drinks claim ORAC values far superior to other antioxidants, are they comparing serving to serving? Probably not. In many cases, they have extended the numbers out to give the ORAC values in a liter/quart of mangosteen juice and then compared that to one-ounce servings of other liquid antioxidant supplements. To get the true value per recommended one-ounce serving, you would have to divide by 32, which takes you down to a more reasonable 500–600 ORAC units per serving. Don't get me wrong: I like mangosteen and use it in some of my own formulations, but I don't think it's useful to exaggerate the numbers. And besides, as discussed above, since antioxidant levels in the blood are tightly regulated by your body, there are probably no health benefits to numbers over 3,000–5,000 ORAC units per serving of a single antioxidant anyway.

And when it comes to capsules, most capsules are 500 milligrams, which means it would take 56 capsules of an unconcentrated extract to equal an ounce of a food-based source of the antioxidants. In other words, it would take over 200 capsules to give you the same volume as a four-ounce serving of the same antioxidant-rich whole food. That means the ORAC value of the capsule needs to be 200 times more concentrated than the whole food in order to give you an equivalent value. This can be done by removing the water and fiber, which have no ORAC value. Grape skin extract, for example, has a much higher ORAC value than the whole grape skins, but this does not mean that from a standpoint of cost, dose, and/or serving that the extract is necessarily superior. But keep in mind, there is the convenience factor. Isn't it worth paying a premium to easily supplement with a full-spectrum antioxidant that works throughout the entire body and on all types of free radicals—an antioxidant that makes up for the fact that you aren't including all necessary beneficial foods in your daily diet? Most definitely.

## THE ULTIMATE ANTIOXIDANT

There is no such thing as an ultimate antioxidant, but look for a formula that incorporates something approximating the scope listed below and that approximates the levels of each ingredient as listed. It may contain more of any particular ingredient, but if it contains substantially less, it's merely there as label dressing (or "pixie dust" as we say in the trade).

- **Beta Carotene (5,000 IU)**—Carotenoids are phytonutrients that protect plants from damage caused by ultraviolet (UV) radiation and other environmental factors. In humans, they have been shown to inhibit the proliferation of various types of cancer cells, such as those affecting the lungs, stomach, cervix, breast, bladder, and mouth. They also have been proven to protect against atherosclerosis, cataracts, macular degeneration, and other major degenerative disorders. Probably the best known of the carotenoids, beta carotene is converted by the body into vitamin A as needed to strengthen the immune system and promote healthy cell growth. In addition, beta carotene is a potent antioxidant, offering particular benefits to the immune system and the lungs. Note: Synthetic beta carotene, which is made from acetylene gas,[1] is to be avoided at all costs.

- **Alpha Carotene (400 IU)**—Recent studies have shown that alpha carotene is one of the most powerful carotenoids and has a strong inhibitory effect on cancer. It works by allowing normal cells to send growth-regulating signals to premalignant cells. It is usually found as part of a natural beta carotene complex

- **Lutein (8 mg)**—In addition to being specific for the prevention of macular degeneration (lowering the risk by over 50 percent), lutein has also been shown to have strong anti-cancer properties. Its antioxidant effect is significantly enhanced by the presence of zeaxanthin and bilberry. When combined with vitamin C, these three antioxidants have been shown to significantly decrease the risk of cataracts.

- **Lycopene (6 mg)**—Derived primarily from tomatoes (cooked with olive oil, not raw), lycopene appears to be one of the best defenses against prostate and bladder cancers. When used by itself, study results are mixed, but when used in conjunction with vitamin E (d-alpha-tocopherol) and green tea extract, studies indicate that lycopene inhibits prostate cancer proliferation by 90 percent. (Studies aside, if you decide to supplement with the lycopene/vitamin E combination, I would strongly recommend using a full-spectrum natural vitamin E with all the tocotrienols and tocopherols, not just the d-alpha fraction.)

- **Zeaxanthin (300 mcg)**—Lutein and zeaxanthin are both part of a group of carotenoids known as xanthophylls, which are extremely beneficial to the eyes and help significantly in the prevention of macular degeneration.

- **Selenium (75 mcg, methylselenocysteine)**—Selenium is synergistic with glutathione and the enzyme catalase in helping to protect the integrity of cell membranes. It stops the growth of tumors, and it protects the liver. Low levels of selenium have been linked to death from heart disease and cancer of all kinds. Some studies have shown that selenium may be 50–100 times more powerful than any other anti-carcinogen known.

- **N-Acetyl-Cysteine (NAC) (225 mg)**—One of the keys to a healthy immune system is maintaining high levels of glutathione in the body. Unfortunately, supplementing with glutathione directly doesn't really help, but there are alternatives. Supplementation with N-acetyl-cysteine has been proven to substantially raise the body's glutathione levels. In addition, NAC supplementation is mandatory for all smokers and big-city dwellers as it protects against toxic aldehydes that enter the body through cigarette smoke and pollution.

- **L-Methionine (225 mg)**—An essential sulfur-containing amino acid, methionine is a powerful antioxidant and liver detoxifier, where it assists in the normal detoxification processes. As an antioxidant, it provides powerful protection in the colon. Methionine is also involved in the synthesis of choline, adrenaline, lecithin, SAMe, and vitamin $B_{12}$.

- **Quercetin (150 mg)**—Quercetin is in a class of antioxidants known as bioflavonoids. A prime role of quercetin is to protect the integrity of cell walls from free-radical damage. In addition, quercetin prevents the release of histamines into the bloodstream, thereby helping to control food and pollen allergies.

- *Ginkgo Biloba* **(150 mg, 24 percent ginkgo flavone glycosides and 6 percent terpene lactones)**—Known as the brain antioxidant, ginkgo has been shown to increase brain functionality, which makes it useful in helping to improve concentration and memory. This makes it a specific for Alzheimer's disease, where it has the added benefit of helping to significantly reduce depression. In addition, ginkgo oxygenates the blood, increases circulation, and strengthens blood vessels. Its anti-inflammatory, lung-relaxant properties have proven useful in the treatment of asthma, where it eases coughing and reduces tissue inflammation.

- **Curcumin (120 mg)**—Curcumin is what gives the spice turmeric its yellow color. Studies have shown that it can inhibit colon cancer cells by 96 percent in a matter of hours. It appears to have great potential in countering the effects of prostate and breast cancers. In a sense, curcumin can be thought of as natural chemotherapy, with the ability to selectively kill cancer cells while at the same time leaving normal cells alone. Note: Curcumin and green tea strongly reinforce each other.

- **Green Tea Extract (120 mg, 95 percent polyphenols)**—Green tea antioxidants are of the same family as grape seed and pine bark extracts. They are polyphenols, chief of which are the flavonoids called proanthocyanidins. In green tea, the main proanthocyanidins are the catechins, and the most powerful of the catechins is epigallocatechin gallate (EGCG), found in the highest concentration in green tea. It works to prevent tumors from developing the blood vessels they need to survive (anti-angiogenesis) and it has been shown to inhibit metastasis. It is the first known natural telomerase inhibitor, eliminating the "immortality" of cancer cells, which is what makes them so deadly. Green tea is particularly effective in destroying the causes of leukemia, prostate cancer, and breast cancer. It has also been shown to be effective in regulating blood sugar, reducing triglycerides, and in reversing the ravages of heart disease. (Incidentally, the Japanese, who drink large amounts of green tea, have some of the lowest rates of cardiovascular disease in the world.) Green tea seems to almost totally prevent cancer from causing DNA damage in smokers—a possible explanation as to why the Japanese, who are among the world's heaviest smokers, have such a low incidence of lung cancer. Finally, green tea has great benefits for the brain as well, serving as an effective monoamine oxidase (MAO) inhibitor, and protecting against brain-cell death. The net result is that there are strong indications that green tea extract may play a major role in protecting against both Parkinson's and Alzheimer's disease.

Note: the consumption of casein from dairy products can completely block the absorption of the main catechins found in green tea. In other words, drink your tea without milk, and take your green tea supplements separate from any dairy in your diet. Or, even better, just think of this as another reason to eliminate dairy from your diet.

- **Bilberry (120 mg, 25 percent anthocyanins)**—The anthocyanosides found in bilberry are known for their ability to help nourish and repair the tiny capillaries within the eye. In addition, bilberry bioflavonoids are beneficial to the connective tissue that lines blood vessels and binds ligaments throughout the body.

- **Alpha-Lipoic Acid (100 mg)**—Sometimes called the "mother" antioxidant, alpha-lipoic acid (ALA) plays a major role in helping recycle vitamins E and C so they can be used again by your body. ALA is one of the main boosters of glutathione levels in body cells and a key co-factor involved in generating energy in the cells' mitochondria. Finally, ALA has also been shown to significantly rejuvenate the cognitive skills of people as they age. Note: If you use R-lipoic acid, only 50 mg is required.

- **Superoxide Dismutase (SOD) (75 mg, water-dispersible granules as opposed to oil based)**—Superoxide dismutase works along with glutathione to neutralize reactive oxygen molecules in the body. SOD specifically targets the superoxide radical, which, as we discussed earlier, attacks cell mitochondria. When mitochondria are destroyed, the cell loses its ability to convert food to energy and dies. SOD also works in the cytoplasm of the cell to prevent the hydroxyl radical from attacking enzymes, proteins, and the unsaturated fats in cell membranes.

- **Tocotrienols (75 mg)**—Derived from rice bran or palm oil, tocotrienols are a unique vitamin E fraction that is forty times more powerful than standard d-alpha-tocopherol vitamin E. Most tocotrienol formulations are also rich in the gamma-tocopherol fraction of vitamin E, which strongly inhibits both the estrogen-responsive and the non-estrogen-responsive breast cancer cells.

- **Grape Skin Extract (60 mg, 50 percent stabilized resveratrol)**—For several years, grape seed extract was all the rage. As it turns out, grape skin extract, also known as resveratrol, is equally powerful. In controlled studies, resveratrol has been shown to reduce skin cancer tumors by up to 98 percent and to stop production of leukemia cells.[2] In addition, it works as a cyclooxygenase (COX) inhibitor, thus halting the spread of cancer throughout the body. And new studies indicate it may significantly slow down the aging process and prolong life.[3]

- **Grape Seed Extract (60 mg, 84–93 percent oligomeric proanthocyanidins)**—Similar to green tea, the active ingredients in grape seed extract are proanthocyanidins (although in a different combination and ratio). The importance of the proanthocyanidins in grape seed extract is that they are water-soluble and highly bioavailable. Grape seed extract is known as a defender of the circulatory system: it improves peripheral circulation, revives declining capillary activity by up to 140 percent, and increases vascular response by 82 percent.[4] It repairs varicose veins and aids in the prevention of bruising. In addition, grape seed extract is synergistic with vitamin C, vastly increasing vitamin C activity and strengthening collagen activity, including in the connective tissue of the arterial wall and the skin.

- **Chaparral Extract (300 mcg)**—The active antioxidant in chaparral, a lignan called nordihydroguaiaretic acid (NDGA), has been shown to specifically target virtually all forms of herpes virus. Studies of a derivative of NDGA have proven to be even more effective than acyclovir, the prescription drug of choice, at inhibiting the replication of the herpes simplex virus. And maybe even more important, there was no rapid buildup of drug resistance as happens with acyclovir.[5] It is an effective counter to radiation-induced free-radical damage. There are also strong indications that chaparral extract is an effective aid in the prevention of Alzheimer's disease and rheumatoid arthritis.

- **Catalase (300 mcg)**—Glutathione perioxidase, superoxide dismutase, and catalase are the three primary enzymes produced in the body as an antioxidant defense. Catalase is specific for protection against tumors.

## Other Antioxidants

There are other antioxidants that are also well worth taking, but because of the quantity needed to be effective, they need to be taken separately.

- **Red Raspberry (40 mg, active ellagitannins)**—Scientific studies have proven that supplementation with 40 mg per day of red raspberry ellagitannins prevents the development of cancer cells.[6] (It takes a full cup of red raspberry puree to get 40 mg of active ellagitannins.) At low concentrations, it slows the growth of cancer cells; at higher concentrations, it forces cancer cells to self-destruct. Note: There are a number of supplements with ellagic acid, but this form does not work as well as the full ellagitannin complex and may produce side effects such as high blood pressure.

- **Pomegranate (500 mg ellagitannins)**—In the past few years, studies of pomegranates have shown components that inhibit skin and breast cancers, high blood pressure, and atherosclerosis. Pomegranate juice is an antioxidant powerhouse, packed with both the polyphenols that make red wine and green tea effective and the ellagitannins that produce the health benefits of red raspberries. According to an article in the *Journal of Clinical Nutrition*, people who drank just two ounces of pomegranate juice a day for a week increased antioxidant activity by 9 percent.[7] Supplementation with pomegranate extract makes sense if you are looking at cancer prevention, maintaining a healthy heart, reducing LDL ("bad") cholesterol, lowering blood pressure, and protecting against free radicals and aging. In fact, use both red raspberry and pomegranate: the mix of ellagitannins in the two foods appear to be both different and complementary.

- **Noni Leaf (500 mg; or noni fruit extract concentrated 5:1)**—The active biochemical in noni powder, proexeronine, is readily converted in the body to xeronine, an alkaloid that is necessary in virtually every cell in the body. Raising the levels of xeronine to optimum levels can produce profound health effects, and noni appears unique in its ability to accomplish this. It also triggers the release of nitric oxide from the body's cells, a key component in optimizing blood pressure, alleviating erectile dysfunction, fighting viral, bacterial, and parasitic infections, and inhibiting the development of tumors. It is also associated with optimizing learning, memory, and sleep, and reducing the pain associated with inflammation and rheumatoid arthritis.

- **Goji (500 mg, 40 percent polysaccharides)**—Studies have shown that goji berry can induce an immune response and may possess potential therapeutic efficacy in cancer.[8] Other studies have demonstrated that goji induces a remarkable adaptability to exercise load, enhanced resistance, and accelerated elimination of fatigue.[9] And finally, goji has demonstrated the ability to prevent and reverse the effects of free-radical damage.[10]

- **Mangosteen (500 mg)**—Mangosteen contains a unique group of antioxidants called xanthones. Xanthones, particularly beta and gamma mangostin, maintain the immune system, support cardiovascular health, optimize joint flexibility, are naturally antibiotic, antiviral, and anti-inflammatory, and are some of the most powerful antioxidants found in nature (over 14 times the ORAC value of red raspberries). In addition, recent studies have confirmed that gamma mangostin is a potent cyclooxygenase (COX) inhibitor, an important factor in reducing inflammation, pain, and fever.

- **L-Carnosine (500–1,500 mg)**—L-carnosine is a naturally occurring combination of two amino acids, alanine and histidine, that can actually reverse the signs of aging. It works as an antioxidant to protect cellular protein from attack by carbonyl groups and prevents the oxidation of sugars in the body. Supplementation with carnosine represents one of the most powerful things you can do to hold back the ravages of old age.

- **Vitamin E (500 mg of mixed tocopherols and tocotrienols)**—We have talked a good deal about the health benefits of vitamin E already. Just make sure you use a complete vitamin E complex that contains all four tocopherols and all four tocotrienols. Don't settle for just d-alpha, because, at best, it's only the sixth most beneficial component.

- **Vitamin C (500–1,000 mg)**—The antioxidant benefits of vitamin C are invaluable. The trick is that almost all of the vitamin C sold today is in an isolate form that is extremely harsh on the body. You need 500–1,000 mg of vitamin C a day, but try to find it in a "living-food matrix," that is, bound to food so your body can effectively utilize it.

# A NOTE ON HOMOCYSTEINE

Homocysteine is a toxic amino acid that is present in everyone. Although technically not a free-radical problem, high levels of homocysteine in the blood can lead to similar kinds of damage to the cardiovascular system and other parts of the body as happens with free radicals. Homocysteine is neutralized through a process called methylation (the exchange of methyl groups in the body). As we age, our body's ability to provide methyl donor groups declines. The bottom line is that everyone should be on a supplement that provides these methyl donor groups and prevents homocysteine buildup, which can damage the cardiovascular system and DNA and cause cancer and deterioration of the brain. S-adenosylmethionine (SAMe) is a popular supplement that does this (200–400 mg a day). A less expensive option would be to purchase a supplement that contains trimethylglycine (500 mg), vitamin $B_6$ (50 mg), folic acid (800 mcg), and vitamin $B_{12}$ (500 mcg, the best form is methyl-cobalamine).

## ANTIOXIDANT FOODS

Certain foods are high in antioxidants and should be a regular part of the diet. In fact, the U.S. Department of Agriculture recently rated a large number of foods according to their ORAC values. Remember, the higher the number, the more powerful the antioxidant effect. All ratings were based on 3.5 ounces of the tested food. As a reference, carrots (high in the carotenoids) had a 207 rating.

- Broccoli, 890
- Brussels sprouts, 980
- Spinach, 1,260
- Strawberries, 1,540
- Kale, 1,770
- Blueberries, 2,400
- Raisins, 2,830
- Prunes, 5,770

Don't forget that these foods contain other phytonutrients that go well beyond their antioxidant value. Do not eat according to ORAC values alone. They each work in different areas of the body and on different free radicals. Eat as many of them as you can, as often as you can.

## GENERAL RECOMMENDATIONS

Over the years, I have created a number of antioxidant formulas for supplement companies. In fact, this is my specialty—the design of cutting-edge nutritionals using standardized herbs and isolates. On the other hand, I have also become known as a strong advocate for the use of whole herbs and food complexes in all formulations. Why the apparent contradiction? Nature packages nutrients in food complexes and, in general, it is best to design supplements using only whole-food complexes. Antioxidants, however, provide one of the few exceptions to that rule, as long as a few provisos are followed.

The reason for the exception is that antioxidants are specialists, not generalists. No single antioxidant works on all free radicals and in every area of the body. For example, glutathione protects and repairs the liver, whereas bilberry works to defend the eyes. You need to combine a number of antioxidants in one supplement in order to offer an effective defense. In fact, many antioxidants reinforce and/or recycle each other.

For maximum protection, it is vital that you get an antioxidant complex that provides a full-spectrum defense. This is the only real defense against free-radical devastation. For this reason, it is impossible to even come close to fitting the variety you need (at adequate levels) into one supplement, unless you use some standardized herbs and isolates. The trick is to:

- Use only natural isolates, no synthetics.

- Get as complete a complex as you can, even when using isolates.

- Take advantage of the synergistic effect that a number of the antioxidants share with each other. For example, zeaxanthin and lutein reinforce each other, as do curcumin and green tea.

A good antioxidant formula should play a key role in your health supplement regimen. Find a formula you like and use it daily. Remember, it is a supplement program—use it to supplement an antioxidant-rich diet.

That covers basic nutrition and supplementation. In the next chapter, we'll look at the use of enzymes for digestion and also for boosting the immune system's ability to fight infection.

# CHAPTER 11

# *Enzymes = Life*

- **Why We're Lacking in Enzymes**
- **The Benefits of Taking Digestive Enzymes**
- **The Case for Proteolytic Enzymes**

nyone who has any understanding of health has got to be taking enzyme supplements with every meal they eat. Unfortunately, most people think of enzymes (if they think of them at all) as necessary only if they have some kind of digestive problem. And, yes, it's true that people suffering from digestive problems, hiatal hernias, acid reflux, ulcers, and the like, have benefited greatly from using enzyme supplements. But if that's all you think enzymes are for, you've missed the point. In fact, a person's life span may be directly related to the exhaustion of their enzyme potential. The use of food enzymes decreases that rate of exhaustion, and thus results in a longer, healthier, and more vital life.[1] While that statement is a bit of an oversimplification, it's more right than not.

Enzymes are proteins that speed up (catalyze) chemical reactions in living organisms. They are required for every single chemical action that takes place in your body. All of your tissues, muscles, bones, organs, and cells are run by enzymes. Your digestive system, immune system, bloodstream, liver, kidneys, spleen, and pancreas, as well as your ability to see, think, feel, and breathe, all depend on enzymes. All of the minerals and vitamins you eat and all of the hormones your body produces need enzymes in order to work properly.

Enzymes allow many chemical reactions to occur within the constraints (temperature, oxygen levels, acid/alkaline balance, etc.) of a living system. As organic catalysts, they are involved in, but not changed by, chemical reac-

173

tions, and they do not alter the equilibrium of those reactions. Like all catalysts, enzymes work by providing an alternative pathway of lower activation energy for a reaction. By bringing the reactants closer together, enzymes can help make chemical bonds weaker, thus helping reactions proceed faster than without the catalyst (many millions of times faster). This is important since these "reactions" govern every function in your body, not to mention the destruction of viruses, bacteria, and cancerous cells.

Without enzymes, metabolism would progress through the same steps, but would go too slowly to serve the needs of the cell. In addition, enzymes often work together in a specific order, creating pathways. After each enzyme reaction, the product of that reaction is passed on and used as the raw material (substrate) for another enzyme to work on. And then another and another, thus creating what is called a "metabolic pathway." Metabolic pathways control cell metabolism, the process (or really the sum of many individual processes) by which living cells take in nutrients, eliminate waste, and maintain life.

In essence, enzymes are the stuff of life. By allowing reactions to happen at far lower energy thresholds, they make life happen where otherwise there would be none. In the movies, Victor Frankenstein used electricity to create life; he probably would have been better served using enzymes.

But where do enzymes come from? As it happens, they are produced both internally—in every cell in your body, but most notably in the pancreas and the other endocrine glands—and they are present in all of the raw foods that we eat. The basic digestive enzymes produced in the body are protease to aid in the digestion of protein, amylase for the digestion of starches and carbohydrates, lipase to digest fats, cellulase for breaking down fiber cellulose into smaller units, and lactase, which works in the digestion of dairy products. At birth, we are endowed with a certain potential for manufacturing enzymes in our bodies, an enzyme "reserve," if you will. Nature intended that we continually replenish that reserve through proper nutrition and eating habits. Unfortunately, for most of us, that just doesn't happen.

## WHY WE'RE LACKING IN ENZYMES

Most people believe that when you eat a meal, it drops into a pool of stomach acid where it's broken down, then it goes into the small intestine to have nutrients taken out, and then into the colon to be passed out of the body. In fact, the truth is a bit more complex. What nature intended is that you eat enzyme-rich foods and chew your food properly. If you did that, the food would enter the stomach laced with digestive enzymes. No stomach acid would be present. Your meal would then be churned around by the action of the stomach, and the enzymes that were present would "pre-digest" your food for about an hour—actually breaking down as much as 75 percent of your meal.

Only after this period of "pre-digestion" is hydrochloric acid, produced by the parietal cells in the stomach wall, introduced. The acid inactivates all of the food-based enzymes, but begins its own function of breaking down what is left of the meal. The digestive enzyme pepsin is also introduced by the stomach at this point. Unlike food-based enzymes, pepsin thrives in the high-acid environment produced by stomach acid. Eventually, the nutrient-rich food concentrate that results from the action of enzymes and stomach acid moves into the small intestine. In the small intestine, the acid is neutralized in the duodenum and the pancreas reintroduces digestive enzymes to the process. As digestion is completed, nutrients are passed through the intestinal wall and into the bloodstream. That's what nature intended, but unfortunately most of us don't live our lives as nature intended.

Processing and cooking destroy enzymes in food. Man is the only animal that cooks his food. In fact, any sustained heat of approximately 118°F to 129°F (48°C to 54°C) destroys virtually all enzymes. This means that, for most of us, the food entering our stomachs is severely enzyme deficient. Actually, there are some enzymes added from our saliva, but the amount is minuscule because we chew our food only about 25 percent as much as is required. The result is that most of our meals enter our stomachs woefully devoid of enzymes.

The food then sits in the stomach for an hour, like a heavy lump, with very little pre-digestion taking place. That makes it impossible for the normal amount of stomach acid to completely break down the meal, which means that what's left of it enters the small intestine largely undigested. At this point, the pancreas and the other organs of the endocrine system are put under tremendous stress since they have to draw reserves from the entire body in order to produce massive amounts of the proper enzymes. The less digestion that takes place before food reaches the small intestine, the greater the stress placed on the endocrine glands. Recent studies have shown that virtually all Americans have an enlarged pancreas by the time they are forty. (The ever-increasing intake of refined carbohydrates is also a major

## RAW OR COOKED?
## THE POTTENGER CAT STUDY

F. M. Pottenger, M.D., and D. G. Simonsen conducted a series of studies with cats to determine what, if any, impact cooked food had on health. They divided the cats into several groups on controlled diets, identical except that in one group the food (milk, cod liver oil, and meat) was 100 percent raw. The other groups got varying combinations of cooked and raw food. The results were astounding: the group on pure raw food maintained normal good health throughout the experiments and showed no sign of degenerative diseases, but the groups on mixed raw and cooked food (and especially the group eating all cooked food) showed an astonishing breakdown of health in all the animals, including:

- Incomplete development of the skull and other bones
- Bowed legs
- Rickets
- Curvature of the spine
- Paralysis of the legs
- Seizures and convulsions
- Thyroid abscesses
- Cyanosis of the liver and kidneys
- Enlarged colon
- Degeneration of motor nerves throughout the brain and spine

By the fourth generation, the cats on cooked food had totally died out.

contributing factor.) Is it any wonder that the incidence of diabetes is exploding in the developed world?

## THE BENEFITS OF TAKING DIGESTIVE ENZYMES

Regular supplementation with digestive enzymes takes stress off the pancreas (and the entire body) by providing the enzymes required for digestion. In other words, digestive enzyme supplements may be one of the best insurance policies increases, it's easy to see that the level of bioavailable testosterone will only continue to decrease over time.

Most women in modern society have, at some point in their lives, taken birth control pills. But one study showed that contraceptive use was associated with elevated SHBG levels and reduced bioavailable testosterone, even after discontinuing use.[3] In fact, women who were taking contraceptives at the time of the study had SHBG levels four times higher than those seen in women with no contraceptive exposure. Women who had stopped taking them for six months were still two times higher in SBHG than the women who hadn't taken the Pill. Earlier research had shown increases in SHBG levels with oral contraceptive use to be associated with a concomitant 40–60 percent decrease in free testosterone levels. Keep in mind that lowered levels of free testosterone are believed to play a major role in women's sexual problems and could place women at risk for decreased sexual desire, decreased arousal, decreased lubrication, and increased sexual pain.

## Herbal Options

The good news is that bound testosterone can easily be freed, with a little help. The use of herbs such as saw palmetto, wild oats and nettles, and puncture weed can reverse the binding process, increasing free testosterone levels an astounding 105 percent on average. And the benefits for both men and women are enormous.

### Saw Palmetto

It's normal for men to have a lot of testosterone and for women to have some. In both men and women, testosterone is converted into a more potent, potentially harmful form called DHT (dihydrotestosterone). DHT is the hormone that stimulates hirsutism, the loss of hair on the head where you want it and hair growth where you don't (including the back and ears for men and the face and legs for women). If you can reduce DHT, you reduce hirsutism, getting rid of hair from the less desirable places and restoring it on top of your head.

Saw palmetto (*Serenoa repens*), a member of the palm family, appears to reduce DHT in three different ways:

1. Inhibits DHT production

2. Inhibits the binding of DHT to its cell receptors

you can give your body so you can enjoy a long and healthy life. You will also experience a number of short-term benefits from taking digestive enzymes:

- A significant reduction in indigestion and heartburn problems resulting from too much acid in the stomach. If there are insufficient enzymes in your food, your body tries to break down your meal through overproduction of stomach acid. Using digestive enzymes drops acid production back to normal levels.

- Since complex carbohydrates are now being substantially digested before they enter the intestinal tract, you should experience relief from gas and bloating. (Note: Some people may actually notice an increase in activity for several days as their digestive systems come alive.)

- Look for improved digestion of dairy products.

- Diminished food allergies due to more complete protein digestion.

- Since the digestion of enzyme-deficient food is an extremely energy-consuming task, within a few days of enzyme supplementation you should notice an increase in energy levels.

- Relief from many of the symptoms of hiatal hernia.

- Relief from acid reflux.

- Relief from ulcers. Digestive enzymes help digest so much of your meal during the 40–60 minutes of pre-digestion that your body requires less acid in the actual digestion phase. This means that taking digestive enzymes will help lower the levels of acid in your stomach. (Those who suffer from chronic low levels of acid need not worry. Digestive enzyme supplements help here, too, by breaking down so much food in the pre-digestion phase that less acid is actually required. And over time, decreased demand results in increased reserve capability.) Second, protease will begin breaking down the protective coating of the *H. pylori* bacteria responsible for so many ulcers. In other words, it will actually begin to digest it. However, for those with a severe existing ulcer, the protease may begin to digest damaged stomach lining tissue because its protective coating is missing. This can cause noticeable discomfort for several days. To avoid this, start with very small amounts of the supplement with your meals and build up slowly.

## AN ENZYME EXPERIMENT

There is a fun experiment that you can perform with any good digestive enzyme formula. It will actually let you see the benefit of enzyme supplementation in just a few minutes.

Make two bowls of instant oatmeal (it needs to be the instant kind). Mix the contents of a couple of digestive enzyme capsules into just one of the bowls of oatmeal. Mixing thoroughly is crucial as it simulates the action of chewing, swallowing, and mixing in the stomach. Then wait 45 minutes.

Now, check the oatmeal. If the formula you are using is any good, there should be a pronounced difference in the two bowls. The untreated bowl should be as expected: a congealed, lumpy, stick-to-your-ribs consistency. The bowl with the enzymes, however, will look quite different. It will be "digested" and have the consistency of watery gruel.

Which oatmeal would you rather have working through your body: the one that's stuck to the bowl like cement or the enzyme-treated oatmeal that's pre-digested? Which oatmeal do you think is less stressful to digest?

## What to Look for in a Digestive Enzyme Formula

You'll benefit from any good vegetarian-based enzyme supplement, but look for one that contains several protein digesters such as protease and papain (from papaya), amylase for starches and carbohydrates, lipase and bromelain (if you are not allergic to pineapple) to digest fats, cellulase for breaking down fiber, and lactase for digesting dairy. Avoid formulas that contain extra ingredients, such as herbs, vitamins, and probiotics. It's not that they're bad, it's just that there's only so much space in a capsule.

Be suspicious of any enzyme formula that lists only the milligrams of enzymes present as opposed to the activity level of each enzyme. Activity level is what you're interested in. Two batches of the same enzyme of equal weight can have wildly different activity levels. For example, 1,000 milligrams of an enzyme that's been exposed to high heat might have an activity level of zero. When it comes to enzymes, weight measurements are just not useful and can be downright misleading. The internationally recognized and accepted standard for measurement is by Food Chemical Codex (FCC) Units. This is usually expressed in different activity units for each type of enzyme. For protease, HUTs (hemoglobin units, tyrosine basis); for amylase, SKB (named after the creators of the test, Sandstedt, Kneen, and Blish ) or DU (used in the brewing industry); for lipase, LU (which stands for lipase units). The bottom line is that when comparing enzymes, you need to compare activity levels.

Another ingredient you will sometimes find in enzyme formulations is betaine HCL, a supplementary form of stomach acid (hydrochloric acid). Many people, particularly as they get older, produce insufficient stomach acid for proper digestion. For these people, supplementation with betaine HCL makes sense, but not in an enzyme formula. As we previously discussed, many of the digestive enzymes are neutralized in an acid environment—which is why they do most of their work in that 40–60 minute period of pre-digestion that takes place after eating and before stomach acid is released. If you take betaine, it's best to take it as a separate supplement 40–60 minutes after eating.

## THE CASE FOR PROTEOLYTIC ENZYMES

Proteolytic enzymes or proteases are enzymes that help break down proteins. These include chymotrypsin and trypsin (produced by the pancreas), bromelain, papain, fungal proteases, nattokinase, endonase, serrapeptase, and others. Supplementing with a specially designed proteolytic enzyme formula (sometimes called a systemic enzyme formula) between meals, so that the enzymes can enter the bloodstream and augment the functions of your metabolic enzymes, can confer tremendous health benefits. What do proteolytic enzymes do in the body? Benefits include:

- Reducing inflammation—Inflammation is a natural response of the body to injury, but excessive inflammation retards the healing process. Proteolytic enzymes reduce inflammation by neutralizing the biochemicals of inflammation (bradykinins and pro-inflammatory eicosanoids) to levels where the synthesis, repair, and regeneration of injured tissues can take place. Reducing inflammation can have an immediate impact on heart health, cancer prevention and recovery, and Alzheimer's prevention. It also helps speed up recovery from sprains, strains, fractures, bruises, contusions, surgery, and arthritis.

  Osteoarthritis (OA) may also be reduced through oral enzyme therapy, as demonstrated in one study that compared it to the nonsteroidal anti-inflammatory drug diclofenac in patients with OA of the hip.[2] This study showed no real difference between enzyme therapy and diclofenac, imply-ing an equal benefit relation between the substances. The researchers con-cluded that enzyme therapy may well be recommended for treating OA patients with signs of inflammation as indicated by a high pain level.

- Cleansing the blood of debris—Proteolytic enzymes are the primary tools the body uses to "digest" organic debris in the circulatory and lymph sys-tems. Supplementing improves the effectiveness of the process.

- Dissolving fibrin (a protein involved in clotting) in the blood, thereby reducing the risk of dangerous clots—Certain specialized proteases such as nattokinase and endonase help improve the "quality" of blood cells, optimize the ability of blood to flow through the circulatory system, and reduce the risk of clots. In effect, they help regulate the blood clotting cascade, normalizing the function of this vital defense mechanism. They work not so much as a blood thinner but as a corrector of blood chem-istry and function. They are safe and non-toxic, which is more than can be said for medical options such as warfarin. This is extremely important in reducing the risk of stroke. Consider using proteolytic enzymes just before and after long plane flights to minimize the potential of blood clots in the legs. How big is the problem? One study estimated that one mil-lion cases of deep venous thrombosis related to air travel occur in the U.S. alone every year and that 100,000 of these cases resulted in death.[3] And that was before the recent boom in air travel.

- Maximizing immune system function—The primary vehicle the immune system uses for destroying invaders is enzymes. Macrophages, for exam-ple, literally digest invaders with proteolytic enzymes. Supplementation significantly improves the ability of your immune system to do its job.

- Improving breathing—Some proteolytic enzymes help clear away mucus buildup in the lungs.

- Killing of bacteria, viruses, molds, and fungi—Proteolytic enzymes taken between meals literally go into the bloodstream and digest these invaders. One of the tricks of an invading organism is to wrap itself in a large pro-tein shell that the body would view as being "normal." Large amounts of protease can help to remove this protein shell and allow the body's defense mechanisms to take action. With the protective barrier down, your immune system can step in and destroy the invading organism.

- Optimizing oxygen uptake and improving recovery time for athletes—In a recent study, researchers from the Department of Health and Human Performance at Elon University evaluated the capacity of protease to relieve soft-tissue injury resulting from intense exercise. The enzyme group demonstrated superior recovery of muscle function and diminished muscle soreness after downhill running when compared with those taking a placebo.[4]

- Dissolving of scar tissue—Scar tissue is made of protein. Proteolytic enzymes can effectively "digest" scar tissue, particularly in the circulatory system.

- Reducing symptoms of multiple sclerosis (MS).

- Removing circulating immune complexes (CICs), leading to reduced allergies, elimination of many autoimmune disorders, sinusitis, and asthma—Many large protein molecules that are only partially digested in the small intestine are nevertheless absorbed into the bloodstream. Wheat, dairy, and corn proteins are particular culprits. Once in the bloodstream, the immune system treats these oversized proteins as invaders, provoking an immune response. Antibodies couple with these foreign protein invaders to form CICs. In a healthy person, these CICs may be neutralized in the lymphatic system, but if the immune system is compromised or if the level of CICs is just too high, they will accumulate in the blood, where they initiate an "allergic" reaction. The kidneys can no longer excrete all of them, so the body begins storing them in soft tissue, causing inflammation and triggering an autoimmune disorder. Supplemental proteolytic enzymes taken between meals aid in the elimination of CICs.

## What to Look for in a Systemic Proteolytic Enzyme Formula

It is possible to use a good quality digestive enzyme formula in this regard and receive a significant amount of benefit, but it is far more beneficial to use formulas that are optimized for systemic proteolytic function. Proteolytic enzymes are taken between meals so they can be absorbed directly into the bloodstream. The formula should contain a lot of protease, at least 200,000 HUT. This is far more than you will find in a digestive enzyme formula. Some supplements contain fungal (vegetarian based) protease, which although rendered inactive by stomach acid is not destroyed by it. As soon as it passes into the alkaline environment of the intestinal tract, it reactivates. However, the formula will be more effective if it includes several proteases (papain, bromelain, fungal pancreatin) that work in a variety of pH ranges.

The proteolytic enzyme nattokinase has displayed a remarkable ability to optimally balance the clotting ability of blood. Its ability to control clotting rivals that of drugs such as warfarin, but without any of the side effects or downsides—making it of value to everyone, not just heart disease patients. Obviously, if you are already using blood thinners, you will need to work with your doctor if you decide to incorporate proteolytic enzymes in your health program.

The proteolytic enzyme serrapeptase has remarkable anti-inflammatory and anti-edemic (counters swelling and fluid retention) activity in a number of tissues. It can also reduce pain, and it helps clear mucus from the lungs in patients with chronic airway diseases. However, the quality of serrapeptase tends to be inconsistent, and it can cause intestinal distress. It is also very sensitive to stomach acid, which means it has to be enteric coated. There are better alternatives such as Seaprose-S, Endonase, or Protease-S, which are of consistently high quality, cause virtually no intestinal distress, have been proven more effective than serrapeptase, and are not affected by stomach acid.

Finally, look for a formula that incorporates a pH buffering system. It provides extra protection for the enzymes from stomach acid. It can help optimize the pH of the blood and of all your soft tissues (thereby helping in the removal of CICs). Plus, it can help lessen the chances of osteoporosis.

Some doctors mistakenly believe that proteolytic enzymes cannot be absorbed through the intestinal tract wall because they are too large and that they are instead broken down into their constituent amino acids. This is based on old science and is simply not true. There are hundreds of studies showing that enzymes are indeed absorbed intact and easily make their way into the bloodstream, where they "hitch rides" on lymphocytes to travel throughout the body.

## GENERAL RECOMMENDATIONS

Enzymes (digestive and proteolytic) are probably the supplements that I personally use more than anything else. They are critically important.

- Use digestive enzymes with every meal. The heavier the meal, the more you want to use. The best time to take the enzymes is just before eating so they have a chance to "emerge" from their capsules quickly before getting coated by the food. However, if you eat a large, dense, cooked meal, you can still benefit if you take the enzymes even an hour or two after eating.

- In the morning before breakfast and at night before bed, take a systemic proteolytic enzyme supplement on an empty stomach. At higher levels, proteolytic enzymes can be used for detoxification, arterial wall repair, removal of CICs, and cancer reversal. At lower levels, supplementation plays more of a daily maintenance role—preventing those things from happening in the first place.

- When beginning an enzyme supplementation program, start slowly. In order to avoid excessive intestinal agitation and discomfort, start by using the lowest possible dosage of your enzyme supplement for the first few days, then gradually build up your dosage to the recommended amount. Gas, bloating, diarrhea, and constipation are all possible when first starting supplementation with enzymes. Stick with it—after about three weeks, your body settles down and you can begin to receive all of the benefits with no downside.

So, we've now covered how to maximize the absorption of the foods we eat by using digestive enzymes. We've also seen how systemic proteolytic enzymes can do everything from helping clean out your arteries to reducing pain and inflammation throughout your entire body. Next, we will look at the benefits of using herbs.

# CHAPTER 12

## *Miracle Herbs*

- **The Problem with Standardization**
- **The Issue of Herbal Quality**
- **Herbal Preparation Methods**
- **More Art Than Science**

*I*f you were to believe the establishment, herbs have little medical value and are often dangerous. Consider the attacks in recent years on the safety of herbs:

- Possible risk of increased bleeding, especially after surgery—Chamomile, dong quai, feverfew, garlic, ginger, *Ginkgo biloba*, ginseng, St. John's wort

- May worsen swelling and/or high blood pressure—Celery, dandelion, elder, goldenseal, guaiacum, juniper

- Interacts with nonsteroidal anti-inflammatory drugs (NSAIDs)—Feverfew, *Ginkgo biloba*, ginseng, St. John's wort, uva-ursi

But the truth of the matter (if you actually look at the claims, at least the ones where there was any validity) is not that the herbs themselves are dangerous, but rather that they heighten the dangerous side effects of prescription medications. And that's a very different matter.

In truth, just because something is herbal or natural does not make it good. Many natural substances are poisonous, such as hemlock. On the other hand, just because something is herbal or natural doesn't make it weak. Ounce for ounce (despite billions of dollars spent to develop artificial military neurotoxins), no poisons are stronger than cobra or black widow venom. Nature can indeed be very strong, very healing, and very effective. I have personally seen many herbal formulas accomplish things in two to three days that prescription medicines cannot accomplish in weeks, if at all. The keys are that the formula has to be well designed, the herbs used have to be of sufficient quality, and you have to use enough of them. Given those three conditions, herbal formulas can perform miracles.

Despite the best efforts of the medical establishment, herbs are now coming into their own: the American public understands that herbs can be beneficial and have been since the dawn of man. Herbs are being featured in cover stories of major magazines such as *Time* and *Newsweek*. Sales of herbs are well into the billions of dollars a year. This is a time for herbalists and alternative healers to celebrate, right? Not necessarily. While many in the alternative health community have fought for recognition from the medical establishment, personally, I have been very wary of it. And now that recognition has come, I believe we are about to pay the price. What specifically is the problem? The answer lies in one word: "co-option"—to take over an independent minority movement through assimilation into an established group or culture.

## THE PROBLEM WITH STANDARDIZATION

Almost everyone now believes that standardized extracts are a good thing. They answer the medical community's need for predictable doses and effects. All of the top herbal manufacturers now promote their use of standardized herbs. To a large degree, though, I believe it's a red herring. Although for some formulas I will incorporate standardized herbs, in general I'm not a big fan of them. Let me explain.

To understand what standardization means, let's take a look at orange juice. The orange juice you buy in the store, either in half-gallon containers or as frozen concentrate, is actually a great example of a standardized product. The manufacturers of these juice products have been able to identify the "active ingredients" of orange juice that are primarily responsible for taste. In the case of orange juice, those key ingredients are sugar (sweetness) and acid (tartness). Now, the way standardization works with orange juice is that if a manufacturer finds that a batch of oranges is not sweet enough, they'll blend the juice from that batch with the juice from a much sweeter batch to bring it up to the "ideal" sweetness. If that same batch is too acidic, they'll blend it with a batch that's less acidic, until their testing shows that it's reached just the right level of acidity. That's why each can or container of orange juice you buy tastes pretty much like the one you bought the week before. That's standardization.

So, what's the problem? Have you ever tasted a can of frozen orange juice or juice from a container that even comes close to the taste of good fresh squeezed? (Don't bother answering this question if you think that SunnyD® tastes better than real orange juice.) While standardization can make one batch virtually identical to the next, it can never make any batch as good as really good, non-standardized fresh squeezed. The reasons are simple. First, for the most part, standardized orange juice starts with mass-produced, lower grade oranges. Standardization is required because you're starting with an inferior product. Second, the taste of orange juice is governed by far more factors than sugar and acid. It is the result of the interplay of dozens of natural flavors, esters, and oils that are beyond the ability of any manufacturer to control. It is a symphony of taste, a symphony that we cannot duplicate by tweaking one or two "active" ingredients. In fact, tweaking is actually often deleterious because it destroys the natural balance of all those factors that are not standardized.

The process for standardizing herbs is a bit different. With herbs, the active biochemicals are extracted from the herbs in liquid form and then "sprayed" back onto a neutral plant base until the desired concentration of active biochemicals is realized. The net result, however, is the same.

The problem with standardization is that it lowers the bar of what we can expect from herbal formulations. Standardized formulas will never match the quality (and healing power) of a non-standardized formula made from the highest quality herbs, because the standardized formula seeks to control a few "identified" active ingredients to a level found in inferior quality herbs at the expense of all the other "active" ingredients. Standardization distorts plant synergy, and it disrupts the natural ratios of ingredients inherent in the plant itself and replaces them with arbitrary ratios.

In addition, our attempt to identify active ingredients is fundamentally flawed. The procedure used is right out of standard drug testing: isolate individual chemical components and test their effects one at a time in a test tube. If a particular biochemical from an herb tests as "non-active," we can eliminate it from standardization of that herb. But what if that component has a different value in the grand scheme of things? What if, although it may do nothing by itself, its presence makes another component truly effective? In that case, you could have a standardized herbal extract that is virtually useless. Green tea is an interesting case in point. Check any label for standardized green tea and it will state the percentages of polyphenols it's standardized for, but what about theanine? Theanine is an important biochemical found in green tea, but it's an amino acid, not a polyphenol. What green tea extract is standardized for that important marker along with the polyphenols?

An obvious question might be: "If what I'm saying is true, then why is 'everybody' standardizing their herbs?" The answer is that standardization is the herbalists' answer to traditional medicine's complaint that herbs are unpredictable. Another way of saying this is that standardized extracts make herbs more like drugs. But herbs are not like drugs. They are not single chemicals but rather a synergistic blend of natural compounds. Once you acknowledge this, the whole idea of standardization is revealed for what it is—co-option.

Is standardization useless? No, it definitely can give an indication of potency, particularly when using concentrated extracts, but it is by no means the ultimate arbiter of herbal quality. So what's the alternative? Well, one thing that we do know about herbs, through centuries of use, is that high-quality herbs have great healing powers. We also know that well-grown herbs are consistently high in all active ingredients—those that we can identify and those that we won't know about for another hundred years. The bottom line, then, is that if you must guarantee something, then why not:

- Use high-quality herbs with their natural ratios of ingredients. This means, of course, that you can't "doctor up" poor quality herbs as you can with standardization.

- Guarantee a minimum level of potency for all active ingredients (as we know them today). This is a level determined by the initial quality of the herb, not by human manipulation of some arbitrary numbers, and, therefore, this keeps the natural ratios of all biochemicals intact.

This strategy provides all of the advantages of standardization and none of the negatives.

## Turning Herbs Into Drugs

Over the last few years, several companies have tried taking standardization to the next level by running herbs through the same laboratory tests that prescription medicines must pass, called bioassays. One company, Pharma-Print, tried this in the late 1990s and proposed taking it even one step beyond that: seeking U.S. Food and Drug Administration (FDA) approval to sell their most effective herbs as prescription drugs. The idea was that this would allow doctors to sell (for a higher price, of course) a "fully tested medicine version" of the same herbs you currently buy in the health food store. Although PharmaPrint succumbed to stockholder lawsuits, the FDA decided that turning standard food grade products into patented, prescription-only drugs was a good idea. In February 2000, it approved a concentrated fish oil capsule as a prescription drug. Is it more concentrated than regular fish oil? Absolutely, but you can get the same result by just using more non-prescription fish oil at a fraction of the cost.

There are several fundamental problems with this whole process of trying to medically standardize herbs:

1. First, as we've already alluded to, no testing process in the world can measure the synergistic effect of all the biochemical components in herbs. No testing process can determine if a compound, even though it may not be biologically active itself, serves to increase the biological activity of another compound. That's why no testing process can match the skill of the professional herbalist in determining the effectiveness of an herb—just as no testing process can match the nose and palate of a professional wine taster.

2. It reinforces the paradigm of herbs as drugs—that is, for symptom X, you should take herb Y. And it puts herbal medicine in the hands of doctors (who, as a rule, have no understanding of herbal medicine) and takes it out of the hands of the herbal professionals.

3. It actually leads to the classification of herbs as drugs, as the FDA has already done for fish oil.

4. It totally ignores the other aspects of herbal quality.

5. It significantly raises costs.

Interestingly enough, this is not a new idea—we've gone down this road before, with disastrous consequences. The modern prescription drug industry was created out of herbal medicine. The word *drug* itself actually comes from the old German/Dutch word *droog*, which was used to describe the process of "drying" herbs in preparation for use. The apparent motive behind the development of pharmaceuticals was to create purer, more potent, and more effective "medicines" than were found in the herbs themselves. Unfortunately, as we now know, the net result was, in many cases, just the opposite—less effective medicines with a whole range of deadly side effects. Pharmaceuticals, however, do offer one major advantage over herbs: they are patentable and, as such, generate billions of dollars in profits for the companies that manufacture them and the medical system that distributes them.

## THE ISSUE OF HERBAL QUALITY

Ninety-nine percent of the herbs used by American companies do not come from the United States. They are imported from Eastern Europe and from many Third World countries such as India, China, and Mexico. Unfortunately, many of these countries use large amounts of insecticides and pesticides in growing their herbs. DDT (dichloro-diphenyl-trichloroethane), banned for over thirty years in the U.S., is still commonly used in Asia, whereas organophosphate nerve-gas-based insecticides are commonly used throughout Eastern Europe. Mexico, incidentally, has cleaned up its act considerably over the last ten years, initiating a program in 1997 to phase out DDT and chlordane.

Also, many of the areas in these countries where herbs are grown are heavily polluted. The herbs are inundated by polluted rain and irrigated by polluted rivers. In the countries that previously comprised Eastern Europe, for example, there had been no environmental laws for decades. Rivers were used as open sewers, with everything from chemical toxic waste to radioactive waste dumped into them.

The reason most American companies use these herb sources, regardless of the problems just mentioned, is that they are cheap. Good quality organic and wild-crafted herbs can cost twenty times as much, or more. My favorite example is ginseng. High-quality, wild-crafted, or organic ginseng will cost $400–$600 per pound, depending on the season. And yet you can buy low-grade ginseng for as little as $5 a pound and stick it in a formula. Both grades are designated "ginseng" on the label, but which grade do you think actually works? Which grade do you think most companies use? Before you use any company's herbal formulations, you should learn where their herbs come from.

## HERBAL PREPARATION METHODS

There are a number of ways herbs can be prepared. In increasing order of potency, they are:

1. Fresh herb.

2. Dried. Dried herbs are more concentrated because the water has been removed. Dried herbs can be ground up and put in pills or capsules.

3. Teas.

4. Commercial tinctures (liquid extracts), the standardized versions found in most stores. Tinctures can provide concentrations of 30:1 over the fresh herb.

5. Commercial liquid concentrate (like a tincture, but with some of the fluid removed).

6. Commercial dried concentrate (no liquid solvent left).

7. High-energy, ultra-potent tinctures and extracts.

## The Barron Effect

Certainly, the quality of the herbs used in a tincture is fundamental to its effectiveness, but it is by no means the only factor. How a tincture is made is of equal importance. It has been known for centuries among herbalists that if you time the "brewing" of a tincture to the phases of the moon, the resulting tincture is stronger. Specifically, if you start brewing your tincture on the new moon and squeeze it on the full moon, it will be 10–15 percent stronger than an "unphased" tincture. This certainly sounds magical and mystical, particularly because no one has ever known why it works. Nevertheless, it has been demonstrated over and over again that those tinctures made in accordance with the phases of the moon are demonstrably stronger. Incidentally, no commercial manufacturer "brews to the moon" because it takes too long (two weeks). Instead, virtually all commercial manufacturers use a three-day or four-day brewing process.

About ten years ago, a remarkable discovery was made. While brainstorming one day with Ron Manwarren, my main herbalist, I hit upon the actual principle behind "moon phase brewing" and came up with an idea for how we could duplicate the "moon effect" when brewing tinctures—independent of the moon, many times stronger than moon phase brewing itself, and in less time. Ron was then able to take these ideas, add in a few of his own, and develop a process that incorporates this "Barron Effect" into the brewing process, at a strength dozens of times stronger than the moon itself. The net result is herbal tinctures that have been tested at 100 percent stronger than anything produced through normal processing, stronger even than tinctures made through traditional moon phase brewing. The process produces more extract from a given amount of herbs, and the tincture is also stronger in the sense that more biological components are now being extracted (components that were previously left behind by other extraction methods). In particular, in addition to extracting the standard alcohol- and water-soluble biochemicals, it also extracts those that are only oil-soluble and that were previously left behind. This process is not only effective for tinctures, but also allows for concentrates of significantly increased potency and effectiveness.

## MORE ART THAN SCIENCE

Another way in which herbs differ from drugs is that, at its most powerful, most effective, and most healing, herbal medicine makes use of herbal formulations as opposed to single herbs. You've probably had someone recommend that if you're anxious, you should take kava kava, or if you have a cold, to take echinacea. That's right out of traditional medicine—turning herbs into drugs. And it's the least effective way to use herbs.

Herbal formulas, on the other hand, not only address particular symptoms, they also support the body as a whole. In addition, they make use of the synergistic effect inherent in many herbs. For example, many of the more powerful herbal formulations incorporate cayenne, not just because of its remarkable healing properties, but because cayenne is a potentiator for many other herbs, helping to energize them, to stimulate them, to "drive" them into the bloodstream. (Bioperene®, a standardized black pepper extract, is now used in many commercial herbal formulas for the same purpose.) Lobelia, on the other hand, is a potentiator for "nerve rebuilding" herbs, both stimulating ones such as *Ginkgo biloba* and soothing ones such as St. John's wort.

But only more experienced herbalists are aware of these synergies and know the proper proportions to use. Putting together effective herbal formulas is much more akin to an art than science. A good herbalist can identify hundreds of herbs and determine their quality by taste, smell, and touch, and as we indicated earlier, no testing equipment comes close to matching the sensitivity of the great herbalists. I understand that this "artistic" approach to formulation drives conventional doctors crazy, but I consider that a side benefit.

## Idiot Formulations

Quite simply, there are many so-called formulators who don't have the slightest idea what they're doing, but are good marketers and convince people to buy nearly useless formulas. Their errors generally fall into one of two categories.

People often send me a formula and say they just purchased it because it looked incredible and they want to know what I think. After all, they tell me, it has everything you need in one formula. Invariably, I'll suggest they do a little math. For example, the dosage for their miracle pill may be 500 mg and it contains fifty different ingredients. Simple math says that if the ingredients are all present at equal weight, the most you can have of any one is just 0.01 gram. Invariably, the ingredients are not present in equal amounts and are weighted to the first two or three ingredients on the list. That means that the bottom 20–30 ingredients in the formula may be present in amounts as small as 0.001 g. The ink used to print the ingredient's name on the label weighs more than the actual ingredient used in the formula. Those of us in the trade call herbs used at that level "pixie dust" because they have no effect on the body and are present merely to be listed on the label (to make you think they're doing something).

Another major problem comes from people who have no direct experience with ingredients they are using and build their formulas from a book. (When medical doctors produce herbal formulas, this is how they usually do it.) They create formulas by opening a reference book and looking up every ingredient they can find that's recommended for a particular purpose and throwing it into a formula. Many formulas on the market are created in this manner, which leads to some very bizarre combinations. Among my favorites are the intestinal formulas that contain both probiotics and goldenseal. If you look them up on the Internet, you will find that both are listed as being beneficial in promoting intestinal health. However, probiotics achieve their benefit by promoting the growth of beneficial bacteria in the intestinal tract. Goldenseal, on the other hand, is an excellent antibiotic and produces its benefit by killing harmful bacteria in the intestinal tract. Unfortunately, with continual use, goldenseal also kills beneficial bacteria. By ingesting formulas that contain both ingredients for intestinal maintenance, you are both pro-moting and killing beneficial bacteria at the same time! That's kind of like using diet root beer and high-fat ice cream when making a root beer float. What's the point?

## GENERAL RECOMMENDATIONS

- Part of the paradigm that is currently being promoted is: "Yes, herbs can be helpful if you have a cold or a headache or want a little more mental clarity, but if you're really sick, you need real drugs." Nonsense! Drug companies are spending hundreds of millions of dollars developing phar-maceutical knock-offs of herb-based phytochemicals. Tests consistently prove that the knock-offs are less effective, have serious side effects, and cost many times more than the herb itself. Nevertheless, doctors prescribe the knock-off, people pay the inflated prices because their doctors pre-scribe it, and everybody suffers the consequences. In these situations, co-option can mean death. Don't fall for it.

- Look for herbal formulations made from organic or wild-crafted herbs.

- Look for formulations designed by real herbalists.

- Look for herbal tinctures manufactured using a high-energy extraction process. (Note: Tinctures are usually made with alcohol because it works as such a great solvent for extracting the bio-active phytochemicals and also helps preserve the extract for years.)

- Look for (and expect) dramatic healing results.

Now that we've explored the areas of diet and supplements, let's look at steps you can take to bring your body's various systems back into balance.

# PART FOUR

# Balancing the Body's Systems

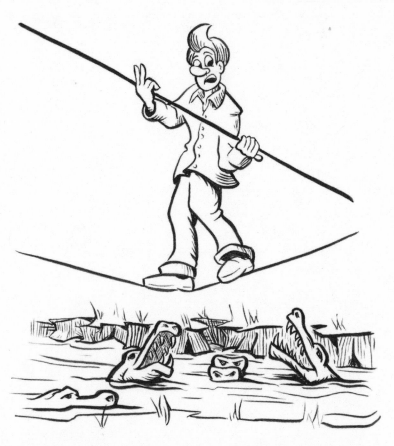

*I don't think this is what Jon meant by balance!!*

# CHAPTER 13

# *Balancing Hormone Levels in the Body*

- **Estrogen and Progesterone**
- **Testosterone**
- **Adrenaline**
- **Growth Hormone**
- **DHEA**
- **Pregnenolone**
- **Melatonin**

*I*n a perfect world, there would be no need to address hormone balance at all, but the world we live in is far from perfect. Diet, stress, and environmental factors are constantly working to throw our bodies out of balance. Due to exposure to chemical estrogens omnipresent in our food, water, and air, the vast majority of men and women already suffer the effects of estrogen dominance by the time they are in their early thirties. Also, due to diet and lifestyle, most men and women find that much of their testosterone has become "unavailable" by this age as well. For men, that problem is compounded by the fact that what testosterone they do have is being converted into dihydrotestosterone, an active form that can contribute to baldness, prostate enlargement, and cancer. In fact, levels of all of our hormones (DHEA, melatonin, growth hormone) start changing and are subject to imbalance and deficiency as we age.

For years, I have been leery of recommending the use of formulas that modify the body's hormonal balance—and certainly the misuse of hormone-altering formulas by athletes and medical doctors (using hormones that are not bioidentical) in the last decade has not helped change that point of view.

Nevertheless, once you throw out all of the preconceptions and look at the issue objectively (and look at the real results, both short and long term), the case for selectively altering your hormonal balance becomes compelling—with a few caveats:

- Only selected hormones should be "adjusted" without a doctor's guidance.

- Use only natural hormones (or hormones that are chemically identical to the natural hormone). Hormones are produced from many different sources: some are derived from animals, some from plants, some are created in laboratories, and some are created through changing the DNA of bacteria or single-celled plants so they produce the desired hormone. As it turns out, for hormones, the source is not the real question. The real question happens to be: is the hormone a perfect match for the hormone found in our bodies? As we will see, things are not always what they seem.

- Use only therapeutic or homeopathic doses. Therapeutic doses mimic the amount of hormone your body normally produces. Pharmacological (or medicinal doses) are substantially higher than therapeutic doses and are often accompanied by significant side effects. Never use pharmacological doses without a doctor's guidance.

## ESTROGEN AND PROGESTERONE

Every woman between the ages of 13 and 113 needs to seriously consider supplementation with a natural progesterone cream. Why? Because virtually every woman who lives in an industrialized country (the United States, in particular) is at high risk of estrogen dominance because of exposure to xenoestrogens. Xenoestrogens, which are mostly petroleum-based synthetic estrogens, are now present in massive amounts in our food chain, water supply, and environment.

Some high-potency estrogens (such as estrone and estradiol) are produced by the body itself. But the greatest problem comes from the powerful and destructive petrochemical-based xenoestrogens. Not only are these xenoestrogens omnipresent, they are considerably more potent than estrogen made by the ovaries—some are even potent in amounts as small as a billionth of a gram.

At one time, our diets afforded some protection. Fruits, grains, and vegetables (in their natural state) provide low-action phytoestrogens for the body. These phytoestrogens fill the body's estrogen receptor sites, making them unavailable for use by the more potent estrogens (both natural and synthetic). Unfortunately, today's diets are dominated by processed foods, which are stripped of these beneficial phytoestrogens. The net result is that virtually all of the body's receptor sites are ready and waiting for the far more intense estrogens.

It is important to understand what role estrogen plays in the body. In addition to promoting the growth of female characteristics at puberty, the estrogen hormones also promote cell growth. It is the estrogens, for example, that stimulate the buildup of tissue and blood in the uterus at the start of the menstrual cycle. The problem comes when high levels of estrogen (natural and synthetic) are unopposed by sufficient amounts of natural progesterone. This leads to continuous, unrestrained cell stimulation, which can lead to the following problems:

- Endometrial cancer

- Increased risk of breast cancer

- Loss of bone mass

- Increased risk of autoimmune disorders such as lupus

- Fibrocystic breasts

- Fibroid tumors

- Depression and irritability

- Pre-menstrual syndrome (PMS) symptoms (cramping and bloating, depression, and irritability)

- Menopausal symptoms (hot flashes, night sweats, depression, and irritability)

- Decreased sex drive

- Increased body hair and thinning of scalp hair

- Migraine headaches

- Impaired thyroid function, including Graves' disease (a form of hyperthyroidism)

- Increased body fat

- Increased blood clotting

- Impaired blood sugar control

- An acceleration of puberty in young girls, from an average age of fourteen or fifteen to now as young as eight or nine, with 1 in 100 girls now showing signs of puberty by the age of three.[1]

- Declining male sperm production and an increase in testicular and prostate cancers

## Out of Balance

Once we understand the problem, it is easy to see that for the vast majority of women, hormone replacement therapy with conjugated estrogens such as Premarin® and the current favorite, ethinylestradiol, is not the answer. In fact, it may be a major contributor to the problem. The primary issue with these estrogens is that they contain no estriol. Premarin contains estrone and estradiol, and ethinylestradiol contains only a synthetic form of estradiol. This is significant because research has shown that the average ratio of serum estrogen in the female body is 90 percent estriol, 7 percent estradiol, and 3 percent estrone. (This includes the various estrogen metabolites, such as hydroxyestrogen and the 16a-hydroxylated estrogens.) The ratios are important once you understand that both estrone and estradiol are pro-carcinogenic, whereas estriol is anti-carcinogenic. So, why would you want to use an estrogen supplement that has only the pro-carcinogenic estrogens and not a single drop of the anti-carcinogenic estrogen that normally represents 90 percent of the body's total?

In those cases where estrogen supplementation is warranted, insist that your doctor give you either "true triple estrogen" (and insist that it be in a ratio similar to the 90-7-3 mentioned above) or use pure estriol cream. Studies have shown that the higher the ratio of estriol in the body versus the amount of estrone and estradiol together, the lower the risk of breast cancer.

That said, you have to wonder why more doctors don't ask, "If estrogen dominance got you there in the first place, then why would you want to add a powerful estrogen complex with no protective estriol in it to your body?" Of course, you wouldn't, and yet Premarin was, for many years, the most frequently prescribed drug in America.

## A Natural Alternative

The only natural balancer to excessive estrogen in the body is natural progesterone, not more estrogen. This has been clearly detailed in books such as *What Your Doctor May Not Tell You About Menopause* by Dr. John R. Lee.

Natural progesterone is the only known substance that mitigates virtually all of the problems associated with estrogen dominance and with virtually no side effects of its own.

Synthetic progesterone, such as Provera®, often recommended by doctors, is not the same thing. Progesterone is a natural substance, and as such cannot be patented, so pharmaceutical companies have to modify it slightly. They do this by creating a new molecule, called medroxyprogesterone, that does not exist in nature. This "slightly" modified, artificial progesterone is what most doctors prescribe when they tell you they're giving you progesterone. This synthetic form of progesterone carries a whole range of serious

## A BOGUS WARNING ABOUT PROGESTERONE

Over the last couple of years, warnings have started to appear on products containing natural progesterone stating that they contain a substance known to cause cancer. This is nonsense that is based on bogus science. The warning was triggered by the state of California, which mandated that any product sold in the state that contained natural progesterone had to contain the warning, and since everyone sells in California, the warning became ubiquitous. But why the warning?

In 2004, the California Office of Environmental Health Hazard Assessment published the results of a review of studies (human, animal, and in vitro) that lumped together natural progesterone, synthetic progestins, and other "progesterone-like" compounds. All of the data from the studies of these compounds were mixed together. This would be equivalent to studying the safety of the friendly bacteria acidophilus and lumping it together with studies on *Staphylococcus*, salmonella, and *E. coli,* and concluding that acidophilus was deadly based on those mixed numbers. Absurd! Plus, the majority of studies that included progesterone (either natural or synthetic) involved combinations with synthetic estrogens, compounds that are known carcinogens. And none of the studies used progesterone in transdermal cream form, but rather involved oral, injected, and suppository forms of the hormone—at dosages as much as 10,000 times the recommended amount.

Requiring a warning label on natural progesterone creams based on this data is embarrassing to the medical community and shameful to the state of California. It isn't worth the time it takes to read it.

# SYNTHETIC VS. NATURAL HORMONES

Consider the fact that the testosterone molecule and the estrone molecule are virtually identical, except for the fact that the positions of the oxygen atom and the OH atoms change places. This slight "modification," however, happens to be enough so that one hormone makes men and the other women.

Even closer is the similarity between DHEA and estrone. The molecules are actually identical except for the location of some of the double bonds between carbon atoms. You cannot get closer, and yet the function of DHEA and estrone could not be more different.

And now look at the difference between natural progesterone, Provera, and drospirenone (the synthetic progesterone of choice in the newest birth control pills).

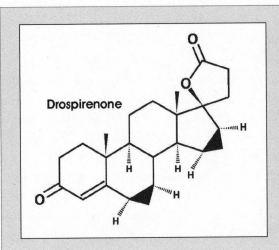

Drospirenone

The bottom line is that progestins such as Provera and drospirenone are not natural. They are synthetic forms of progesterone with a range of serious side effects.

side effects, including depression, birth defects, increased body hair, acne, risk of embolism, decreased glucose tolerance, and allergic reactions. In exchange for these significant side effects, Provera does offer some protection against endometrial cancer and a very modest, short-term increase in bone formation.

On the other hand, supplementation with natural progesterone, when used as directed in small amounts, has no known side effects. It is best utilized by the body when administered transdermally with a skin cream that contains approximately 500 milligrams (mg) of natural progesterone per ounce and offers the following potential health benefits:

- Improve bone formation. According to Dr. John R. Lee, natural progesterone may significantly improve bone formation by as much as 15 to 35 percent. This is unique to natural progesterone—estrogen supplementation does not increase bone formation but merely slows the rate of loss for a five-year period around the time of menopause. And synthetic progestin only mildly increases bone formation.

- May help protect against endometrial and breast cancers.

- Relieve symptoms of PMS and menopause.

- Normalize libido.

- Improve the body fat profile.

- Improve sleep patterns.

- Help relieve migraine headaches.

Every woman living in the industrialized world should seriously consider supplementation with natural progesterone. Whether you're still going through your menstrual cycles (or whether you're pre-menopausal, menopausal, or postmenopausal), you need to seriously consider supplementation. The benefits are extraordinary and the risks minimal. And the risks of not supplementing potentially include an increased chance of getting breast cancer, endometrial cancer, and osteoporosis.

If you decide to begin a regimen of natural progesterone supplementation, look for a premium quality balancing cream that contains a minimum of 500 mg per ounce of 100 percent pure, USP-grade progesterone, preferably in a natural, vegetarian formula that uses no artificial or synthetically derived fragrances, parabens, or preservatives.

There is one cautionary note about progesterone cream: if you use more than directed, or don't cycle on and off as instructed, levels will build up in your fat tissue. If done over an extended period of time, it has the potential to affect the balance of the adrenal hormones such as DHEA, cortisol, and testosterone. After using progesterone cream for any length of time, it's probably a good idea to have your body levels checked.

## Men and Estrogen

As we've already mentioned, men are also exposed to the effects of xenoestrogens. In addition, as their testosterone levels drop with age, there is in many cases a concomitant rise in estradiol levels—the major reason that many older men develop breasts. Just as with women, estradiol stimulates cell growth in men and is potentially carcinogenic. This is one of the main factors involved in the dramatically increased incidence of prostate cancer. Estradiol stimulates the *BCL2* gene, which is responsible for stopping cell death. What at first glance sounds like a positive is, upon closer inspection, not. When cell death in prostate tissue is blocked, cell growth continues unabated, becoming a major contributing factor in the enlargement of the prostate and the development of prostate cancer. In other words, any man over thirty years old would be well advised to supplement with a natural men's progesterone cream.

## TESTOSTERONE

A growing body of evidence suggests that testosterone levels drop as much as 40 percent in men between their early forties and early seventies. And for 10 to 15 percent of all men, those levels will dip below normal even as early as their thirties if they have to deal with stress, depression, personal life changes, or medications. This causes a decrease not only in sexual desire and performance, but also in the competitive drive to succeed and accomplish something meaningful in life. In women, excessive estrogen in the body causes a reduction in testosterone levels, which leads to a similar decline in sexual desire and performance and a similar reduction in "life drive."

Both men and women need and produce testosterone in their bodies, although in differing amounts. Testosterone (in both men and women) is responsible for:

- Pumping up energy levels

- Firing the need to succeed

- Bonding us with our mates

- Fueling our sexual desires and elevating our levels of sexual satisfaction

- Growing hair on our heads, while at the same time keeping us from going bald

- Building muscle and burning off fat

- Facilitating better blood circulation

Unfortunately, once we reach our thirties, available testosterone levels for both men and women begin diminishing with age. However, it's not actual testosterone production that decreases as we age but rather the amount of free circulating (bioavailable) testosterone, as more of it gets bound to both albumin and a natural substance called SHBG (sex-hormone-binding globulin). SHBG plays the biggest role in testosterone binding when testosterone levels are low, while albumin plays the dominant role at higher levels.[2] The important point is that when "bound" (particularly to SHBG), testosterone becomes unavailable for use by the body. This means that although total testosterone levels may remain essentially unchanged as you age, only a small fraction of that total is actually "available" to enter a cell and activate its receptor. And considering that as we age the amount of SHBG steadily

3. Promotes the breakdown of DHT

In fact, it appears that one of the primary mechanisms through which saw palmetto works in the body is that it inhibits 5-alpha-reductase, the enzyme that converts testosterone into DHT. Supplementation with extracts of the saw palmetto fruit lowers DHT, thereby reducing hirsutism and increasing available testosterone.

### Nettles and Wild Oats

Extracts of wild oats (*Avena sativa*) and nettles (*Urtica dioica*) can safely help increase testosterone levels in the body. German researchers have identified a biochemical found in nettle root, known as (+/-)-3,4-divanillyltetrahydro-furan, that has a high binding affinity to SHBG, actually describing the affinity as "remarkable." These researchers also suggested that the beneficial effects of plant lignans (such as found in flaxseed oil) on hormone-dependent cancers may be linked to their binding affinity to SHBG.[4] The most potent known lignans in this respect are constituents of nettle root. In addition to SHBG binding, at least six constituents of nettle root inhibit aromatase, reducing conversion of androgens to estrogens and thus increasing available testosterone.

There are no formal studies testing the effect of wild oats on humans, but there are significant amounts of anecdotal clinical observations, particularly with younger men who had low testosterone levels for their age. Supplementation with *Avena sativa* results in dramatically increased testosterone levels. The key to the effectiveness of wild oat supplements lies in the quality of the extract, because active avenacosides provide the potency. If you're going to use a supplement that contains wild oats, make sure it comes from a reputable supplier.

### Puncture Weed

Puncture weed (*Tribulus terrestris*), also known as yellow vine and goat head, is a flowering plant found in Europe, Africa, southeast Asia, and Australia. It doesn't just free up testosterone, it also boosts production of testosterone in the body. *Tribulus* enhances testosterone levels by increasing levels of luteinizing hormone (LH), which is responsible for "telling" your body to produce testosterone.

## The Benefits of Testosterone Balancing

Surprisingly, women are far more vulnerable to testosterone level changes than men. The reason is that they have so much less to work with (and even less if on the Pill). So, when even a small amount of their available testosterone gets bound to SHBG, the results include a loss of energy and motivation, less interest in their spouse and loss of libido, decrease in muscle and significant increase in body fat (a prime reason women start to gain weight in their forties), hirsutism, and a significant increase in the risk of breast cancer since bound SHBG is no longer available to lock up excessive estrogens. Regular use of a women's testosterone-balancing formula can help to significantly reverse and/or prevent all of these conditions.

It should be noted that SHBG binds not only to testosterone, but to all of the sex hormones including estradiol (an "active" form of estrogen). Normally, this binding serves as a storage system for excess hormones, but in men there is a problem: SHBG also has an affinity for prostate tissue. In effect, because of its affinity for both, SHBG can bind estrogen to cell membranes in the prostate, which causes an increase in prostate-specific antigen (PSA) secretion, a prime factor in prostate problems, including cancer. The wild oats and nettles found in most men's testosterone-balancing formulas work together to reverse this binding process, thereby reducing the likelihood of prostate problems. Saw palmetto also has been proven to inhibit the 5-alpha-reductase enzyme, which causes testosterone to be converted into DHT, again stimulating the growth of prostate tissue. Regular use of formulas that contain saw palmetto, wild oats, and nettles can help reduce enlargement of the prostate, tone the bladder (improve urinary flow and relieve strain), decrease urinary frequency (especially during the night), and reduce inflammation of the bladder and prostate.

The ingredients found in testosterone-balancing formulas work naturally in both men and women to enhance sexual desire, sensation, and performance. The effect on human sexual appetite can be powerful. Both men and women can feel a boost in sexual desire, sometimes after only a few hours (more often, though, in about 7–10 days). And both men and women can experience an increase in frequency of orgasms when taking quality extracts of wild oats and nettles.

## ADRENALINE

Although not directly related, adrenal exhaustion (low adrenaline levels) and low testosterone levels share some key similarities. For most people, their impact is felt starting around the same time in life—in their thirties—and many of their symptoms are similar, including exhaustion, reduced sexual vitality, and loss of zest for life. Adrenaline is produced in the adrenal glands and is probably best known as the body's "fight or flight" hormone—the hormone that stimulates your body's response to stress (tells the heart to speed up and the blood vessels to narrow). Unfortunately, the body was simply not designed to deal with "fight or flight" on the 24/7 basis of modern urban life. By definition, "fight or flight" refers to exceptional circumstances, such as the sudden appearance of a Bengal tiger. Eventually, under constant stress, the adrenal glands run down and can no longer produce sufficient adrenaline. In response, we tend to use stimulants such as coffee or "energy drinks" to force the adrenal glands to pump even when exhausted. But there's only so far you can push the adrenals, and eventually they reach a state of total exhaustion in which they can no longer produce sufficient adrenaline no matter how many stimulants you use.

Fortunately, there is a class of herbs known as adaptogens that work well with the testosterone-balancing herbs so that it's possible to supplement with formulas that do double duty. By definition, an adaptogen is an herb that helps the body adapt to stress. As such, they naturally help to rebuild adrenal gland function and restore hormonal balance. Foremost among the adaptogens is ginseng. There are three main types of ginseng that you'll find in formulas: American, Asian, and Siberian. American and *Panax* (Asian) ginseng are used primarily for their ability to energize the body and improve sexual function. Siberian ginseng, also known as *Elutherococcus*, is not really a true ginseng but more of a distant relative. Nevertheless, it has the most powerful adaptogenic qualities—helping the body adapt to stressful conditions, improving athletic performance, and reinforcing the immune system. In the end, though, the type of ginseng used is probably less important than the quality. As mentioned previously, high-quality, wild-crafted, or organic ginseng costs $400–$600 per pound, depending on the season. Low-grade ginseng costs as little as $5 a pound. Obviously, there's a difference in efficacy, yet both grades are designated "ginseng" on the label. Make sure you trust the company you buy your ginseng from. Regular use of a high-quality ginseng has been shown to increase stamina, revitalize the body, counteract chronic fatigue, improve resistance to stress, and enhance immune function. For these reasons, ginseng is useful for combating adrenal exhaustion.

## GROWTH HORMONE

The rejuvenating powers of growth hormone (GH) are no secret to the wealthy: for the last 30–40 years, GH has been available from doctors, required two injections a day, and cost up to $1,800 a month. Over the last few years, however, several alternatives for the rest of us have become available. And while I could never recommend the injections (for a variety of reasons), I can endorse the alternatives.

Many fantastic claims are made for the effects of growth hormone, even claims of "almost" eternal youth. Would that it were so! Although the effects are more subtle for most people, they are nevertheless wide ranging:

- Fat loss (14 percent on average after six months, without dieting)

- Elimination of cellulite

- Higher energy levels and enhanced sexual performance

- Regrowth of heart, liver, spleen, kidneys, and other organs that shrink with age

- Greater heart output and lowered blood pressure

- Improved cholesterol profile, with higher HDL ("good") cholesterol and lower LDL ("bad") cholesterol

- Superior immune function

- Increased exercise performance

- Better kidney function

- Stronger bones

- Faster wound healing

- Younger, tighter skin

- Hair regrowth

How exactly does GH produce these results? First of all, as we detailed in our discussion of progesterone, it is important to understand that hormones are the body's chemical messenger system—they tell the body what to do and when. Growth hormone is produced in the pituitary gland and released in a series of microscopic "pulses" throughout the day (mostly in the evening). It signals a number of body functions relative to aging and the production of other hormones, such as DHEA and melatonin, and various parts of the endocrine system, including the hypothalamus (considered to be the "master gland"). Interestingly enough, the release of GH at pulse levels stimulates the pituitary to produce even more GH.

However, it's most important function is telling the liver to produce insulin-like growth factor 1 (IGF-1), the main key to anti-aging. Specifically, the benefits of GH can be measured in terms of how much it increases the body's production of IGF-1 (above a 20 percent increase starts to be significant in terms of effectiveness).

There is some concern that, because it increases IGF-1 levels in the body, GH may increase the risk of prostate cancer. This is based on a couple of in vitro studies that showed IGF-1 may stimulate tumor cell growth, a study out of the Harvard School of Public Health that equated high levels of IGF-1 with an increased risk of prostate cancer, and the fact that human "giants" (who are, in fact, large because of abnormally high GH levels) have a higher risk of cancer. A simple reality check, however, calls these observations into question. First, both GH and IGF-1 levels decline as we age, yet the incidence of prostate cancer increases as these levels decline—the exact opposite of the expressed concern. In addition, in numerous studies involving thousands of patients receiving growth hormone over many years, there were no observed increases in prostate cancer. In fact, based on real-life observation, there is evidence that growth hormone supplementation may reduce the risk of prostate cancer.

## Supplementing with Growth Hormone

Most supplement formulas will increase IGF-1 levels by a minimum of 20 percent, with some even approaching 100 percent. Keep in mind, however, that one 30-minute aerobic session can easily increase IGF-1 levels by 100 percent, and a solid session of weight training can increase levels by an incredible 400–800 percent. Injections, on the other hand, which work directly on the liver (almost like a massive "pulse"), can increase IGF-1 production by only 20–40 percent. A downside to injections, in addition to cost, is that they can give too much GH to the body, shock the body, and can stop the pituitary from producing its own GH. This may explain why injectable GH produces more immediate results, yet ultimately plateaus in terms of effectiveness.

Incidentally, you can no longer actually buy true HGH or human growth hormone. Technically, only growth hormone actually taken from human beings can be called "human" growth hormone. Thirty years ago, the sole source of growth hormone was human cadavers, but that was abandoned when it turned out that growth hormone taken from people had a major downside (in addition to cost)—it occasionally caused the human equivalent of mad cow disease.

Fortunately, at around the same time, recombinant DNA technology came into its own and scientists learned how to alter the DNA of a single-cell yeast plant so that it would produce large amounts of growth hormone (molecularly identical to real HGH), safely and inexpensively. Because this growth hormone is identical to HGH, people often use the terms *growth hormone* and *human growth hormone* interchangeably, but it should be referred to as a "plant-based growth hormone."

Given this good, inexpensive source of growth hormone, another problem remained: the growth hormone molecule is so large (containing 191 amino acids) that it cannot be absorbed orally. That meant it could only be administered by injection, which required a doctor and was very expensive. Because of the cost, growth hormone injections became known as the secret youth formula of movie stars and the very rich.

For years, the only alternatives to this have been the amino acid–based precursor formulas (also called GH secretagogues). Typically, such formulas contain ingredients such as glutamine, tyrosine, GABA, arginine, and lysine. Although not as powerful as growth hormone injections, these formulas can be quite effective, provided your pituitary is functioning well, and carry none of the downside of injections. Within the last few years, two alternatives have appeared that use real (plant-based) growth hormone. One is homeopathic GH, which makes use of real GH diluted down to homeopathic levels. It appears to work about as well as the GH secretagogues. In the late 1990s, a new form of GH that could be sprayed into the mouth and absorbed orally was introduced. Again, this works about as well as a GH secretagogue for most people. Its advantage is that it will work for people whose pituitaries are dead and no longer capable of producing HGH. However, it can be expensive and there is a wide variation in the quality of HGH sprays.

## DHEA (DEHYDROEPIANDROSTERONE)

In animal studies, DHEA supplementation bordered on the miraculous. It seemed to extend life by 50 percent; protect against heart disease, cancer, autoimmune diseases, obesity, and diabetes; boost the immune system; and reverse the effects of stress. The reality for human beings turned out to be somewhat less.

I am not a big fan of DHEA supplementation (at least without a blood workup) for several reasons. First of all, oral DHEA is composed of particles that are too big to be directly used by the body, so it has to be sent to the liver to be broken down. Unfortunately, since the liver is unaccustomed to receiving DHEA in this form, it ends up converting most of it into androgens (sex hormones). It is these androgens that can cause the growth of facial hair in women and may contribute to prostate disorders in men. The second problem with standard oral DHEA supplementation is that there is strong evidence that it reduces the body's own production of DHEA. Also, DHEA supplementation (usually in doses greater than 10 mg a day) is often accompanied by side effects that include acne and excessive skin oiliness, growth of facial and body hair in women, irritability or mood changes, and overstimulation and insomnia.

There has been a lot of debate as to whether DHEA contributes to prostate problems or not. As with growth hormone, once you step back, you see that most of the debate makes no sense. The argument is that since DHEA can be converted into testosterone and dihydrotestosterone (hormones believed to stimulate prostate tissue), it is counterproductive in those who have prostate gland enlargement or prostate tumors. But actual experience does not support that conclusion. The only case I know of that showed a definite link was one in which the patient was receiving DHEA doses of 700 mg a day—much higher than the usual dose of 2–50 mg a day. At low dosage levels, DHEA may actually work to block androgen receptor sites in the body—making them unavailable to the more potent androgens—thus serving to protect the prostate.

## Supplementing with DHEA

As mentioned earlier, the oral DHEA commonly available is composed of particles that are too big to be directly used and are sent to the liver, which ends up converting most of it into androgens. What's left is converted into 7-Keto DHEA, the useful portion. Supplemental 7-Keto DHEA is now available and seems to provide most of the benefits of regular DHEA. But since it isn't converted to active androgens (testosterone and estrogen), it is much safer and has minimal side effects. If you're looking to supplement with DHEA, 7-Keto probably makes the most sense.

Many people use supplements containing Mexican wild yam (*Discorea villosa*) as a DHEA supplement. The theory is that wild yam contains diosgenin, a DHEA precursor that your body uses to produce its own DHEA. Unfortunately, there is no evidence that your body converts any wild yam into DHEA. All benefits related to wild yam appear to be from its phytoestrogen effect.

## PREGNENOLONE

Pregnenolone is the ultimate hormone precursor. Virtually every hormone can be produced by your body from pregnenolone. As with the other hormones, pregnenolone levels decline precipitously as you get older. The prime benefit of pregnenolone supplementation is that it helps balance out your other hormone levels as required. In addition, it also provides specific health benefits:

- Memory enhancement and improved cognitive performance
- Supports the adrenal glands
- Anti-fatigue agent
- Significant benefit in rheumatologic and connective tissue disorders (rheumatism, osteoarthritis, scleroderma, psoriasis, lupus, and spondylitis)
- Repair of the myelin sheath structure protecting the nerves
- Improved immune function
- Reduced PMS and menopausal symptoms

Use of pregnenolone has shown no serious side effects, even at very high doses (up to 700 mg a day). However, at a high dosage level, there has been some occurrence of minor side effects, including overstimulation and insomnia, irritability, anger or anxiety, acne, and headaches.

## MELATONIN

Melatonin is a natural hormone made during sleep in the pineal gland, a pea-sized gland located in the brain. The trigger for production of melatonin is total darkness—any light in the room will inhibit your body's production.

Today, however, living in a world with nightlights in the bedroom or street-lights sneaking through the window, we actually have an epidemic of people with insufficient melatonin production, even at a very young age. The problem doesn't just come from light falling on our eyes while we sleep, but from light falling on any part of the body. Even if you wear an eye-mask, if light is falling on your arms or chest or feet, that's enough to slow melatonin production. Without artificial light, we would normally be in total darkness 8–12 hours a night, producing melatonin during all of those hours. Living in a city or suburban area may cut the hours of total darkness to six or less, and in many cases, zero. Melatonin levels also decline significantly as we age.

Since its discovery in 1958, melatonin has been studied extensively and shown to be widely beneficial to the body. The benefits of supplementation include:

- Better Sleep—Lowered levels of nighttime melatonin reduce the quality of sleep, resulting in the need for more sleep. If your pineal gland does not produce adequate melatonin early enough in the evening, both the quality and quantity of your sleep may suffer. Lack of melatonin may make it difficult for you to fall asleep or may cause you to wake up too soon. Too much melatonin and you will feel exhausted or "drugged" throughout the day. By taking melatonin instead of other sleep aids, rapid eye movement (REM) sleep (dreaming) is not suppressed, nor does it induce "hangover" effects when used as directed.

- Enhanced Immune Function—Many people report that supplementation with melatonin has significantly reduced their incidence of colds and infections. The exact way in which melatonin affects the immune system is not known. However, since much of the activity of the immune system takes place at night, some researchers have proposed that melatonin interacts with the immune system during sleep, helping to buffer the adverse effects of stress. It has been proposed by some that the increased incidence of cancer we see today is partially due to the extended time we are exposed to artificial lighting. This is reflected in the fact that melatonin levels in breast cancer and prostate cancer patients are half of normal.

- Powerful Antioxidant Capabilities—Melatonin is one of the most powerful antioxidants produced in the body. In addition, since it is both water- and fat-soluble, melatonin can reach almost every cell in the body. However, since it cannot be stored in the body, it must be replenished daily.

- Mood Elevator—Nighttime melatonin levels are low in people with major depressive and panic disorders. Individuals with mood swings or who are melancholic also have lower melatonin levels. Both seasonal affective disorder (SAD) and cyclic depressions are related to the peaks and valleys of melatonin levels.

## GENERAL RECOMMENDATIONS

### Estrogen and Progesterone

Women who are still going through their menstrual cycles or are pre-menopausal, menopausal, or post-menopausal should seriously consider supplementation with an all-natural progesterone cream. Make sure you and your doctor avoid all synthetic forms of progesterone. The benefits can be profound, and the risks of not supplementing potentially include an increased risk of breast cancer, endometrial cancer, and osteoporosis. For men, since they are not immune to the effects of xenoestrogens, low levels of natural progesterone supplementation can help with depression, relieve prostate problems, and prevent prostate cancer.

In most cases, estrogen supplementation is not called for. The problem is usually related to a lack of progesterone, not estrogen. But in those cases where it is required, make sure your doctor uses either all-natural triple-estrogen in the normal body ratio (approximately 90 percent estriol, 7 percent estradiol, and 3 percent estrone) or a pure estriol cream. As we discussed earlier, this is the exception, not the rule, and most doctors are unaware of the difference.

### Testosterone

Extracts of saw palmetto, wild oats, nettles, and *Tribulus* can safely help increase testosterone levels in the body by releasing the bound testosterone already there and helping to prevent conversion of testosterone to dihydrotestosterone in men. For men, zinc supplementation of approximately 50 mg a day is also advisable to help prevent production of dihydrotestosterone.

### Growth Hormone

Supplementation with a secretagogue, a homeopathic growth hormone formula, or the new sublingual polymer matrix growth hormone makes sense for anyone over thirty-five. All of these are fine to use on a daily basis as they do not suppress the body's own production of GH. You also might want to increase your exercise levels: both aerobic exercise and weight training can significantly boost GH levels in the body.

## DHEA

I do not recommend supplementation with DHEA without constantly monitoring DHEA levels in the blood. Supplementation with 7-Keto DHEA at 25–50 mg a day (up to 200 mg can actually be used to promote weight loss) bypasses virtually all potential problems with DHEA. Also, supplementation with pregnenolone and/or growth hormone will help raise DHEA levels in the body. If you choose to supplement with regular DHEA, 5–25 mg makes sense (up to 50 mg if blood levels are monitored), but do not use it daily, as supplementation may suppress your body's own production of DHEA.

## Pregnenolone

Start with 5 mg a day of pregnenolone and increase by 5 mg a day (to a maximum of 30 mg) until you feel really good. Then try backing it down to the lowest level that still produces that same feeling. Finally, start backing off on the days that you use it until you are using it only two to three times a week (so as not to suppress your body's own production). As you age, you can increase the days and dosage. The final recommended dosage is age dependent: if you're younger than fifty, consider dosages in the range of 10–20 mg two to three times a week; if you're over fifty, the dose should typically be 15–30 mg daily.

## Melatonin

Melatonin in small doses several times a week (so as not to suppress your body's own production) makes sense as a supplementation program. Dosage varies according to what your body needs, ranging from 0.3 mg to 20 mg a day. The correct dosage is the one that helps you sleep but lets you wake up without feeling "drugged." Start with 0.5 mg and increase by 0.5 mg a night until you find what works for you. Note that the effects of supplementation often carry over several nights, so you may need to supplement only every other night or every third night. As you get older, you can increase the amount and frequency of supplementation as needed. Also, consider using black-out curtains in the bedroom and turn off any nightlights in order to get the bedroom as close to total darkness as possible. This will help increase your body's own melatonin production. And when you wake up in the morning, expose yourself to sunlight immediately to cut melatonin production and wake yourself up.

## Precautions

There are several precautions that should be observed when supplementing with hormones.

- Pregnant or nursing mothers should not supplement without guidance from their doctors. Likewise, women trying to conceive would be advised to check with their doctor first.

- Anyone being treated for a pre-existing condition should check with their doctor. This would include conditions such as autoimmune diseases, cancer, and mental illness or depression.

- Anyone on prescription steroids should check with their doctor first.

- Athletes should, of course, be careful as most hormone supplements are considered "performance enhancers."

In fact, it makes sense to check with an antiaging specialist before starting a program of hormone supplementation. Yes, there are now antiaging specialists, but keep in mind that these specialists are still medical doctors and thus prone to the same paradigm blindness that afflicts many doctors.

Now that we've covered the issue of balancing hormones, let's take a look at ways to optimize your immune system.

# CHAPTER 14

# *Optimizing Your Immune System*

- **The Amazing Immune System**
- **How We Build Immunity**
- **Potential Problems with the Immune System**
- **Antibiotics and Antibiotic-Resistant Infections**
- **How to Optimize Your Immune System**

Your immune system plays two vital roles in your body. It responds to foreign organisms by producing antibodies and stimulating specialized cells that destroy those organisms or neutralize their toxic products. In this manner, it defends against foreign invaders: germs, viruses, bacteria, fungi, and parasites. Also, it stands guard over the cells of your body to ensure they are not abnormal or degenerating. Normally, there are anywhere between 100 to 10,000 abnormal cells floating around in our bodies at any point in time—produced as part of the normal metabolic processes.

## THE AMAZING IMMUNE SYSTEM

In many ways, your immune system is the most awesome system in your body, easily rivaling the brain in terms of complexity, subtlety, and "self-awareness." Your immune system is capable of identifying every single cell in your body and recognizing each one as friendly—as belonging to your "self." Conversely, it's also capable of singling out and identifying foreign invaders, ranging from bacteria and viruses to fungi and parasites.

Once it has identified an invader, your immune system then quickly develops a customized defense weapon that specifically targets the invader's weak spot. It then begins building factories that produce these weapons in massive quantities sufficient to totally crush an invader. Then, once the invader has been defeated, the immune system has the awareness to "shut itself down."

As amazing as all of this is, we haven't yet come to the three most amazing aspects of the immune system—the ones that highlight its intelligence. First, once it has defeated an invader, your immune system "remembers" that invader and the defense that was used to defeat it. If that invader ever makes another appearance, even years later, your immune system can launch its defense instantly. In addition, your immune system can identify when a cell in your body has changed, has "gone over to the enemy" as it were. This is a stunning level of sophistication. Out of the trillions of cells in your body, your immune system can tell when a single one has mutated and become cancerous—and, in most cases, move in and destroy it before it can do any harm. In fact, it does this thousands of times a day.

But most amazing of all, your immune system is in total communication with each and every part of itself. "So what's the big deal?" you might ask. "The brain does the same thing." Yes, but remember, the billions of cells of the immune system are not in physical contact with each other. To paraphrase Albert Einstein, at its core, the immune system resembles nothing so much as a great thought.

## Cells of the Immune System

In the following paragraphs, I'm going to summarize the function of the immune system. While a full discussion would take several volumes, I would like to provide a brief overview, a sense of how this marvelous system works.

All blood cells, both red and white, begin as stem cells in your bone marrow. These undifferentiated cells begin to assume individual characteristics and become either red cells (the oxygen carriers) or white cells (the cells of the immune system). Further differentiation divides the white cells (also called leukocytes) into four main types of cells: lymphocytes, phagocytes, granulocytes, and dendritic cells.

### Lymphocytes

Lymphocytes are white blood cells that serve as the key operatives of the immune system. In a healthy body, not under attack, they number about one trillion. There are three main classes of lymphocytes.

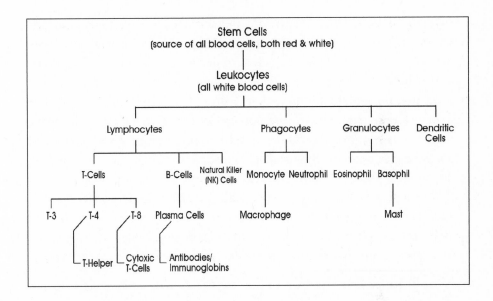

- B-Cells—Each B-cell is programmed to make one specific antibody to defend against a specific invader. An antibody is a soluble protein produced by B-cells that's capable of binding to and destroying or neutralizing a foreign substance (antigen) in the body. Antibodies belong to a particular family of nine proteins called the immunoglobulins. So, one B-cell produces an antibody to defend against a particular strain of flu, whereas an entirely different B-cell produces the antibody for the strep bacteria, and so on. B-cells work primarily in the fluids of the body, defending against "foreign" invaders and toxic molecules. They are not capable of defending against the body's own cells that have "gone bad." Once a B-cell encounters the particular invader that it is built to defend against, it produces many large plasma cells, "factories" that produce millions of specific antibodies and release them into the bloodstream. Once the invader has been eliminated, the B-cells stop production of the plasma cells.

- T-Cells—Although B-cells are capable of recognizing invaders on their own, primarily that function falls to the T-cells. T-cells are smarter than B-cells; they've been to school, as it were. After being produced in the bone marrow, T-cells make their way to the thymus gland, where they are educated in how to distinguish between the cells of the body and invading cells, and how to distinguish between normal healthy cells and mutated rogue cells. T-cells that cannot make this distinction are eliminated so they do not make their way into the body and begin attacking it. Every T-cell carries a marker (T-3), a distinctive molecule on its surface that affects how it behaves.

In addition, some T-cells carry a T-4 marker. These are known as the helper T-cells, which serve the purpose of identifying foreign invaders, then activating B-cells, other T-cells, natural killer (NK) cells, and macrophages to attack the invader. And some T-cells carry a T-8 marker. These are cytotoxic T-cells (also called "suppressor cells"), which identify rogue mutated cells in the body or cells that have been invaded by viruses and compromised. Once they've identified the enemy, cytotoxic T-cells attack the cells that have been infected or are malignant and destroy them. This process is often referred to as the cell-mediated immune response.

• Natural Killer (NK) Cells—Unlike cytotoxic T-cells, NK cells do not need to recognize a specific invader to act. They attack a whole range of microbes and to tumor cells. Also, they kill enemy cells on contact by delivering lethal bursts of potent granular chemicals that "burn" holes in target cells, causing them to leak and burst.

### Phagocytes

Phagocytes are the large white cells that eat and digest invading pathogens, primarily through protease enzyme activity. There are several kinds of phagocytes: monocytes, neutrophils, and macrophages. Macrophages have a number of functions in the immune system. Not only do they attack foreign invaders, they also play a key role as scavengers by "eating up" worn out cells and other waste in the body. Once macrophages have "digested" an invader, they then present the key identifying molecules, or antigens, to the T-cells to initiate the immune response. Macrophages play a key role in fasting. When you are not eating and creating new metabolic waste in the body, macrophages get a chance to get ahead in terms of cleaning up debris. Fasting time becomes "spring cleaning" time for macrophages.

### Granulocytes

Granulocytes include eosiniphils, basophils, neutrophils (neutrophils are classed as both phagocytes and granulocytes), and mast cells. Granulocytes destroy invaders by releasing granules filled with potent chemicals.

### Dendritic Cells

Dendritic cells have long threadlike tentacles that are used to wrap up antigens and expended lymphocytes and carry them to the lymph nodes for removal from the body.

## Organs of the Immune System

We've already discussed two key immune system organs, the bone marrow (which produces the cells of the immune system) and the thymus (which trains the T-cells). Other key organs include the lymph nodes, spleen, tonsils and adenoids, and the appendix. Although you can survive without some of these organs, they are vital and irreplaceable. The spleen, for example, serves as both a staging area for the white cell defenders and as a blood filtration plant for removing worn out blood cells. There is some evidence to indicate that the only organs in the body that can produce a defense against polio are the tonsils and adenoids. As for the appendix, it plays two important roles. First, it is rich in lymphoid cells, which suggests it helps in training immune cells. More significantly, though, recent studies indicate it serves as a haven for useful bacteria when they otherwise might be flushed from the intestinal tract.[1]

## The Complementary Immune System

If the initial lymphocyte (cell-mediated) immune response is overwhelmed, the "complementary immune system" (the complement system) kicks in. This secondary system is comprised of approximately twenty-five proteins and enzymes that activate in a cascading sequence and end with what's called the "membrane attack complex." As its name implies, this complex attacks the cell walls of invaders. A secondary function of the complementary immune system is to help rid the body of CICs (circulating immune complexes). If the overload on the complement system is great enough, severe inflammation of tissue, caused by the activity of albumins, can result, and the body's tissue begins to attack itself. That is, we now have an autoimmune condition.

## How Your Immune System Communicates

We now have a sense of how the immune system works, how it identifies invaders and mounts a response, but how does it communicate with itself? The answer lies in a set of powerful chemical messengers called cytokines, secreted by the cells of the immune system. You've probably heard of several of these cytokines, including interferon and tumor necrosis factor (TNF), but it is the interleukins that swarm through the body like billions of tiny messengers. They activate the B-cells and T-cells, "train" cells and promote the rapid growth of "trained" defenses, shut down defenses when the threat is gone, and control the inflammation response. In short, they provide a remarkable set of intelligent checks and balances on the immune system—guiding it, training it, regulating it, marshaling it as required, and resting it when no longer needed.

## HOW WE BUILD IMMUNITY

Whenever T-cells or B-cells become activated by an invader, some of those cells become memory cells—they encode a "memory" of the particular antigen associated with that invader so the next time they encounter the same antigen, the immune system can respond without delay. There are a number of factors that affect the level of immune response we are capable of mounting. Genetics certainly plays a role, as some individuals are born with stronger immune systems than others. Diet, lifestyle, and environment can also enhance or erode the immune system. In addition, strength of immune response and the duration of immune memory are strongly influenced by the type of antigen and how much of it originally entered the body.

When we are born, we have weak immune systems. Whatever immunity we have is given to us by our mothers. Almost immediately, however, if we are nursing, that immunity begins to grow. The first "milk" we receive from our mothers is, in fact, not actually milk but a substance called colostrum, which is primarily for boosting our immunity. Colostrum is packed with natural immune boosters, such as immunoglobulins, lactoferrin, alkylglycerols, and transfer factor. In addition, nursing helps build the cultures of "friendly bacteria" in the digestive tract, which also support immune function. Children who are put on formula are denied these benefits. Not only are formula-fed children more liable to experience colic, ear infections, and colds, but there is significant evidence that their immune systems never fully "catch up."

### Vaccines

In the wisdom of modern medicine, we have created vaccines to "pre-build memory" for our immune systems—memories of significant diseases we have never had, such as measles, mumps, polio, diphtheria, and smallpox. Vaccines contain a weakened, sterilized version of microorganisms (or proteins from those microorganisms) that is capable of producing an immune response in the body without inducing a full-blown onset of the disease itself. Although vaccines have played a significant role in helping reduce the number of deaths among children, this benefit has not come without cost.

I'm not going to dwell on this issue, because I have a strong emotional attachment to it, which makes it impossible for me to be objective. My youngest brother was one of those "small percentage" of children who responded badly to the series of three immunization shots he received back in the early 1960s. Each time he received one of the shots, he ran a high fever and cried all night, the last time literally screaming for several hours. Each time, my mother called the pediatrician, who reassured her that it was nothing to worry about. As it turns out, the doctor was wrong: my brother, along with thousands of other children, had an allergic reaction to the shots. Each shot caused a small brain hemorrhage, ultimately leaving him severely retarded. Although the manufacturer of the vaccine had indications that this was a possibility, it had not been made clear to the pediatricians who used it. Also, before 1990, doctors were not legally obligated to report adverse reactions to vaccines to the U.S. Centers for Disease Control (CDC); even with the current legal obligation, it's estimated that only 10 percent of doctors report the damage they see to the CDC.

This sort of reaction to a vaccine and this sort of irresponsibility by a pharmaceutical company are not as anomalous as you might think. The polio vaccine given to children in the 1950s and 1960s was not as sterilized as originally thought. In fact, when better test equipment was later used, it was found that there were over 140 live viruses in early versions of the vaccine. One of those viruses, SV40, is strongly implicated in brain cancer. Jonas Salk testified before a U.S. Senate subcommittee that, since 1961, except for a few importations from other countries, all cases of polio were caused by the oral polio vaccine. In fact, there is strong evidence that the original polio epidemic itself in the late 1940s was caused (or at least greatly exacerbated) by another vaccine. The early triple vaccine against diphtheria, whooping cough, and tetanus has been shown beyond doubt to cause paralytic polio in some children. The incidence of polio in children vaccinated with this shot was statistically greater than in unvaccinated children. This scandal broke in Britain during 1949, an epidemic year for polio; other reports soon followed from Australia.

In 1986, the U.S. government quietly set up a National Vaccine Injury Compensation Program to compensate those harmed by vaccines. To date, over $1.5 billion has been paid out. In addition to the "active" constituents, vaccines include substances such as ethylene glycol (antifreeze), formaldehyde (a known carcinogen), aluminum, and thimerosal, a mercury-based preservative.

I'm not saying vaccines should be eliminated, only that we should use a little more discrimination than we are at the moment. Eventually, it's possible that new techniques of genetic engineering, by totally isolating the offending antigen, may be able to offer a safer form of vaccine. But for now, we need to remember that whatever benefit vaccines provide comes at a cost, and we need to decide, on a case-by-case basis, whether or not we wish to pay that cost. It's also worth noting that one of the reasons parents can "safely" opt their children out of vaccinations at the moment is because most children are in fact being vaccinated. That means that the risk of exposure to childhood diseases such as diphtheria and whooping cough is almost nonexistent. If, however, enough children go unvaccinated, the chances of those diseases reappearing at epidemic levels begins to climb exponentially. When it comes to vaccines, it may be a "damned if you do, damned if you don't" situation.

As for adult vaccines, the options are only slightly better. Take the flu vaccine, for example. First, since it has to be produced in advance of the flu season, it is based on last year's flu strains, which makes its effectiveness in any given year less than optimal since it's not designed to work with the current flu strains. Using the most optimistic figures from the CDC, the flu vaccine prevents the flu in about 70 to 90 percent of healthy adults twenty to sixty-five years old. But it's just 30 to 70 percent effective among the elderly, chronically ill, and very young. However, among the most vulnerable, the flu shot is estimated at 50 to 60 percent effective in preventing hospitalization or pneumonia and 80 percent effective in preventing death. But those are the optimistic numbers. Less optimistic numbers place its effectiveness as low as 0 percent. In fact, since 1980, death rates from influenza in the over sixty-five age group have been increasing, at the same time flu vaccination rates have increased from 33 to 65 percent. Flu shots have also been linked to Alzheimer's disease in adults, and the flu drugs Tamiflu and Relenza have been linked to delerium, suicidal events, and convulsions in children.[2]

## POTENTIAL PROBLEMS WITH THE IMMUNE SYSTEM

A number of problems can occur that compromise the immune system.

- The immune system is overwhelmed by too many invaders.

- The immune system becomes weakened and vulnerable to attack.

- The immune system becomes misprogrammed and loses the ability to identify invaders or mutated cells.

- The immune system becomes misprogrammed and begins to mistakenly identify healthy body cells as the enemy and attacks them (autoimmune diseases).

- The immune system is compromised or missing some key component at birth.

Of these problems, the first four are, in most cases, correctable. Only when the body is born without the ability to produce a key component are our options truly limited, but not necessarily hopeless.

## ANTIBIOTICS AND ANTIBIOTIC-RESISTANT INFECTIONS

In a moment, we will discuss how to maximize your immune function, but we first need to explore how modern medicine's approach to dealing with immune system problems has led us to the brink of disaster. Antibiotics are chemical compounds that inhibit the growth of microorganisms such as bacteria, fungi, and protozoa. They are the primary drugs doctors use to support the immune system. Until recently, they were considered one of modern medicine's greatest achievements. Unfortunately, their usefulness is rapidly diminishing, and, as it turns out, they may ultimately be responsible for creating some of mankind's greatest plagues. How did this happen?

Penicillin, the first modern antibiotic, was discovered by Dr. Alexander Fleming in 1928. But just four years after drug companies began mass-producing it in 1943, microbes began appearing that could resist it. Since then, we've seen penicillin-resistant strains of pneumonia, gonorrhea, and hospital-acquired intestinal infections join the list. And it's not just penicillin—bacteria resistant to most of the other antibiotics of choice have also proliferated.

Antibiotic resistance to synthetic drugs is almost impossible to stop since it is the result of the simple rules of evolution. Any population of organisms, bacteria included, naturally includes variants with unusual traits—in this case, the ability to withstand a particular antibiotic's attack. When this antibiotic is used and kills the defenseless bacteria, it leaves behind only those bacteria that can resist it. These renegade variants then multiply, increasing their numbers a millionfold in a single day, instantly becoming the dominant variant. In other words, the very act of using an antibiotic creates the opportunity for resistant strains to flourish.

It's important to understand that antibiotics vary in the way they kill microbes. Penicillin, for example, kills bacteria by attaching to their cell walls and then breeching those walls, thus killing the bacteria. Erythromycin, tetracycline, and streptomycin, on the other hand, kill bacteria by attacking the structures inside the bacteria (ribosomes) that allow them to make proteins, thus also destroying the bacteria. Because each antibiotic is a single compound and one-dimensional in its approach, it's not that hard for microbes to "evolve" around such attacks. For example, microbes resistant to penicillin have developed cell walls that prevent the penicillin from binding. Similarly, other variants prevent antibiotics from binding to ribosomes, thus neutralizing the effect of those antibiotics.

Where it gets really frightening, though, is that bacteria swap genes like politicians swap favors—which brings us to vancomycin, the antibiotic of last resort. When all other antibiotics failed, doctors knew they could count on vancomycin. But then vancomycin resistance was discovered in a common hospital microbe, enterococcus. By 1991, thirty-eight hospitals in the United States reported the variant. Just one year later, vancomycin-resistant staph bacteria were observed with the same gene. What this means is that not only are bacteria programmed to "evolve" defenses against antibiotics, but once they produce such a defense, they are also programmed to rapidly share that defense with other strains of bacteria, thus rapidly spreading the resistance.

## What Can Be Done?

It was briefly thought that alternating the most commonly used antibiotics might stop the spread of antibiotic resistance. But a new model shows that this practice of cycling, alternating between two or more classes of antibiotics as often as every few months, probably will not work. The latest theory is that mixing cocktails of antibiotics may help. And, in fact, this is closer to the way natural substances avoid the resistance problem, but it cannot match the sophistication displayed by those same natural substances.

When you think about how quickly pathogens evolve around antibiotics, it's more than amazing that they have been unable to do so against most natural antipathogens, such as garlic, olive leaf extract, and oil of oregano, even given tens of thousands of years to do so. What is their secret? Actually, it's quite simple—or more accurately, quite complex. While drugs are essentially one-dimensional, which allows microbes an easier way around them, natural antipathogens often contain dozens of biochemicals. Not all of them are "active," of course, but many of the so-called inactive components potentiate the active ones and offer therapeutic combinations numbering in the thousands. This presents a complexity that makes it virtually impossible for microbes to work around.

Take garlic, for example. For a long time, many people thought there was only one active component in garlic, allicin (in fact, many supplement companies still promote that concept). However, researchers now know that allicin is rapidly oxidized, breaking down into more than 100 biologically active, sulfur-containing compounds. (While allicin still serves as a marker of garlic's potency, S-allylcysteine and other compounds are the most therapeutically active ingredients.) How many possible therapeutic combinations can you get from garlic's 100 biologically active compounds? Thousands and thousands—the complexity is far more than simple pathogens can evolve around. And that's the secret: when you combine several natural substances in one formula, the combinations of compounds are beyond counting, and microbes are defenseless.

The widespread use (and misuse) of pharmaceutical antibiotics has led us to a world filled with growing numbers of drug-resistant "superbugs," all capable of unleashing a devastating worldwide plague at any time. At the moment, natural antipathogens offer the only viable first line of defense. But for those antipathogens to be truly effective, we also need to optimize our own internal defenses.

## HOW TO OPTIMIZE YOUR IMMUNE SYSTEM

Since the purpose of the body's immune system is to defend against attack and help initiate repair, the better it does its job, the healthier we are. To facilitate this process, we need to address the two key areas of immune function we've already identified:

1. Improve overall immune function to allow the body to better defend itself.

2. Specifically target (kill/destroy) invading bacteria, viruses, microorganisms, and other related pathogens to help take some of the load off the immune system.

Scientists have known for years that it is possible to improve the functioning of the immune system. The conventional medical approach has been to use expensive, proprietary drugs, including concentrated cytokines such as interleukin and interferon. The world's miracle doctors, on the other hand, have adopted a more holistic approach using natural substances to:

- Stimulate and strengthen your immune system

- Fight infection

- Strengthen tissue against assault by invading microorganisms

- Stimulate macrophage capability

- Increase T-cell production and protect helper T-cells

- Complement the action of interferon and interleukin-1

- Assist the cell-mediated immune response

## Immune Boosters

Not only are natural immune boosters safer than the drug-based approach (having fewer side effects), they are also far more powerful than their pharmaceutical counterparts. Let's take a look at some of the more powerful immune boosters available.

### Echinacea

Echinacea (purple coneflower) is truly a miracle herb. It was "discovered" in the late 1800s by a traveling salesman named Joseph Meyer, who learned about it from the Plains Indians while traveling out West. He brewed it up as an alcohol tincture and sold it as a cure-all—demonstrating its effectiveness by letting rattlesnakes bite him and then drinking his tonic. Needless to say, he never got sick, from whence comes the phrase "snake oil."

How does echinacea work? First, it contains echinacoside, a natural antibiotic comparable to penicillin in effect, which can kill a broad range of viruses, bacteria, fungi, and protozoa. This makes it invaluable in wound healing and in the treatment of infectious diseases. Research has also reported echinacea's efficacy in treating colds, flu, bronchitis, and tuberculosis. Echinacea also contains echinacein, a biochemical that protects against germ attack by neutralizing the tissue-dissolving enzyme hyaluronidase, produced by many germs. Among the many pharmacological properties reported for echinacea, macrophage activation has been demonstrated most convincingly.[3] One study showed that echinacea extracts can boost T-cell production by up to 30 percent more than immune-boosting drugs.[4]

There are two primary varieties of echinacea: *Echinacea purpurea* and *E. angustifolia*. They are similar, but also have complementary properties. Formulas that use both are more likely to be effective. It's also worth noting that potency runs from seed (greatest potency) to root to leaf to almost none in the flower. And, of course, herb quality is paramount.

Over the last few years, there have been several studies that claimed to debunk echinacea's ability to boost the immune system and fight colds. Suffice it to say that the studies were either flawed in design (reviews of previously flawed studies), used the wrong parts of the echinacea plant (flowers and leaves rather than roots and seeds), or used it at the wrong strength. Forget the studies—echinacea still stands as one of the best immune boosters available.

## Pau d'arco

Pau d'arco (*Tabebuia avellanedae, impetignosa, and heptaphylla*) is a tree that comes from the rain forests of Brazil and other areas of South America. It is the inner bark of the tree that provides the medicinal function.

This amazing herb nourishes the body's defense system and helps protect against pathogenic organisms. It has been used for centuries to improve immune function, detoxify, and reduce pain throughout the body, especially in the joints. Research has shown that it contains a natural antibacterial agent, has a healing effect on the entire body, cleanses the blood, and kills viruses. Pau d'arco has been used as a treatment for AIDS, allergies, infections and inflammations, anemia, asthma, arthritis and rheumatism, arteriosclerosis, bronchitis, cancer, candidiasis, colitis, cystitis, diabetes, eczema, fistulas, gastritis, gonorrhea, hemorrhages, Hodgkin's disease, liver disease, leukemia, lupus, multiple sclerosis, osteomyelitis, Parkinson's disease, prostatitis, psoriasis, skin sores, snake bites, ulcers, varicose veins, warts, and wounds.

## Suma

Natives of the Amazon jungle have used suma root (*Pfaffia paniculata*) for at least the last 300 years. It wasn't until 1975, however, that Suma was tested at the University of São Paulo, Brazil. The studies concluded that although it was not a cure, suma nevertheless brought significant relief for cancer, diabetes, and gout sufferers, with no undesirable side effects. Since then, studies at the American College of the Healing Arts have indicated that consistent use of suma may help combat fatigue (including treatment of chronic fatigue and low-energy conditions), prevent colds and flu, speed healing, regulate blood sugar, and stimulate the sex drive.

The key working ingredients in suma are pfaffic acid (prevents the spread of various cell disorders), pfaffocides and other saponins (help stop diseases already in progress), plant hormones sitosterol and stigmasterol (prevent cholesterol absorption and improve blood circulation), alantoin (helps accelerate healing), and germanium. Suma has one of the highest concentrations of germanium sesquioxide (Ge-132) of any plant known. Discovered about thirty years ago, Ge-132 can apparently invigorate the body, restore sexual function, protect against miscarriages, heal burns, reduce pain, treat circulatory disorders, and shrink cancers.

## Medicinal Mushrooms

Many of the compounds found in reishi, maitake, and cordyceps mushrooms are classified as host defense potentiators: it is believed that combinations of these compounds target and strengthen the human immune system, as well as aid in neuron transmission, metabolism, hormonal balance, and the transport of nutrients and oxygen. Through a host-mediated (T-cell) immune mechanism, they help the body regulate the development of lymphoid stem cells and other important defense responses.

- Reishi (*Ganoderma lucidum* or *lingzhi*)—The anti-cancer and immune-enhancing effects of the reishi mushroom are thought to be largely due to its mucopolysaccharides, which the body incorporates into cellular membranes, making them resistant to viruses and pathogenic bacteria. The polysaccharides appear to activate macrophages, the white blood cells that "consume" viruses, bacteria, and other large particulate matter.

- Maitake (*Grifola frondosa*, also known as sheep's head and hen of the woods)—Maitake mushrooms have a very high concentration of a unique polysaccharide compound called beta-1,6-glucan, which researchers consider to be one of the most powerful immune stimulants and adaptogens known. One study showed that maitake produced a 64 percent inhibition of breast cancer and tumor activity and a 75 percent inhibition of skin cancer and tumor activity.[5] Also, laboratory studies conducted at the U.S. National Cancer Institute (NCI) and the Japanese National Institute of Health showed that maitake extract kills the human immunodeficiency virus (HIV) and enhances the activity of helper T-cells.[6] In fact, the NCI researchers reported that the maitake extract was as powerful as AZT (a commonly prescribed AIDS drug) but without the toxic side effects.

Research has demonstrated that maitake stimulates the production of a variety of immune cells, including macrophages, NK cells, and T-cells, and it increases their effectiveness by increasing the production of interleukin-l, interleukin-2, and lymphokines. Further, maitake has been confirmed to have a multifaceted benefit for treating cancer and tumors: it protects healthy cells from becoming cancerous, helps prevent the spread of cancer (metastasis), and slows or stops the growth of tumors. Maitake works in conjunction with chemotherapy by lessening the negative side effects (by as much as 90 percent).

- *Cordyceps*—*Cordyceps* has properties similar to those of ginseng and has been used to strengthen and rebuild the body after exhaustion or long-term illness. It is one of the most valued medicinal fungi in Chinese medicine. It has also been used traditionally for impotence, neurasthenia, and backache. Recent research with extracts of *Cordyceps* has yielded a protein-bound polysaccharide with activity against tumors, as well as immunological enhancement. Cordyceps is widely employed to treat upper respiratory problems, impotence, and weakened immune systems, and also by athletes to increase endurance.

- AHCC (Active Hexose Correlated Compound)—AHCC is a proprietary dietary supplement rich in polysaccharides and fiber derived from mushrooms. Studies have shown that it can be effective in stimulating the production of NK cells, killer T-cells, and cytokines (interferon, interleukin-12, and TNF-alpha). In Japan, it is used extensively in hospitals in combination with chemotherapy treatments to reduce the adverse side effects of those treatments.

## Astragalus

*Astragalus membranaceus* has been a foundational herb in traditional Chinese medicine for hundreds of years. It is one of the important "*Qi* tonifying" adaptogenic herbs from the Chinese materia medica. Current research on astragalus focuses on the immune-stimulating capacity of its polysaccharides. It also appears to be useful in dealing with cancer and in increasing stamina. First and foremost, though, it is an immunostimulant used in the treatment of chronic viral infections, hepatitis, edema, common cold, and flu. Astragalus increases the interferon response to viral infection and works synergistically with interferon. It also increases phagocytic activity and antibody levels and improves the functioning of natural killer cells.

## Aloe vera

The polysaccharide component of aloe vera, acemannan, possesses significant immune-enhancing and antiviral activity. Supplementing with acemannan has been proven to increase lymphocyte response to antigens by enhancing the release of interleukin-1. In addition, acemannan has been shown to increase macrophage levels and have a positive effect on T-cell activity. Look for whole-leaf aloe extract, which is two to three times more potent than the gel/juice. Why? The greatest concentration of active ingredients is at the interface of the rind and the inner gel. If your extract doesn't come from the whole leaf, you lose large amounts of the active biochemicals.

## Alkylglycerols

Alkylglycerols (AKGs) are lipids naturally manufactured in the body and found in mother's milk, the liver and spleen, and bone marrow. They play a major role in the production and stimulation of white blood cells. They also help to normalize bone marrow function. The immune-supportive effect of AKGs helps our bodies protect against bacterial, fungal, and viral infections. The most potent supplemental source of AKGs in the world is shark liver oil.

## Colostrum and Lactoferrin

Colostrum is the clear, yellowish, pre-milk fluid produced from the mother's mammary glands during the first seventy-two hours after birth. It provides both immune and growth factors essential for the health and vitality of the newborn. Obviously, supplementation with human colostrum is not an option, but researchers have found that bovine colostrum is virtually identical, except that the immune factors are actually several times more concentrated.

The immune factors in colostrum have been shown to help the body resist pathogens such as viruses, bacteria, yeast, and fungi. In addition, colostrum contains a number of antibodies to specific pathogens, including *E. coli*, salmonella, rotavirus, *Candida*, streptococcus, staphylococcus, *H. pylori*, and cryptosporidia. Proline-rich-polypeptide, a component of colostrum, works as an immunomodulator, boosting a low immune system and balancing an overactive immune system. Another key group of components of colostrum are the transfer factors, small molecules that transfer immunity information from one entity to another. In effect, they transfer immunity "memory," thereby giving you instant resistance to a number of diseases.

Colostrum is also a potent source of lactoferrin, a globular protein produced in the body. It is found anywhere that is especially vulnerable to attack, such as in the gut, eyes, ears, nose, throat, and urinary tract. Lactoferrin has been shown to inhibit virus replication (including AIDS and herpes viruses), limit tumor growth and metastasis, directly kill both bacteria and yeast (including *Candida*), and activate neutrophils. Supplementation with lactoferrin can significantly boost the immune system and help the body recover from any existing infection. Maintaining healthy levels of intestinal flora through the use of probiotic supplements allows the body to produce its own lactoferrin.

## Glutathione

Glutathione is a tripeptide molecule found in human cells. In addition to being a powerful antioxidant, glutathione works to support the active functioning of the immune system and is a key component of all lymphocytes. In fact, all lymphocytes require sufficient levels of intracellular glutathione to function properly. It also plays a major protective role against the damaging effects of the whole range of pathogens and carcinogens. For many people, glutathione supplements are upsetting to the stomach. Alternatives include the glutathione precursors L-cysteine and L-glutamate and specially formulated whey products.

## Mangosteen

Mangosteen (*Garcinia mangostana*) is a tropical evergreen tree whose fruit contains a unique group of antioxidants called xanthones. Xanthones, particularly beta and gamma mangostin, work to maintain the immune system, support cardiovascular health, optimize joint flexibility, are naturally antibiotic, antiviral, and anti-inflammatory, and are some of the most powerful antioxidants found in nature. In addition, recent studies have confirmed that gamma mangostin is a potent COX inhibitor, an important factor in reducing inflammation, pain, and fever. Now, while it is true that the immune-boosting abilities of mangosteen have not yet been proven in human studies, the number of in vitro studies (backed by significant anecdotal evidence) supports its listing here.

### Beta-glucan

Beta-glucan is a natural complex carbohydrate (polysaccharide) found in cereal grains such as oats and barley. However, it is found in its greatest concentration primarily in the cell walls of yeast and in medicinal mushrooms. Beta-glucan as a supplement, however, particularly beta-1,3/1,6-glucan extracted from yeast cell wall, is a potent and proven immune response potentiator and modulator—stimulating antitumor and antimicrobial activity by binding to receptors on macrophages and other white blood cells and activating them.

### Perilla frutescens

*Perilla frutescens* (also known as shiso and beefsteak plant) is a member of the mint family and native to southeast Asia. Perilla extract can help restore healthy helper T-cell function, thereby enhancing your body's immune system and minimizing the possibility of autoimmune disorders. The essential oil is extracted from the perilla leaves by steam distillation, and it is available as either a bottled oil, with a taste resembling dark sesame oil, or in capsules. It provides omega-3 fatty acids with none of the digestive problems of flax or fish oils. Beyond that, however, perilla is traditionally used in Chinese medicine and has been shown to stimulate interferon activity and, thus, the body's immune system.

## Pathogen Destroyers

Pathogen destroyers represent an alternative, complementary route to assisting your immune system. They don't build immune function as the immune boosters do. Instead, they "free up" immune function by directly destroying pathogens in the body that would otherwise occupy the attention of your immune system. They function as natural antibiotics and antivirals.

## Olive Leaf Extract

The olive tree (*Olea europaea*) is native to the Mediterranean region. Olive leaf extract has a long history of use against illnesses in which microorganisms play a major role. In more recent years, studies of olive leaf extract (containing oleuropein, calcium elenolate, and/or hydroxytyrosol) have shown that it is effective in eliminating a broad range of organisms, including bacteria, viruses, parasites, and yeast/mold/fungi.[7]

## Oil of Wild Mountain Oregano

Oregano (*Origanum vulgare*) is a perennial herb native to Europe, the Mediterranean, and central Asia. Oil of wild mountain oregano is antiviral, antibacterial, antifungal, and antiparasitic. It also has strong antioxidant and anti-inflammatory effects. The key components, isomeric phenols, in dilutions as low as 1 to 50,000, destroy a wide range of pathogens, including *Candida albicans*, aspergillus mold, staphylococcus, *Campylobacter*, klebsiella, *E. coli*, giardia, pseudomonas, and proteus. Another phenol constituent of oregano, thymol, helps boost the immune system.

## Grapefruit Seed Extract

Grapefruit seed extract is a broad-spectrum antipathogen. Internally, grapefruit seed extract can help with gastrointestinal disorders, diarrhea, food poisoning, parasites (single and multi-celled), *Candida* infections, oral infections, colds and flu, sore throats, and sinusitis. Externally, grapefruit seed extract is used for many skin conditions as well: acne, athlete's foot, cold sores, warts, cuts, wounds and infections, rashes, dandruff, nail fungus, and chickenpox. Physicians have observed that the herpes simplex virus becomes inactive just ten minutes after the application of grapefruit seed extract.

There are dozens of studies published over the last thirty years supporting grapefruit seed extract's antipathogenic properties. For example, a study by the U.S. Department of Agriculture found it effective against three animal viruses (foot and mouth disease, African swine disease, and swine vesicular disease).[8] Other studies have proven its effectiveness against *E. coli*, salmonella, and *Staphylococcus aureus*. In fact, it is used in a number of hospitals around the world for its antimicrobial properties, to sterilize hospital laundry and carpets and, in higher concentrations, to disinfect operating rooms.

There are several articles on the Internet indicating problems with grapefruit seed extract—primarily that it doesn't work, it's not natural, and that it contains highly toxic synthetic compounds produced in manufacturing. None of these concerns hold up under examination, but the main complaint is that all its benefits come from added preservatives. This is based on a single study out of an obscure university in Germany. In fact, the results of this study are countermanded by dozens of other studies published over the last thirty years proving the exact opposite—that grapefruit seed extract does indeed have strong antipathogenic properties.

### Habanero and Horseradish

Habanero (*Capsicum chinense* Jacquin) and horseradish (*Armoracia rusticana*) are stimulants that quicken and excite the body. They energize the body, stimulating its defenses against invading viruses, and help carry blood to all parts of the body. They are also diaphoretics and thus help raise the temperature of the body, which increases the activity of the body's immune system.

Horseradish, in particular, contains volatile oils that are similar to those found in mustard: glucosinolates (mustard oil glycosides), gluconasturtiin, and sinigrin. In test tubes, the volatile oils in horseradish have shown antibiotic properties, which may account for its effectiveness in treating throat and upper respiratory tract infections. At levels attainable in human urine after taking the volatile oil of horseradish, the oil has been shown to kill bacteria that can cause urinary tract infections; one early trial found that horseradish extract may be a useful treatment for people with urinary tract infections.[9]

### Liquid Zinc

Like colloidal silver, liquid ionic zinc is antibacterial and antiviral, but without the potential toxicity issues found with silver. The mineral zinc is found in all body fluids, including the moisture in the eyes, lungs, nose, urine, and saliva. Proper zinc levels offer a defense against the entrance of pathogens. In the 1800s, surgeons used zinc as an antiseptic/antibiotic after surgery, and they noted its amazing healing properties: wounds would heal, at times, as quickly as twenty-four hours after an operation, without swelling, and scarring was barely noticeable after a short period of time. Because zinc moves through all the fluids in the body, it creates a defense against infection-causing bacteria and viruses trying to enter the body and stops bacterial and viral replication. In other words, to be effective it must be in a liquid form. If you take zinc tablets, your body must convert it; if you take it in a liquid form, it's already in the form that your body needs.

## Garlic and Onions

Although the previous pathogen destroyers are extremely potent, garlic (*Allium sativum*) is my favorite—for the simple reason that it is the "kindest" to the beneficial bacteria in the intestinal tract. In addition, garlic is one of the best infection fighters available for both bacterial and viral infections. Garlic also possesses the ability to stimulate the activity of macrophages to engulf foreign organisms, such as viruses, bacteria, and yeast. Furthermore, garlic increases the activity of the helper T-cells. Garlic may be particularly effective in treating upper respiratory viral infections, due to its immune-enhancing properties and its ability to clear mucus from the lungs. It is also effective against streptococcus and staphylococcus bacteria.

Everything that's been said about garlic goes for onions too. Onions and garlic share many of the same powerful sulfur-bearing compounds that work so effectively as antiviral and antibacterial agents.

## Colloidal Silver

Colloidal silver is a suspension of submicroscopic metallic silver particles in a colloidal base. Although colloidal silver can be an effective antipathogen, I have several concerns. Concentrations can vary wildly in supplemental forms, and in many products, the silver particles are too big and not a true colloidal suspension, meaning that, over time, they drop out of suspension and the concentration in the liquid lessens. When it is at sufficient strength to be effective, colloidal silver is indiscriminate—that is, it kills the good intestinal bacteria as well the bad. And it can, if taken in sufficient quantity, cause argyra, an irreversible blue/gray discoloration of the skin. (Although rare as the result of using colloidal silver, it has nevertheless been documented.)

My bottom line recommendation (and I know this will anger many colloidal silver advocates) is to restrict colloidal silver to external use except for special occasions. In other words, do not use it on a daily basis and be sure to follow any internal use with a good probiotic supplement.

## Immunomodulators

Immunomodulators are nutraceuticals that can regulate your immune system, boosting a weak system or calming down an overactive system. If a person with low immune function takes an immunomodulator, it will help raise that immunity. Likewise, if a person with a hyperactive immune system takes an immunomodulator, it will tend to calm down their immune system and normalize it. It appears that they accomplish this, to some degree, by naturally increasing the body's production of messenger molecules to regulate the immune system. By using immunomodulators such as L-carnosine, cetyl myristoleate (CMO), and colostrum, you can retrain the immune system to respond more efficiently and to not overreact (as happens in the case of people with autoimmune disorders).

---

## NEW SCOURGES: BIRD FLU, MRSA, AND EXTREME DRUG-RESISTANT TUBERCULOSIS

### Bird Flu

In August 2005, I published a newsletter focused on avian (bird) flu. I indicated that although the threat was not particularly imminent, the press would turn it into a major story. They did. I also stated that, despite the press, there was nothing indicating a bird flu pandemic was more likely in the next couple of years than it was over the last ninety, when we saw the last such pandemic. It's been over two years, and it hasn't happened yet.

That said, the threat is real, and at some point, we will have a major pandemic. When it happens, there are several things you should know. Don't count on having access to a reliable vaccine because no vaccine has proven effective at stopping the current strain of avian flu, let alone the eventual mutation that will truly threaten humans. Yes, it will be a related strain, but as experience has shown, when it comes to flu vaccines, "related" is not close enough. If you don't have a vaccine for the actual strain causing the pandemic, the odds are not good that a "related" vaccine will help. Also, don't count on relief from antivirals such as Relenza and Tamiflu—neither has shown much benefit in helping those infected with avian flu. Even normal flu viruses are adapting to them, and they are becoming less effective by the month.

Which leaves you with the solution proposed by most alternative health experts: build up your immune system to fight off the virus. But that's a questionable tactic with bird flu. In fact, it may amount to a death sentence for most people, at least if not accompanied by the use of pathogen destroyers. It's essential that you understand that death from bird flu is most likely to come from a cytokine storm triggered by your own immune system, not from the flu itself. This is the same situation we saw in the great influenza pandemic of 1918. Over-reaction by immune systems played a primary role in the high death rate in the 1918 Spanish flu pandemic, and it is playing a similar role in human cases of bird flu today.[10]

What this means is that, along with using immune boosters, you absolutely must use pathogen destroyers to reduce the viral load and eliminate the chances of a cytokine storm. If you do that, you've effectively turned the bird flu into a regular flu, easily handled by a good immune system.

## MRSA

*Staphylococcus aureus* (*S. aureus* or staph) is a type of bacteria commonly carried on the skin and in the noses of healthy people without causing infection. This is known as bacterial colonization. However, when *S. aureus* organisms invade the body, they can cause serious infections. Most staph infections can be treated easily with antibiotics, while others are resistant to antibiotics such as methicillin (methicillin-resistant *S. aureus* or MRSA). *S. aureus* survived as a relatively undistinguished microbe until the mid-twentieth century. The introduction of the first antibiotic, penicillin, in 1941 set the bacterium on its path of deadly mutation. It took just two years for the first reports of the bacterium's newfound resistance to start trickling in.

In the early 1960s, doctors deployed a new antibiotic, methicillin, against the disease. The first signs of resistance to methicillin appeared in less than a year. MRSA quickly became ingrained in hospitals in Europe, Australia, and the United States. By the early 1990s, MRSA infections had become the leading cause of hospital-acquired skin infections in the U.S. Recent studies have shown that this kind of staph bacterium has also colonized hospitals in Egypt, Taiwan, and South America.

For decades, antibiotic-resistant staph infections were found only in hospitals, where the constant use of different antibiotics, including methicillin, made the bacteria resistant to many of the most powerful antibiotics. In the last few years, however, MRSA has popped up in health clubs, high school gyms, sex clubs, jails, and schools—just about anywhere bacteria can grow. It has affected everyone from athletes to school children to newborn babies. It has become a growing problem that is largely unknown by the general population. Researchers at Olive View–UCLA Medical Center in Sylmar, California, analyzed skin infections that showed up in their emergency room, and the results were nothing short of alarming: in 2002, MRSA caused 29 percent of those infections, but just two years later, the rate was 64 percent. A national health study (the 2001–2002 National Health and Nutrition Examination Survey) estimated that as many as 2 million people in the U.S. alone may be infected with methicillin-resistant staph infections. And in its most severe form, MRSA can turn into a fatal flesh-destroying scourge.

Again, as with bird flu, along with using immune boosters, you need to use pathogen destroyers—in this case, to destroy the bacteria that one-dimensional antibiotics cannot reach.

### XDR-TB

As serious as MRSA may be, it's probably not the most immediate threat we face. That honor probably belongs to extreme drug-resistant tuberculosis. Although it's been around for a few years, in just the last year XDR-TB has begun to make its presence known in virtually every country in the world. If you thought bird flu was deadly, XDR-TB is virtually 100 percent fatal. As its name indicates, no known drugs are effective against it. On the other hand, natural remedies such as garlic, olive leaf extract, oil of wild mountain oregano, and grapefruit seed extract are likely to be beneficial. So, as with bird flu and MRSA, it makes sense to stock up with natural pathogen destroyers and immune builders to protect against any and all mutations. Since no known drugs can help, you have nothing to lose.

## GENERAL RECOMMENDATIONS

Too many people think of the immune system as something existing in isolation. That's a huge mistake. As we noted in Chapter 2, your body is composed of a series of integrated systems and, as such, is the sum of those systems—and it is only as strong as the weakest of them. Let's take a quick walk through the Baseline of Health Program and see how each system impacts the immune system.

- How good can your immune system be (even taking all the supplements you want) if your colon is packed with pounds of old fecal matter? A substantial portion of your immune system then has to combat the effects of self-toxicity. Clean up your intestinal tract and you free up your immune system.

- Beneficial bacteria in the gut (if they're present) manufacture potent immune boosters, such as transfer factor and lactoferrin, right in your intestinal tract. If you use a good probiotic supplement, you substantially boost your immune system by increasing internal production of powerful immune factors.

- Supplementing with digestive enzymes significantly reduces the incidence of circulating immune complexes (CICs), thus taking enormous stress off the complementary immune system and reducing the chances of autoimmune disorders.

- Proper diet and nourishment boost your immune system. Each immune cell in your body is manufactured from the food you eat, so a nutritionally deficient diet means functionally deficient immune cells. A good vitamin/mineral supplement enhances the production of your body's immune cells.

- A full-spectrum antioxidant boosts the immune system in multiple ways. Just one example is the spice curcumin: it can increase white blood cell count by 50 percent in just twelve days.[11]

- Every tenth of a point that your blood and/or tissue pH falls below its optimum dramatically impacts both your primary immune system and the complement system. Low pH and disease, including cancer, go hand in hand.

- Cleaning out the liver with an effective flush and rebuilding program improves its ability to produce immune factors and remove bacteria from the blood. Cleaning out the blood with an herbal blood cleanser and balancing your blood's pH also helps to improve immune function.

- Daily use of supplement formulations comprised of the herbs and nutraceuticals discussed in this chapter can significantly enhance the immune system across the board.

- Make sure you have several pathogen destroyers on hand for use at the

first sign of oncoming illness. It is much easier to stop a viral or bacterial infection during the incubation stage (when you are experiencing the
first symptoms) than if you wait until it's full blown.

- Remember to use the immunomodulators L-carnosine, *Cetyl myristoleate*,
  and colostrum.

- Keep in mind that the primary entry point for most pathogens is via your
  eyes, nose, and mouth through contact with your hands. Your hands pick
  up potential threats by virtue of contact with other people (shaking hands,
  for example) and with objects (touching doorknobs and telephones). Regular washing of the hands throughout the day, with regular soap and water,
  can take a considerable amount of stress off the immune system. Avoid
  antibacterial soaps, which merely serve to foster the growth of "super"
  bacteria and viruses.

- One of the primary benefits of regular exercise is an optimized immune
  system. However, overly strenuous exercise actually has the reverse effect,
  so don't overdo it. High-performance athletes often have trashed immune
  systems and require a constant intake of antibiotics to avoid getting sick.

As you can see, virtually every system in the body impacts the immune system. You truly are only as strong as your weakest link. The Baseline of Health
Program is designed to enhance the immune system at every level and in
every system in the body.

In this chapter, we covered the basic aspects of the immune system. In the
next chapter, we will explore ways to optimize your energy levels.

# CHAPTER 15

# It's All About Energy

- **Healing Energy**
- **Direct Application**
- **Reflected Energy**
- **Antennas**
- **The Laying On of Hands**
- **Embedding Energy**
- **Energizing Water**

All life is energy. Every nerve impulse in your body is an electric current, your muscles are powered by chemical energy, and every cell in your body is a mini-battery pumping out 70–90 millivolts, when healthy. The steak and potatoes you eat for dinner are really just fuel for the fire, like throwing coal in a furnace. Digestion is a slow form of burning that produces energy for your body to live on. In fact, death itself is defined as the absence of electrical activity in the brain.

## HEALING ENERGY

Optimize that energy and you optimize your health. Energy is neither good nor bad; it just is. The same electricity that is used by a chiropractor or a physical therapist to stimulate your muscles and promote healing with a TENS (transcutaneous electrical nerve stimulation) machine is the same electricity used in prisons to execute people in electric chairs. So, is electricity good or bad? Again, the answer is neither—it's just a question of what frequency and amplitude you use and how you use it.

If you charge your body with the right frequencies, you can prevent disease.

For the most part, other forms of energy are no different than electricity. The same laser light that is used by the Department of Defense as a weapon is also used by an eye doctor to improve your vision via Lasik surgery or a plastic surgeon to remove facial hair and wrinkles. Again, the difference is merely one of frequency and amplitude. The proper use of energy in the healing arts has a long and significant history, from the TENS machines and laser surgery to the use of sound waves to break up kidney stones, from x-rays and magnetic fields to see into the body to the use of light to clean the blood. That said, some forms of energy and some delivery systems are more effective than others.

The use of healing energy merely involves pairing the right frequency and amplitude with the right delivery system. There are essentially five different ways that you can apply healing energy to the body:

- Direct application of energy to the body, such as with a TENS machine or a scalar chamber.

- Using specially designed materials to selectively concentrate and reflect back healing frequencies generated by the body itself.

- Wearing or using a device that functions as an antenna and draws selected healing frequencies out of the "ether."

- The laying on of hands.

- Embedding energy in a supplement, pendant, patch, etc.

## DIRECT APPLICATION

This is the easiest method to understand and potentially the most powerful. The TENS machine, which uses electric current to stimulate and relax muscles directly and a magnetic field to improve blood flow and block pain, is an example familiar to many people.

Another far more controversial example is the Rife Machine and its descendents. Back in the 1920s, Royal Rife (1888–1971) found that by applying select frequencies to the human body he could destroy most viruses, bacteria, and even aberrant cells. The key to making this work was a microscope of his own invention that allowed him to identify the exact frequency that worked on each particular problem. That was the key—the frequencies were very specific.

He achieved spectacular results, so much so that on November 20, 1931, forty-four of the nation's most respected medical authorities honored Rife with a banquet billed as "The End to All Diseases." He was subsequently attacked by the government authorities, discredited in the press, and his laboratory sabotaged and burned. Today, updated versions of his machines are available that attempt to work around the fact that we no longer have Rife's ability to identify for each individual the exact frequency needed. This is usually done by having the device cycle through a number of frequencies, the idea being that one will be the frequency needed to destroy your particular problem. Do these devices work? Some do (or have) very well. The problem is that the ones that work the best tend to attract the attention of government and medical authorities when word of mouth stories of cancer cures begin to spread, which, of course, gets the companies shut down. Do these machines cure cancer? Not really, but the best of them can throw a cancer into remission. And as long as you keep using the device, they keep the cancer in check, for a time. However, if you don't take care of the underlying health issues responsible for the cancer, it will tend to come back at some point and no longer respond to the machine.

Another device is the scalar-generating watch used to block unhealthy artificial electromagnetic fields (EMFs). It works by using a special chip that generates an 8-hertz standing wave that helps reinforce your body's own bioelectric field, protecting it from damage caused by disruptive EMFs, such as the alternating current powering homes and offices or the frequencies generated by your cell phone. These watches work, and you can verify improvements in the immune system while wearing the watch. The problem is that they are restricted to one healing frequency (at least as they are now manufactured), whereas there are actually a number of healing frequencies, each helping the body in a different way.

Yet another device is the far-infrared blanket, which is woven of fabrics that incorporate ultra-small far-infrared radiating ceramic crystals (actually, crystal "dust"), such as tourmaline and serpentine, in their weave. These crystals, energized by heat from the body, emit far-infrared light. Far infrared is just beyond red on the light spectrum, and although it cannot be seen by the human eye, it has the ability to penetrate skin and warm the flesh and organs underneath. In doing so, it promotes better circulation and accelerated detoxification. An even more powerful version is the far-infrared sauna, which I highly recommend.

Probably the strongest and most effective way (but not the most convenient or least expensive) is to find a health practitioner who has a scalar energy chamber that you can use for thirty minutes or longer, once or more a week, for a direct high-intensity application of healing energy. Not only do these chambers provide greater intensity, but most allow for adjusting frequencies for different healing effects.

## REFLECTED ENERGY

One of the more interesting delivery systems is seen in a number of "energy" pendants. The principle is simple: at all times, your body is generating a complete spectrum of energies and frequencies, from the very beneficial to the not so beneficial. What the reflecting devices do is selectively block a pre-chosen beneficial frequency from escaping your body, focus and concentrate it, then feed it back into the body. Does this work? Several years ago, I was given a metal pendant that I wore on a chain over my chest. Within three days, I found that my lungs were irritated under the pendant and that I was coughing constantly. I took it off and put it away, and the condition cleared up immediately. Three times over the next couple of months I repeated the experiment, each time with the same result. My body may not have liked it, but it was definitely affected by it.

So, yes, it absolutely is possible to concentrate and reflect the body's own energy to promote healing (subject, of course, to the effectiveness of the particular device). But as with everything else mentioned above, it has to be the right frequency. Incidentally, that's why so many devices use the 8-Hz resonant frequency of the earth, known as the Schumann resonance. This frequency absolutely works, is beneficial, and always offers a "safe" choice. But you miss many positive results if you never explore any of the other beneficial frequencies. On the other hand, a company producing a device needs to know what it's doing before it selects frequencies. A bad selection can produce short- or long-term negative results.

## ANTENNAS

Theoretically, the idea behind antenna devices is that there are energies and subatomic particles around us at all times, and by using/wearing the right kind of antenna, we can selectively extract, concentrate, and focus these beneficial energies into our bodies. Several devices on the market claim to do this, such as Tachyon devices, which claim to "restructure certain natural materials at the sub-molecular level, creating permanent Tachyon antennas that are able to focus Tachyon energy." I have several problems with this explanation. First of all, tachyons are only theoretical particles with theoretical properties proposed several decades ago by physicists. They have never actually been seen. (In 1973, one physicist claimed to have identified one such particle in an experiment that has never been duplicated.) In fact, most physicists have now abandoned the concept of tachyons. For those who still believe, it is supposed that tachyons exist within cosmic rays and that they can be produced from high-energy particle collisions.

So, we have Tachyon collection plates that you can buy, treated with a secret process that allows them to capture particles never seen by physicists and channel them into the body to produce healing benefits. That's a stretch. But do they work? Yes, they appear to provide some benefit. And this brings up a problem that we see with many healing energy devices: the explanations surrounding them are often confusing, disjointed, illogical, and, in some cases, nothing more than mumbo jumbo. But that doesn't mean that some of the devices don't work to some degree—just that they may not work in the way explained. The unfortunate thing is that mainstream debunkers use the dubious explanations to throw the baby out with the bathwater. A more likely explanation for how they work is that they either are embedded with energy or work as reflecting devices.

## THE LAYING ON OF HANDS

Stories about healers, healing hands, and healing energy go back centuries, to the beginning of recorded history. If it's a myth based on a placebo effect, it certainly has remarkable staying power. Why?

Let's begin our exploration of that question with four concepts that are easier to understand before we make the giant leap to "healing hands."

1. Every substance or object (animate or inanimate) absorbs and radiates energy in its own unique way. That is to say, every substance has its own unique energy fingerprint. This is even easier to understand when it comes to living beings because, at every level, we are fundamentally energy beings. Our entire body is built of a complex of electrical systems, and every single cell in our bodies functions as a miniature battery.

2. Some frequencies are beneficial, others are harmful. Some levels of intensity are beneficial and others are harmful.

3. People who are healthy tend to exhibit/radiate more of the beneficial

frequencies at higher levels of intensity, whereas people who are ill tend to exhibit/radiate fewer of those frequencies and at lower levels of intensity.

4. We are indeed affected by energy applied to the body. A TENS machine demonstrably relaxes muscles; a high-voltage charge kills.

Since every human body can generate and accept energy, it is possible for bodies to pass energy from one to the other. Even better, everyone can do it. But it's a little like hitting a baseball: some people have no innate talent for it and never work at it, some have no talent but work at it and develop some facility for it, some have an innate talent but never develop it, and some have talent and work to develop it. These latter people we call "healers." Now, there isn't any peer-reviewed, definitive proof, but some studies have indicated that it works, and others have come to the opposite conclusion. Nevertheless, there are some strong suggestions as to its validity.

Anyone who makes the effort can learn to both feel and manipulate energy. At that point, it's no longer theoretical, at least to the person who experiences it. But if it's so easy to feel, how come we all don't feel it, all of the time? How can something that's supposed to be in all of us be real and yet never experienced by the vast majority of us? The answer is very simple: we tune it out. Actually, this happens far more frequently than you might think. Our brains are bombarded with millions of bits of information every day. If we didn't screen out "non-essential" information, we would be overwhelmed by it. In fact, I'm going to train you right now to "re-observe" an aspect of light that you have tuned out all of your lives and never been aware of, to rediscover an innate ability that most have lost.

Because color temperature is non-essential information for most of us, we tend not to see it. Our brains filter out color temperature information and make all color temperatures look the same. But artists and color photographers don't have that luxury—they have to turn off the filter to "see" what their eyes see. Most people are not aware that their skin color changes wildly as color temperature changes. I'm now going to teach you to be aware.

On the next sunny day, I want you to step out in the mid-day sunlight and look at the skin on your arm. Notice the blue tones. Then, immediately go inside and look at your arm under the light of an incandescent light bulb. Notice that the skin has now picked up a strong red/orange color. Most times, you could walk indoors or out and never notice the change in color because your brain filters it out as non-essential. You've probably experienced this color change millions of times but never noticed it before. The concept didn't even exist in your reality. But once you become aware of how to look for it, you can see it, and what was once non-existent is now easy to see.

Feeling energy moving in and out of your body is no different. The experience is there all the time, but we're just shut down to it—we filter it out. To those who are oblivious to it, it's easy to dismiss. Once you become sensitive to it, its reality is as unquestionable as seeing the world of color you were once oblivious to.

In conclusion, there's nothing about healing hands that falls outside of what we already know about energy and healing. Again, as with patches or pendants, there are many claims made by different people—some may be completely valid, some marginally valid, and some are total nonsense. But I have seen enough to be convinced that some people definitely have "healing hands." In the end, I would recommend being open to the possibility, but skeptical of any claims you hear from any particular healer until you find out for yourself.

## EMBEDDING ENERGY

It's actually quite easy to "embed" a healing frequency in a product or object. If you use scalar energy, the frequency will tend to stay in the object indefinitely (unless overridden by a stronger frequency). This can be done with objects you wear and supplements you ingest. In fact, we do this with the products I formulate for Baseline Nutritionals. The main disadvantage of this kind of delivery system is that the frequency is pre-set, not variable. But in exchange, it has three advantages: convenience; delivery, day in and day out; and cost effectiveness.

Some of the new healing "patches" currently available probably work in this way. It should be noted that charges hold better in products that contain living matter and minerals. In other words, patches containing amino acids and supplements containing "foods" or ionic minerals are suitable for charging. Dead, synthetic products are virtually useless at holding a charge. Another variable to keep in mind is that some forms of energy—scalar energy, to be precise—work better when it comes to embedding energy.

### What is Scalar Energy?

We are about to talk about some things that are probably brand new to you.

This topic is not inherently difficult to understand, but it likely represents a total paradigm shift in how you look at health and nutrition. In order to explain everything, we will touch on some very esoteric areas, such as higher mathematics and subatomic particles. Don't panic. It won't be too involved, and I will summarize and tell you the key points you need to remember.

All of the energy we normally think of is characterized by both particle and wavelike properties. The waveform of all these energies can be graphed as a Hertzian wave (either in the form of a sine wave or a step wave). We're talking about everything from electricity to light to sound. The only difference between all of these forms of energy is how fast the waves rise and fall (their frequency) and how intense those rising and falling motions are (their amplitude).

However, there is a different kind of energy that sits alongside electromagnetic energy. It is called scalar energy, and it has some unusual properties that make it remarkably useful for healing applications. It was in the mid-1800s that the existence of scalar energy was first proposed by the Scottish mathematician, James Clerk Maxwell. It was almost a half century later before the inventor and electrical engineer Nikola Tesla (1856–1943) was able to demonstrate its existence. When Tesla died, he took the secret of scalar generation with him, and it took many years before science was once again able to demonstrate the existence of scalar energy and begin an exploration of its potential.

Scalar waves are created by a pair of identical (or replicant) waves (usually called the wave and its anti-wave) that are in phase spatially but out of phase temporally. That is to say, the two waves are physically identical but out of phase in terms of time. The net result is that scalar waves are a whole different animal from normal Hertzian waves. They even look different, like an infinitely projected mobius pattern on axis.

Scalar energy is different from standard Hertzian electromagnetic energy in a number of important ways. First, it's more field-like than wavelike. Instead of running along wires or shooting out in beams, it tends to "fill" its environment. This becomes very important in terms of developing the technology for embedding products with scalar energy. For many of the same reasons, it is capable of passing through solid objects with no loss of intensity. In fact, that is exactly what Tesla demonstrated over 100 years ago when he reportedly projected a scalar wave through the earth with no loss of field strength. Again, this is vital in the development of technology capable of embedding scalar energy in products.

Scalar energy implants its signature on physical objects. This is actually the heart of the issue. All electric fields can implant their signature on objects, but not to the degree that scalar energy can. This becomes extremely important in the mechanics of embedding an energy field in products and then transferring that charge from the products into every cell of your body. Scalar energy can regenerate and repair itself indefinitely, which has important implications for the body. In other words, once the charge is implanted, you can keep it there, unless it is "overwritten" by another charge.

The right scalar frequencies have a whole range of profound beneficial effects on the human body. In the New Age community, there has been much talk of the energy benefits of things like tachyons, radionics, pyramids, and so on. Analysis shows that these are all, at heart, scalar-generating devices.

Scalar waves can be generated in many ways: electronically, magnetically, physically, or optically (by the movement of phased patterns on a computer monitor). For that matter, everything that generates an electromagnetic field also pumps out a scalar footprint, from your tabletop radio to the reactor on a nuclear submarine. One of the most interesting technologies for generating scalar waves is the use of computer programs to cause both a computer CPU to oscillate at pre-determined frequencies and emit scalar energy, while at the same time generating scalar charges off of the computer monitor by running very precise hieroglyphic patterns on the screen. To create what is called a charging chamber, several monitors are aimed (precisely aligned with lasers) at an amplifying device in the center of the room. The entire room then becomes a scalar charging chamber. This produces a high-intensity charge and an ability to regulate frequencies that makes it extremely effective. Any individual standing or sitting in the room is charged, and, as it turns out, so is any product or object, up to its ability to hold the charge. I have also experimented with variations of this technology that have the ability to erase any pre-existing frequencies in an object before embedding a new frequency. This, theoretically, can produce a cleaner healing energy.

## Embedding Scalar Energy in Nutritional Products

For the most part, we've already covered how to get the charge into a nutritional product, but that still leaves an unanswered question: how do the charges make their way from the product into your body? The first issue is where do these charges embed in the human body? Since all life is fundamentally energy based, all living beings have numbers of structures capable of holding a scalar charge. In point of fact, the very same structures that allow the scalar charge to be embedded in plant-based products also allow that same charge to be transferred to the human body from those products. For example, there are crystalline structures in every cell wall capable of holding a charge. There are also liquid crystal structures in the collagen network comprising all of the space between cells that can hold a charge. And then there's your DNA: quantum mechanical models in physics describe subatomic particles, such as excitons, plasmons, and solitons, that can store and carry biological information along helix macromolecules in response to low-level scalar energy. In other words, scalar energy is capable of imprinting itself on your very DNA.

Before we move on to the benefits of scalar energy for your health, it would be worth dwelling for a moment on what proof exists that everything I'm talking about is real. It is indeed possible to measure scalar fields, but most people don't have the required equipment. Therefore, let's turn to a form of proof that we can see right now—Kirlian photography. A Kirlian photograph is merely a specialized kind of photography that images the bioelectric field that surrounds all objects, particularly living objects.

*U.S. News and World Report* ran an article a number of years ago calling Kirlian photography a hoax. To quote from the article: "Controlled experiments have shown that the Kirlian photos (captured by passing an electric current through the subject, whose 'energies' are then recorded on special photographic plates) are the result of moisture and pressure, not spiritual vitality."[1] And that's absolutely true, as far as it goes. The simple fact is, though, that it's absolutely possible to set up a hermetically sealed environment where moisture and pressure are constant, and therefore not influencing the outcome of the pictures. And yet, even in those controlled environments, it's possible to produce startling and revealing photos.

For example, following are two pictures of lentil sprouts—identical, except for the fact that the lentil on the left has been soaked in very hot water for a minute or so. According to the *U.S. News and World Report* article, since it has more moisture in it, it should conduct more electricity than the unblanched lentil on the right and produce a brighter field.

As you can see, the exact opposite is true. And that's why the National

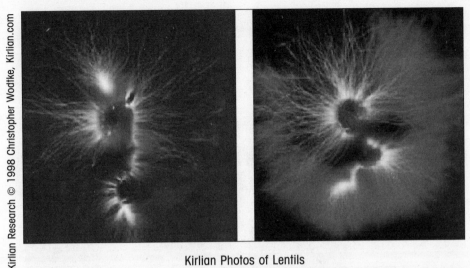

**Kirlian Photos of Lentils**

Institutes of Health and Cambridge University, among other major institutes, have studied Kirlian photography. In fact, newer Kirlian cameras are based on gas discharge visualization and record their images digitally, totally bypassing film emulsions. Research supports both their effectiveness and their validity.[2]

What can we learn about scalar-enhanced products through Kirlian photos? The most important thing is that the scalar charge is, unquestionably, embedding itself in the products. Here, we reprint examples of products before and after embedding.

These photographs are revolutionary in their implications. They clearly tell us that the more alive something is (the more organic it is), the bigger its energy field will be. They also tell us that scalar-enhanced products demonstrate a bigger field.

## Benefits of Scalar Energy for Health

What health benefits are there to consuming scalar-enhanced products? As it turns out, there are many. First, enhanced products are more assimilable by the body, absorbed better and faster. Enhanced products can be assimilated so quickly by your body that they can transform your bioelectric field in as little as ten seconds. Following are images as registered through biofeedback devices that measure galvanic skin response and body temperature

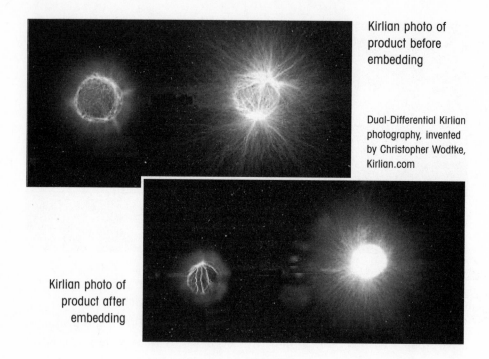

Kirlian photo of
product before
embedding

Dual-Differential Kirlian
photography, invented
by Christopher Wodtke,
Kirlian.com

Kirlian photo of
product after
embedding

and then interpret that data to create representations of the body's bioelectric field. First, you see the field before taking any product and then the change in the field just ten seconds after taking the enhanced product.

Beyond what you can see, though, enhanced products carry a whole range of benefits inherent in the charge itself and independent of the product. In that sense, the product functions as a carrier of the healing charge. There are at least a dozen major health benefits that come from this charge, and they are profound. Regular intake of enhanced products can:

- Eliminate and nullify the effects of artificial frequencies in the human body.

- Increase the energy level of every cell in the body to the ideal 70–90 millivolt range native to most cells.

- Increase the energy covalent level of every hydrogen atom in the body as verified by spectrographs. This is significant because covalent hydrogen bonds are what hold your DNA together. In other words, consuming scalar-enhanced products can protect your DNA from damage.

- Improve cell wall permeability, thus facilitating the intake of nutrients into each cell and the elimination of waste from each cell. (As a result of the

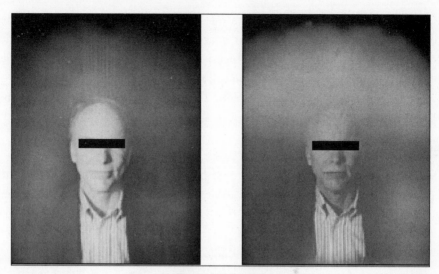

Bioelectric Photos

high transmembrane potential mentioned above, enhanced products effectively cause every cell in your body to detoxify.)

- Decrease the surface tension of the embedded products, thereby significantly reducing the time required for your body to assimilate those same products.

- Increase overall body energy levels.

- Cleanse the blood, improving chylomicron levels (protein/fat particles floating in the blood), triglyceride profiles, and fibrin patterns.

- Improve immune function by as much as 149 percent.

- Improve mental focus.

- Balance out the two hemispheres of the brain as measured by EEG readings, thus optimizing both your analytic and creative skills.

- Work as an antidepressant since it inhibits the uptake of noradrenaline by nerve cells.

- Fight cancer. Cancer cells are, almost without exception, low-voltage cells. While the optimum cell voltage for most cells is in the 70–90 millivolt range, cancer cells are almost exclusively in the 15–20 millivolt range. It has been theorized that as cell voltage starts to drop into the range where the survival of the cell may be in question, the cell begins to proliferate uncontrollably in an attempt to guarantee the "survival" of its genetic code. If you raise cell voltage (which is exactly what can happen when you consume enhanced products), the cell no longer needs to proliferate wildly and it can become "normal" again. The implications in cancer treatment could be profound.

## ENERGIZING WATER

No discussion of healing energy would be complete without discussing the energy/water connection. Water is a miraculous substance, but not all water is alike. There are so many things that can be done in order to enhance its

## CONVENTIONAL MEDICINE AND SUBTLE ENERGY

Curiously enough, although the conventional medical community has a particular antipathy when it comes to New Age healing energy devices, it uses similar devices itself with gay abandon. What is radiation therapy but the direct application of high-intensity energy to the body to achieve a specific healing result? Ultrasound is the same thing, just a different form of energy with a different frequency for a different medical purpose. How interesting that when the medical community uses energy for healing, it's considered "science," but when alternative healers do the same thing, it's called "quackery."

Now researchers at Harvard Medical School are experimenting with using electromagnetic pulses to treat depression. Called transcranial magnetic stimulation (TMS), it involves holding a figure eight–shaped wand near a person's head while generating a strong magnetic field to induce electric currents in brain cells. The researchers believe that TMS works by normalizing disturbed brain activity. In experiments at Beth Israel Deaconess Medical Center in Boston, TMS lifted the spirits of depressed patients who were resistant to antidepressant drugs.[3]

Can't you just hear the conventional medical community's commentary on this device if it had been first used in an alternative health clinic? It would have been dismissed out of hand as mumbo-jumbo quackery. But that thought aside, the key point is that we have the ultimate statement from medical researchers that subtle energy fields, transmitted through the "ether," can directly affect our bodies and our biological functions.

potential in the human body that it is almost mind-boggling. One of the things that can be done to water involves applying energy—everything from magnets to lasers to heat to sound—to give the water new properties. Others involve adding substances to the water, to change its structure or pH, and using the water to carry set frequencies. Here, I'll touch on just a couple of things that can be done with energy.

Terms such as *structured water* and *clustered water* have been loosely thrown around and used in ways that have little connection with reality. In the end though, the concept is simple, easily implemented in a number of ways, and can make a profound difference in the state of your health. Water molecules contain electrical forces that cause the molecules to cluster together. (In fact, the overall charge of the water molecule is neutral, but the charge is not uniform over the entire molecule, meaning that it tends to create an electric dipole, carrying a positive charge at one end and a negative charge at the other.) This is easily seen in the way water beads up on the surface of a car after you wash it. If you disrupt those electrical forces, fewer molecules cluster together, which means the water clusters are smaller. This makes them better able to move in and out among the fibers of your clothes, for example, so that the water cleans better, or to move in and out through the cell walls in your body so that the water carries nutrients in and waste out better.

Making water "wetter" can be done chemically (with surfactants in your laundry detergent or by adding micelle to your drinking water), by applying magnetic fields, electrical charges, or sound waves to the water, and even by heating and cooling the water in the right way. All can cause the water molecule groupings to become smaller ("wetter").

Despite claims from the scientific community that this is all nonsense, that water is totally unaffected by energy, real world results do not support those claims. In some ways, this is like the apocryphal story of the scientists who proved that bumblebees cannot fly. As the story goes, some years ago, scientists used scientific analysis to prove that the ratio of body weight to wingspan is disproportionate in bumblebees, which in theory makes it aerodynamically impossible for them to fly. But, of course, they can and do fly. This is using pure scientific analysis to "prove" the opposite of something that we actually know to be true.

The only difference when it comes to debunking "wetter" water is that it's not being done as a joke. There are thousands of examples of how water is affected by energy. A simple one you may have tried when you were younger

# HOMEOPATHY: AN ENERGY MEDICINE

A discussion of what homeopathy is and how it works is worth an entire book in itself. What I want to deal with here is why the medical community considers it quackery. According to Stephen Barrett's Quackwatch website:

"Homeopathic products are made from minerals, botanical substances, and several other sources. If the original substance is soluble, one part is diluted with either nine or ninety-nine parts of distilled water and/or alcohol and shaken vigorously (succussed); if insoluble, it is finely ground and pulverized in similar proportions with powdered lactose (milk sugar). One part of the diluted medicine is then further diluted, and the process is repeated until the desired concentration is reached. Dilutions of 1 to 10 are designated by the Roman numeral X ($1X = 1/10$, $3X = 1/1,000$, $6X = 1/1,000,000$). Similarly, dilutions of 1 to 100 are designated by the Roman numeral C ($1C = 1/100$, $3C = 1/1,000,000$, and so on). Most remedies today range from 6X to 30X, but products of 30C or more are marketed.

"A 30X dilution means that the original substance has been diluted 1,000,000,000,000,000,000,000,000,000,000 times. Assuming that a cubic centimeter of water contains 15 drops, this number is greater than the number of drops of water that would fill a container more than 50 times the size of the earth. Imagine placing a drop of red dye into such a container so that it disperses evenly. Homeopathy's 'law of infinitesimals' is the equivalent of saying that any drop of water subsequently removed from that container will possess an essence of redness. Robert L. Park, Ph.D., a prominent physicist who is executive director of the American Physical Society, has noted that since the least amount of a substance in a solution is one molecule, a 30C solution would have to have at least one molecule of the original substance dissolved in a minimum of 1,000,000,000,000,000,000,000,000,000,000,000,000, 000,000,000,000,000,000,000 molecules of water. This would require a container more than 30,000,000,000 times the size of the earth."[5]

So, the primary argument against homeopathic remedies is that they are so diluted that they really don't contain even a single molecule of the original substance in them. This argument is absolutely correct, and the numbers cited above are dead on. And if one remains rooted in the world of drugs and drug doses, then based on that argument there can be only one conclusion: homeopathy is a fraud and homeopathic remedies are placebos.

However, if one steps back for a moment and considers everything we've talked about in this chapter, then it's easy to see that homeopathy is based on an entirely different premise. The idea behind making the dilutions is, in fact, not to maintain any of the original substance at all, but rather to transfer the essential frequencies of the original substance (a "memory of the substance") to the water itself. In other words, the entire argument against homeopathy as presented by Dr. Barrett misses the boat. That's not to say that homeopathy works or doesn't work—just that the argument used against it is meaningless because it doesn't address the actual operating premise of homeopathy. It's a bit like saying someone isn't a good doctor because they can't run a four-minute mile: the statement about the doctor's running ability may be true, but it has no relevance to his or her medical ability.

The essence of homeopathy is transferring the frequencies of various substances into water and then using that water to manifest the properties of the original substance. We already know that water can be changed when exposed to electromagnetic forces and that it can remember those forces for a period of time. We know that energy-altered water can significantly change the way irrigated plants grow. Based on those observations, you cannot dismiss homeopathy out of hand.

If scientists want to evaluate homeopathy, they have to evaluate it on those terms. You can't impose your own explanation for how something works and then dismiss it because of the holes found in your imposed explanation. Given that modus operandi, you can easily eviscerate anything, even modern medicine. It's also worth noting that homeopathy has a vast following of people who swear by it. Even if its healing benefits turn out to be due to the placebo effect, homeopathy would nevertheless seem to be a lot more effective and safer than many pharmaceutical drugs.

is to rub a plastic comb on a wool sweater to charge it with static electricity, and then turn on a tap so the water runs in a thin stream. Hold the charged comb close to the water and the water will bend toward the comb. Voila! Proof positive that water is affected by energy fields.

Amazingly, many in the scientific community dismiss the health benefits that hundreds of thousands of people experience drinking "energized" water as mere placebo effect. The world's agriculture industry has been exploring the benefits of irrigating with water exposed to a magnetic field for some time now. Plants, of course, are not subject to the placebo effect. Differences in crops as the result of using magnetized water can only result from changes to the water, not psychological mind games with the plants. Studies have shown that magnetically treating water can increase plant height, branch number per plant, and shoot dry weight as compared to distilled water and rain water.[4] Evidence clearly shows the difference in plant growth using magnets to create "wetter" water.

## GENERAL RECOMMENDATIONS

As you will note, I have avoided making specific recommendations in this chapter. That was deliberate, because there are so many enhanced products, patches, pendants, and supplements now that it's impossible to evaluate them all. I'd rather arm you with information that you can use to evaluate a product or device on your own and make a reasoned assessment. Ultimately, the only relevant question is, "Does it work for you?" If it works for you, then it doesn't matter what I tell you, or for that matter, what your doctor tells you.

And just a note on the placebo effect, which is what most medical researchers ascribe to healing energy devices and techniques. If it comes down to it, which would you rather use—a placebo that costs you pennies and that convinced your mind to heal your body of cancer or a chemotherapy drug, backed by volumes of clinical testing, that costs you thousands of dollars and that in your case didn't work, made you feel terrible in the process, and ultimately killed you? With one, you'd be a sucker that was healed; with the other, a dead rational being. An interesting choice, yes?

In the next chapter, we'll look at how our thoughts can affect our well-being and our capacity to heal.

# CHAPTER 16

## The Thought That Kills

- **The Connection between Thoughts and the Immune System**
- **The Health Effects of Stress and Depression**
- **Pharmaceuticals are Not the Solution**
- **Natural Alternatives for Stress and Depression**

For years, stress and/or depression have been suspected of somehow increasing the risk of contracting numerous infectious diseases. In addition, there is mounting evidence that increased levels of stress and depression also correlate with an increased incidence of cancer. And finally, there is a strong statistical link between stress and depression and death itself. As a result, a relatively new field of research, psychoneuroimmunology, is dedicated to unlocking the connection between thoughts (i.e., our nervous system) and the immune system.

## THE CONNECTION BETWEEN THOUGHTS AND THE IMMUNE SYSTEM

Psychoneuroimmunology researchers have discovered several links between our thoughts and the immune system. For one, we know that when we are stressed, our bodies produce more of the stress hormone adrenaline. While it is true that adrenaline helps to mobilize the body's energy reserves, it also causes a decrease in available antibodies and a reduction in both the number and strength of lymphocytes. We have also learned that the brain is directly wired to the organs of the immune system (the spleen, thymus, lymph nodes, and bone marrow) and that stress and depression affect their performance.

Most interesting of all is the connection between the neuropeptides produced by brain cells and the rest of the body. In much the same way that the immune system uses interleukins to communicate with itself, the brain uses the hormone-like neuropeptides to communicate with itself and the rest of the body, including the immune system. The cells of the immune system carry receptors for the various neuropeptides produced by the brain. When we are happy, for example, the brain produces one kind of neuropeptide and the cells of the immune system have specific receptors for these "up" chemicals. Once received, these neuropeptides cause the immune system to strengthen and build. Correspondingly, when we are depressed, we produce a different set of neuropeptides, and immune cells also have receptors for these "down" communicators, whose net effect on the immune system is to shut it down.

Incidentally, this is by no means a one-way communication. The cells of the brain have receptor sites for the interleukins and interferons produced by the lymphocytes of the immune system. And it turns out that some macrophages and activated lymphocytes are capable of producing their own neuropeptides—to communicate directly with the brain in its own language.

Basically, through the same two systems (the nervous system and the circulatory system) that our minds use to interact with our immune systems, our minds also connect with every organ and cell in our bodies, affecting the performance, functioning, and growth of our bones and bone marrow, glands, heart (everything from heart rate to the heart tissue itself), the walls of our veins and arteries, the functioning of individual cells, and even the very structure of our DNA. The entire body is created and run by the brain, with equal feedback from the organs and cells themselves, again through both the direct wired connections of the nervous system and the neuropeptides traveling through the circulatory system.

## A Deeper Connection

In addition to what medical researchers have been able to verify and explain regarding interactions between the nervous system and the immune system, there are a number of "incidents" that hint at much more.

### Depression, Heart Attacks, and Strokes

A group of medical researchers in Montreal tracked 222 post–heart attack victims, both men and women. The researchers found that those who were depressed (who felt sad, hopeless, and listless) were more likely to die of another heart attack within eighteen months of their first heart attack than those who were not—ten times more likely, in fact.[1] A study of patients with a history of heart disease found that those who were depressed were eight times more likely to develop potentially deadly heart arrhythmia than those who were not depressed.[2] In another study of 194 heart attack patients, those who reported lower amounts of emotional support were nearly three times more likely to die within six months than those with higher levels of emotional support.[3]

A ten-year study was conducted to follow the mortality rates of people who had experienced a stroke. Those who had been diagnosed with either major or minor depression were 3.4 times as likely to have died within the follow-up period. The death rate among depressed patients with few social contacts was especially high—over 90 percent.[4]

## The Monday Morning Blahs

Have you ever wondered when most people die? Statistically, it turns out that people are more likely to die on Monday morning before going to work than at any other time of the week. There has been much speculation as to why this happens, but most people agree it's because they are stressed to be heading back to jobs they can't stand after a weekend off.

## The Placebo Effect

A placebo is an inactive pill, liquid, or powder that has no treatment value. In clinical trials, experimental treatments are often compared with placebos to assess the treatment's effectiveness. Nevertheless, on average, 35 percent of all people who receive a given placebo experience a significant effect. In fact, in a series of trials, 52 percent of colitis patients treated with a placebo reported feeling better. Astoundingly, 50 percent of the inflamed intestines actually looked better when examined with a sigmoidoscope.[5] It seems that a person's beliefs and hopes about a treatment, combined with their suggestibility, have a significant biochemical effect.

## Surgery

For years, it had been suspected by many doctors (and dismissed by many more) that patients under anesthesia could hear their surgeon's comments and that what they heard affected them. There were many anecdotal stories of doctors who, upon opening up a patient, would see a tumor and comment out loud that it looked malignant. And then, even though the tumor would later prove to be benign, the patient nevertheless would fade rapidly and be dead in a matter of days. Well, new studies are now proving that not only is this true, but to a degree far higher than previously imagined. Dr. Henry Bennett, a psychologist from the University of California Medical School at Davis, suggests that, under anesthesia, patients might be especially vulnerable to upsetting remarks they overhear since their normal coping techniques aren't available to them.[6]

Studies that support this statement include a number of patients who were given the suggestion during surgery that one of their hands was becoming warmer and the other cooler. The temperature of both hands changed accordingly.[7] In another study, patients were played a taped message while they were anesthetized during surgery that told them that if they heard the same message later, they should signify this by touching their ears in a post-operative interview. Later, in the interview, all of the patients absentmindedly tugged at their ears, although not one of the patients could recall having heard the message.[8]

During back surgery, which normally causes urination problems for the patients after surgery, researchers suggested to the anesthetized patients that they would be able to relax their pelvic muscles after the surgery, and thus would need no catheter. None of the patients who received the suggestion subsequently needed a catheter.[9]

### Brocq's Disease

In 1952, the *British Medical Journal* reported on an extraordinary case concerning Brocq's disease, a genetic disorder that causes the skin to resemble the scales of a reptile.[10] What was so extraordinary about this case is that although Brocq's disease is a hereditary condition, and considered incurable by the medical community, it was nevertheless cured in this particular case through hypnosis. Under hypnosis, the patient, a sixteen-year-old boy, was able to "go in" and reprogram his DNA. The net result was that within ten days of starting treatment, the boy remained symptom free for at least five years, at which point his therapist lost touch with him.

### Cancer

A now well-known example was reported by Dr. Bruno Klopfer in 1957.[11] A patient of Dr. Klopfer's, whose cancer had metastasized and riddled his body with tumors, had reached the point where all available medical approaches had failed, and he was confined to bed with only a few days to live. Then, just before the end, the patient heard about Krebiozen, an experimental drug then being tested. Desperate, he demanded that his doctors include him in the experimental trials. Believing that the man was as good as dead anyway, and that they therefore had nothing to lose, they put him on Krebiozen. Miraculously, the man's tumors began to melt away. He made a remarkable recovery and was discharged from the hospital.

Two months later, however, reports began to appear that continuing research on Krebiozen had raised serious doubts about the efficacy of the drug. Within a few days of the patient's reading these reports, his tumors had returned and he was once again on the verge of death. At this point, his doctor did something unusual—he lied to his patient and told him that they now had a newer and more potent version of Krebiozen. He then proceeded to inject the man, not with a new and improved version of Krebiozen, and not even with the original drug, but with plain water. Astoundingly, the man's tumors once again began to melt away. As before, the man made a remarkable recovery and went home.

He then remained perfectly healthy, in full remission for seven months, until he saw a news report that declared "Nationwide AMA Tests Show Krebiozen to Be Worthless as a Cancer Treatment." Two days later, the patient was dead.

## THE HEALTH EFFECTS OF STRESS AND DEPRESSION

Stress is your body's response to all of the demands made upon it. The body responds to all stresses, both positive and negative, by trying to get back to normal. Unfortunately, the stressful and fast-paced times we live in are taking their toll. Forty-three percent of all adults suffer adverse health effects due to stress, and 75–90 percent of all visits to primary care physicians are for stress-related complaints or disorders. Stress is said to be responsible for more than half of the 550 million workdays lost annually because of absenteeism.

When a stressor is perceived, the hypothalamus triggers the adrenal glands to release corticosteroids to increase metabolism and provide an immediate increase in energy. Simultaneously, your pituitary releases adrenocorticotropic hormone (ACTH), which causes your adrenal glands to release epinephrine (adrenaline) and norepinephrine, which work to prolong your body's fight-or-flight response. If a stressful situation goes on for too long without any relief, you may feel tired, irritable, depressed, or anxious. Chronic stress can lead to trouble sleeping or eating, and to diseases and disorders such as headaches, insomnia, high blood pressure, kidney disease, ulcers, asthma, heart attack, or stroke. Eventually, your body's energy reserves become exhausted, and your body breaks down. Recent research has confirmed the role of stress in cardio-vascular disease, cancer, and gastrointestinal, skin, neurological, and emotional disorders, as well as a host of disorders linked to immune system disturbances, ranging from the common cold and herpes to arthritis and AIDS.

Depression works on your body in different ways than stress, but the results are the same. Your body is a product of your thoughts. As we've already discussed, the cells of your body, including your immune cells, have receptor sites for the various neuropeptides you produce. When you are happy, you produce a set of neuropeptides that tell your immune system to jack up, which it does. In other words, happy thoughts improve your health. However, when you are depressed, the opposite happens: the neuropeptides your body produces shut down your immune system. In effect, negative thoughts can actually kill you.

## PHARMACEUTICALS ARE NOT THE SOLUTION

The major pharmaceutical companies have developed a set of drugs called selective serotonin-reuptake inhibitors (SSRIs) to "manage the symptoms" associated with stress and depression. You might know them as Prozac®, Zoloft®, Paxil®, and numerous others. Prozac is widely prescribed for chil-dren—many children under the age of three have already been given Prozac. Thanks to millions of dollars in marketing and promotion, and our own marvel-ous tendency to believe in magic bullets, we have become a "Prozac nation."

But not without cost. SSRIs cause mania and delusions of grandeur in one out of every twenty-five children taking the drugs, as cited on the warning label for Luvox in the *Physicians' Desk Reference*. Eli Lilly, the manufacturer of Prozac, had strong indications it caused violence as early as the 1980s, but suppressed the information until it was leaked to the *British Medical Journal* in 2004.[12] In 70 percent of all murder/suicides involving women and chil-dren, the women were on SSRIs.[13] There are many other examples of the detrimental effects of antidepressants and SSRIs:

- In July 2004, Emiri Padron was on Zoloft when she smothered her ten-month-old daughter with a stuffed animal and then stabbed herself.

- Specialized testing during the autopsy of Eric Harris, one of the shooters at the Columbine High School massacre in 1999, showed "therapeutic" levels of Luvox in his blood. In addition, he was also taking cough syrup. The interaction between cough medications containing dextromethorphan (found in Robitussin, for example) and the SSRIs can greatly increase the possibility of a toxic reaction known as serotonin syndrome, leading to reactions similar to those who have PCP (angel dust) reactions.

- Kip Kinkle, who in 1998 killed his parents and two classmates and then wounded twenty-five others at Thurston High School in Oregon, was on SSRIs.

- Brynn Hartmann, the actor Phil Hartmann's wife, was on Zoloft when she shot her husband and then committed suicide in May 1998.

- In March 1998, Matthew Beck went on a bloody rampage at his office, the Connecticut Lottery Corporation headquarters, killing four senior lottery officials before committing suicide. He was on two antidepressants, including Luvox.

- In October 1997, Luke Woodham was on an SSRI when he killed three people, including his mother, and wounded six others in Pearl, Mississippi.

- In April 2007, Seung-Hui Cho shot and killed thirty-two people and wounded a further twenty-nine at Virginia Tech University before committing suicide in the deadliest mass shooting in modern U.S. history. He too was on antidepressants.

The U.S. Food and Drug Administration (FDA) has finally recognized the hazardous effects of antidepressants and recommended that manufacturers add warning labels on their products. The new warning label states: "Antidepressants increased the risk of suicidal thinking and behavior (suicidality) in short-term studies in children and adolescents with Major Depressive Disorder (MDD) and other psychiatric disorders. Anyone considering the use of [drug name] or any other antidepressant in a child or adolescent must balance this risk with the clinical need. Patients who are started on therapy should be observed closely for clinical worsening, suicidality, or unusual changes in behavior."

The FDA should be congratulated for finally taking this step. However, one might ask why it didn't act ten years ago when the evidence was just as compelling. How many have needlessly died because the FDA, and the governmental agencies of most countries, failed to buck the pressure applied by the pharmaceutical companies to downplay the risks associated with antidepressants? The topic of antidepressants is particularly important in terms of overall public safety because the violent side effects caused by some of these drugs impacts more than just those on the drugs. We've already cited examples of children on antidepressants killing teachers and classmates at school and their own family members. Although this obviously does not occur in all cases, and it does not suggest that anyone on an antidepressant will kill their loved ones, there are nevertheless enough cases to cause concern, especially with children.

The new warnings were implemented because of several placebo-controlled studies that involved nine antidepressant drugs (SSRIs and others) in children and adolescents with major depressive disorder (MDD), obsessive-compulsive disorder (OCD), or other psychiatric disorders (a total of 24 trials involving over 4,400 patients). The conclusive evidence showed that patients on antidepressants were at double the risk of suicidal thinking or behavior (suicidality) during the first few months of treatment than those on the placebo. But what the FDA pointedly avoided studying was the well-documented relationship between the use of antidepressants and violence toward others. We've looked at a sampling of some of the more notorious stories in the news, but these are only a fraction of the incidents reported. And keep in mind, those drugs are supposed to "enhance" mood! (I guess it all depends on what your definition of *enhance* is.) With many children under the age of three already on Prozac, we may have only seen the barest hint of where this problem is truly headed.

To be objective, antidepressants are important for some people with severe symptoms who don't respond to alternatives. When symptoms are debilitating, the risks associated with the drugs may be worth it. But for the majority of people who suffer from the typical daily disappointments in life or certain nutritional deficiencies, short periods of depression are common and can usually be eliminated through various natural remedies with minimal side effects. At least, we should think twice before we simply pop a pill. Being a "Prozac nation" is not only sad, it's dangerous.

## NATURAL ALTERNATIVES FOR STRESS AND DEPRESSION

An emotional injury is like a physical injury—it takes time and attention to heal. There are alternatives to try before seeking a prescription for antidepressants. Nutritional deficiencies can be corrected, amino acids supplemented, herbal remedies used, and hormones balanced.

## Vitamin and Mineral Therapy

Vitamin and mineral deficiencies can cause depression, and correcting these deficiencies is often a safe, fast, and inexpensive way to find relief. Alcohol, smoking, stress, and excess sugar accelerate the depletion of many key antidepressive vitamins and minerals from the body, as does depression itself. Deficiencies in any of the following vitamins, minerals, and fatty acids can contribute significantly to depression:

- Vitamins $B_6$ and $B_{12}$
- Folic acid
- Inositol
- Vitamin C
- Magnesium

- Calcium
- Trace minerals
- Omega-3 fatty acids
- GLA (gamma-linolenic acid)

## Amino Acids

Supplementing with amino acids can help relieve depression.

- S-Adenosyl-L-methionine (SAMe)—SAMe is a naturally occurring amino acid found in every cell of the body. It has a wide range of benefits, including protecting the liver and cardiovascular system. In addition, it has antidepressant action equal to and faster than many drugs and is essential for the synthesis of the hormone melatonin. Amounts required may vary from 200 mg to 3,000 mg a day. SAMe also assists with sleep disorders, particularly those that are induced by the side effects of pharmaceutical drugs. Note: SAMe is not appropriate for bipolar disorder.

- Phenylalanine—Phenylalanine is an amino acid that is used by the body to make the neurotransmitter norepinephrine, which is believed to be in short supply in the brains of people who are depressed. There is some evidence that taking in extra phenylalanine allows the brain to make more norepinephrine. There are also several studies that indicate that phenylalanine may work as well as antidepressant drugs.[14] Although the studies are inconclusive, the anecdotal evidence is strong, and there are virtually no known side effects, so it's worth trying. Begin with 100 mg twice daily, and increase gradually to a maximum of 1,000–1,500 mg three times daily. Reduce the dosage if you experience any increase in blood pressure, headaches, or insomnia. Do not use without a doctor's permission and guidance if you are on any medication.

- Theanine—Anxiety is a close cousin to depression, and the two often go hand in hand. Many people report that 100–200 mg of the amino acid L-theanine works as well as prescription anti-anxiety medications, but it is not addictive or habit-forming. Studies have shown that theanine reduces stress and produces feelings of relaxation.[15] It may do this by raising serotonin levels in the brain. Incidentally, theanine is commonly found in tea.

- 5-Hydroxytryptophan (5-HTP)—5-HTP is an amino acid that occurs naturally in the body and is the final step in the production of the neurotransmitter serotonin. It is actually made in the body from L-tryptophan and like tryptophan is converted into serotonin in the brain. As such, 5-HTP can powerfully promote relaxation and counter depression. 5-HTP is special in that it can cross the blood-brain barrier. It is extracted from the seeds of *Griffonia simplicifolia*, a tree grown mostly in Ghana and the Ivory Coast, but it can also be made synthetically. 5-HTP has gained popularity in the treatment of insomnia, depression, and obesity, among other uses. It is considered a safe and effective treatment for these conditions.

- GABA (gamma-aminobutyric acid)—GABA is made in the brain from the amino acid glutamate with the aid of vitamin $B_6$. It works to inhibit the transmission of neural impulses, thus working to balance out neural excitation. As such, it can help reduce restlessness, irritability, insomnia, seizures, and depression.

## Herbal Remedies

For the vast majority of people bothered by stress or depression, formulas made from high-quality herbs can prove remarkably effective. Look for an herbal formula that contains the following herbs:

- St. John's wort (*Hypericum perforatum*)—St. John's wort is licensed in Germany and other European countries as a treatment for mild to moderate depression, anxiety, and sleep disorders. Sometimes called "nature's

Prozac," St. John's wort helps relieve stress, anxiety, and tension. In Germany, it is the most popular antidepressant, outselling Prozac three to one. More than twenty clinical studies have been completed using several different extracts of St. John's wort, and most have shown antidepressant action equal to standard prescription drugs, without the side effects. St. John's wort is now being studied in the first U.S. government–sanctioned clinical trial, a three-year study sponsored by the Center for Complementary and Alternative Medicine, based in Washington, D.C. Probably the greatest testament to its efficacy is how it has been attacked in the press as "dangerous." The case against it is that it seems to heighten the dangers associated with monoamine oxidase inhibitors (MAOIs) if you are currently using these powerful antidepressant drugs. But this is a marvelous piece of propaganda double-speak that transfers the danger from the antidepressants (where they belong) to St. John's wort, which merely brings those dangers to the fore.

- *Ginkgo biloba*—*Ginkgo biloba* extract is currently being used as an alternative for elderly patients with depression resistant to standard drug therapy. This is because depression is often an early sign of cognitive decline and cerebrovascular insufficiency in elderly patients. In one study, forty patients, 51–78 years old, with a diagnosis of resistant depression, were randomized to receive either ginkgo (80 mg three times daily) or placebo for eight weeks. During the study, patients remained on their antidepressant drugs. In patients treated with ginkgo, there was an average decline in the median Hamilton Depression Scale (a standard test) scores from 14 to 7 after four weeks; the average further reduced to 4.5 after eight weeks. There was only a one-point reduction in the placebo group after eight weeks. In addition to the significant improvement in symptoms of depression for the ginkgo group, there was also a noted improvement in overall cognitive function. No side effects were reported.[16]

- Valerian root—For centuries, valerian has been used to treat nervous tension and panic attacks. A wonderful herb, valerian is calming and quieting to the nervous system.

- Kava kava—Kava is the herb of choice to relax the body, relieve stress, combat mild to moderate anxiety, and relieve headache and back pain. Kava is now recognized by many doctors as an alternative to drugs like Xanax and Valium. As might be expected for something that works so well, kava is under false attack for causing liver damage. The issues of kava's safety and efficacy have been studied extensively, including a statistical review of seven human clinical trials, published in the *Journal of Clinical Psychopharmacology*, which indicated no significant adverse effects related to kava use and liver toxicity at normal doses.[17]

- Ashwagandha—Ashwagandha, an Ayurvedic herb, has been used to stabilize mood in patients with behavioral disturbances. In studies, it produced an antianxiety effect comparable to that of the drug lorazepam and an antidepressant effect comparable to that of the drug imipramine.[18]

- Lobelia—Lobelia is an extremely powerful antispasmodic and sedative. It helps improve breathing dramatically by dilating the bronchial tubes—great for asthmatics. It also works to stimulate a relaxation response in the body and to decrease adrenaline levels. As a result, lobelia helps any condition caused by adrenaline stress such as anxiety and panic attacks.

- Passionflower—Passionflower is remarkably effective as a sedative to calm nerves on edge.

- Black cohosh—Black cohosh was first used by Native Americans to soothe the body by reducing the rapidity of the pulse. It also works internally to soothe nervous disease or spasm.

- Skullcap, hops, and catnip—These three herbs have a long history as marvelously effective herbal tranquilizers, sedatives, and sleep aids.

- *Mulungu*—Researchers have validated the traditional use of *mulungu*, from a tree that grows in the Amazon, for anxiety and stress, where it was shown to alter anxiety-related responses.[19]

## Balancing Hormones

The hormone progesterone is particularly important since women experience clinical depression twice as often as men. Over the years, I have recommended progesterone cream to women, and it has picked up a nickname from many of them: "The Happy Cream." Any time progesterone levels drop, such as during the monthly cycle, immediately after giving birth, or all the time if you are in a state of estrogen dominance, depression is a likely result. Using a good progesterone cream can provide an almost instant turnaround in attitude for many people (including men).

This brings us to the subject of postpartum depression. During the weeks leading up to birth, progesterone levels soar to 10–20 times normal. No wonder women seem to glow during pregnancy. But immediately after giving birth, their progesterone levels plunge to almost zero. This is why so many new mothers experience extreme, even psychotic levels of depression. Simple supplementation with progesterone will resolve the depression in over 90 percent of cases. In fact, any doctor who recommends antidepressants for postpartum depression without trying progesterone first should be named as an unindicted co-conspirator, since they truly share the blame for any psychotic incidents that may result.

A growing body of evidence suggests that testosterone levels drop as much as 40 percent in men between their early forties and early seventies. And for 10–15 percent of all men, those levels will dip below normal even as early as their thirties due to stress, depression, personal life changes, or medications. This in turn causes a decrease not only in sexual desire and performance but also in the competitive drive to succeed in life, which is frequently experienced as depression. In women, excessive estrogen in the body causes a reduction in testosterone levels, which leads to a similar decline in sexual desire and performance and a similar reduction in "life drive"—again, frequently experienced as depression.

## The Importance of Sleep

Sleep is a major component of good health. Insufficient sleep can affect everything from your immune system to blood pressure to obesity and even diabetes. But more to the point, lack of proper sleep is a major body stressor and can be a direct cause of depression.[20] Some doctors have called lack of sleep the number one health problem in the world today. So, how much is enough? The standard answer is that adults need seven to eight hours a night, but that's actually a meaningless statement. The quality of sleep you get probably matters far more than the quantity. Which do you think is more beneficial: six hours of deep, restful sleep or eight hours of fitfully tossing and turning while you sleep? In the end, the depth of sleep is crucial.

If you're not sleeping well, what can you do? Unfortunately, sleeping pills, like most medications, don't deal with the cause, only the symptoms of an unaddressed problem. One of the current stories in the news is about people using the drugs Ambien and Lunesta, who find themselves sleepwalking, sleep phone calling, sleep cooking, sleep eating, and sleep driving (no kidding). The FDA has ordered all manufacturers of prescription sleep aids to strengthen their label warnings to include these potential side effects. This news makes it abundantly clear that sleeping pills won't provide the rest you need. In fact, new studies now show that sleeping pills only help you fall asleep about 12 minutes sooner and gain only about 12 minutes extra sleep per night—hardly a big deal.[21]

Unfortunately, there is no simple solution since there can be many underlying causes of poor sleep, including stress, excessive snoring or sleep apnea, medications, hormonal changes, food additives and caffeine, low-grade aches and pains, systemic inflammation, and an uncomfortable bed. Many of these, of course, just go away if you're on the Baseline of Health Program, but there are actions you can take to help things along.

- Avoid alcoholic drinks in the late evening. Although alcohol can help you fall asleep faster, it prevents you from entering stage 3 and stage 4 (delta) sleep. In other words, you may get enough hours of sleep, but it won't feel like it.

- Cut back on coffee, tea, and other sources of caffeine. The half-life of caffeine is about six hours; in other words, it takes about six hours for half its impact on the body to clear. Obviously, any caffeine you have in the evening will have a notable impact on your ability to sleep that night.

- Don't eat a large, late evening meal before going to bed. You may be able to fall asleep, but again, as with alcohol, it will limit your ability to enter delta sleep. Even more important, though, is that it is physically exhausting trying to digest large meals while sleeping: you are likely to wake up in the middle of the night sweating profusely, breathing heavily, and feeling that alien creatures are beating you up from the inside out. The net result is that you are more than likely to feel exhausted in the morning.

- It is also imperative that you address any physical aches, pains, or discomforts, no matter how minor they might be, that could be interfering with your ability to sleep.

- Find a mattress that works for you. Most people use counterproductive sleeping surfaces—mattresses that are either too hard or that don't provide enough support. If you find yourself waking up stiff or with back pain, you need a new sleeping surface. If you have the money, try a memory foam mattress or one of the new adjustable air mattress beds. For less money, you can just use a feather mattress pad on top of a firm-mattress bed. The bottom line is that if you wake up stiff, achy, exhausted, or numb in any part of your body, you probably need to rethink your current sleep system.

- Do some form of vigorous exercise during the day, but gently stretch at night. Or get a massage. If having a regular masseuse is not in the cards for you, pick up a handheld mechanical massage device, such as a thumper type personal massage unit. And if money really is no object, check out some of the newer computer-operated massage chairs.

- If not a massage, try taking a hot bath or shower in the evening. If you've got the money and can afford it, a home far-infrared sauna can help.

- If you're exhausted during the day, you can take a 20-minute power nap; otherwise, avoid napping during the day as it can interfere with your normal sleep pattern.

- If your mind is too active to fall asleep, try meditating or walking to quiet the mind. Even standing barefoot in the grass or dirt for just five minutes can do an amazing job in discharging tension from the mind. (This works much better on a warm summer evening as opposed to standing in a snow-drift in the middle of winter.)

- Try doing three rounds of alternate-nostril breathing before lying down to go to sleep. This is tremendously relaxing. First, close your right nostril with your right thumb and inhale through the left nostril to the count of four. Then close both nostrils (using your right ring finger and little finger to close the left nostril) and hold for a count of sixteen. Now remove your thumb from the right nostril, and exhale through this nostril to the count of eight. This completes a half round. Next, inhale through the right nostril to the count of four. Hold both nostrils closed for a count of sixteen. Then, close the right nostril with your right thumb and exhale through the left nostril to a count of eight. This completes one full round. If you need to, take it down to a count of three, twelve, and six to get started. As you get more comfortable, you can slowly increase the times of inhalation, holding, and exhalation to whatever feels comfortable, but always keep the 1:4:2 ratio. Do not strain.

And, yes, there are supplements that can help.

- Many people find that regular use of a good proteolytic enzyme supplement can help make little aches and pains go away, thus facilitating sleep.

- Taking 100–200 mg of L-theanine at night can significantly reduce stress and facilitate sleep.

- Ashwagandha can also help promote sleep. Dosage depends on the brand you use and the concentration of its bioactive substances.

- Magnesium supplements can help. Keep in mind that calcium excites nerves whereas magnesium calms them down. Calcium makes muscles contract; magnesium helps them relax. Instead of a calcium/magnesium supplement, think of taking a supplement in which the magnesium is dominant. The best form of supplement for this purpose is a powdered one, so that it mixes with warm water and can be rapidly taken up by the body.

- Melatonin can also help. Dosage varies according to your needs, ranging from 0.3 mg to 20 mg a day. The correct dosage is the one that helps you sleep but let's you wake up without feeling "drugged." Start with 0.5 mg and increase by 0.5 mg a night until you find what works for you. Note that the effects of supplementation often carry over several nights, so you may need to supplement only every other night or every third night. As you get older, you can increase the amount and frequency of supplementation as needed.

- Certain herbs can help: valerian, chamomile, kava kava, St. John's wort, lavender, passionflower, hops, and skullcap are possible choices.

- One final note: There are a couple of special situations such as sleep apnea and restless legs syndrome that can affect sleep. Both of these conditions respond favorably to the full Baseline of Health Program.

## GENERAL RECOMMENDATIONS

Casting aside the extreme point of view that all illness originates in the mind, we are nonetheless left with the fact that what we think (and how we think) unequivocally affects our health. Or as Dr. John Christopher, one of America's foremost naturopaths, was fond of saying, "Most people need a colonic between the ears." If you want to make your mind a partner in health, you need to work at it. Make the effort to move your mind out of stress and/or depression and into relaxation. Listed below are ways to begin the process.

- Learn to meditate—If nothing else, just try watching your breath. Sit down, with your back straight, close your eyes, and concentrate on your breathing. Watch as your breath goes in and your lungs fill, and watch as it goes out and your lungs empty. Don't force; just watch. Enjoy the spaces between inhalation and exhalation.

- Learn to visualize—After you've meditated for a few minutes and calmed down, practice a visualization. See your body as made of healing light, and imagine this light penetrating and soothing every cell in your body. If you are sick, focus the light on the diseased area.

- Practice alternate nostril breathing as described in the section above.

- Practice affirmation—What we say matters. We all probably know, for example, someone who uses the word "afraid" all the time. As in: "I'm afraid I won't be able to go tonight" or "I'm afraid I've eaten too much; I'm absolutely stuffed." Is it any wonder that eventually they're afraid all the time? Dr. Bernie Siegel includes several examples of this negative thinking in his book *Love, Medicine, and Miracles*, such as the man who said "he was always considered spineless" and in the end developed multiple myeloma in his backbone to support his contention. Or the woman who had had a mastectomy who kept telling Dr. Siegel that she "needed to get something off her chest."

  Instead of being controlled by the things we say, instead of having our health compromised by idle words, we should put words to work for us. Try repeating to yourself over and over, with each step you take when you walk or while you're driving, something like, "I'm joy. I'm peace. I'm health. I'm light." Or make up your own affirmation—make it short and rhythmic, so that it almost says itself to a walking cadence. It really works magic. I once hiked the John Muir Trail, starting in the Yosemite Valley in California's Sierra Nevada Mountains, about 237 miles in all, silently reciting a similar affirmation every step of the way. By the end of the trip, I had repeated the affirmation over 500,000 times, and I had sailed over 10,000-foot passes and up and down the 14,500 feet of Mt. Whitney.

- Take an herbal/nutraceutical break—Use a nerve tonic formulation that contains herbs such as valerian root, *mulungu*, ashwagandha, passion-flower, chamomile, lavender, bergamot, St. John's wort, and lobelia, and/or nutraceuticals such as phenylalanine and theanine.

• Try using SAMe—200–1,600 mg a day.

As you can see, there are many alternatives to try. Using antidepressants before looking to address possible underlying causes by trying these options first is not a healthy way to go. Only when all other options have been tried first should you turn to pharmaceutical solutions.

In this chapter, we've looked at how our thoughts affect our health. Next, we'll get physical and look at the health benefits of exercise.

# CHAPTER 17

## *Exercise—Move or Die*

- **The Benefits of Exercise**
- **Different Types of Exercise**
- **Nutrition and Exercise**

N o one likes to hear this, but it's true: if you don't move, you die ... eventually. Exercise fundamentally changes every system and function in your body. Unfortunately, very few people now exercise enough. In June 2007, a poll showed that 35 percent of Americans did not exercise at all, or at most once a week,[1] with approximately the same percentage considered clinically obese.[2] Hmm. Throw in another 25 percent who said that they exercised a total of 60–90 minutes a week—the barest minimum of a routine—and you're looking at approximately 60 percent of people who don't get enough exercise, about the same percentage that qualifies as overweight in the United States. You can see a direct correlation between lack of sufficient exercise and excess weight, but the importance of exercise goes far beyond obesity.

## THE BENEFITS OF EXERCISE

Exercise impacts almost every aspect of health. It can:

- Reduce the risk of premature death
- Reduce the risk of heart disease—the heart is a muscle and grows stronger with exercise
- Alleviate high blood pressure and high cholesterol
- Reduce the risks of many cancers, including colon and breast cancer— women who exercise regularly reduce their risk of breast cancer by 72 percent[3]

- Reduce the risk of developing diabetes

- Contribute to the loss of fat and the optimization of body weight

- Promote peristalsis and relieve constipation

- Build and maintain healthy muscles, bones, and joints—exercise increases bone density

- Ease depression and anxiety

- Enhance performance in all aspects of life

Since exercise is so important, let's look at some of these benefits in a little more detail before we explore the different types of exercise to incorporate into your daily routine.

## Circulation

First and foremost, exercise is about circulation—not just blood circulation, but every circulation system in the body. We're talking about blood, lymph, and energy.

- Blood—Exercise definitely improves the flow of blood. Think what this means for a moment. Even if you eat healthy foods and partake of the most powerful supplements in the world, if that nutrition can't easily reach some part of your body because circulation is restricted, then that part will suffer, waste away, and become diseased. If the blockage is total, that part will die. This could be an organ, a group of cells within an organ, or even a single cell. Blood also brings oxygen to, and removes carbon dioxide waste from, every cell and organ in your body. Again, if circulation is restricted, the cell or organ slowly suffocates in its own waste. Finally, blood carries immune cells and pH (acid/alkaline) balancers to every part of your body. Exercise drives your blood through your body, forcing oxygen and nutrition into every nook and cranny.

- Lymph—Previously, we discussed how lymph is your body's sewer system, removing dead cells, waste, toxic matter, heavy metals, bacteria, and so on from body tissue. Unfortunately, the lymph system has no pump (like the heart) of its own—to a large degree, your body depends on muscle movement to press waste through the lymph system. If you don't move, your lymph is stagnant and you end up poisoning yourself.

- Energy—The Chinese call energy *chi*; the yogis of India call it *prana*; others call it "life force." Whatever you call it, it can be seen, measured, photographed, felt, and manipulated. According to Chinese medicine, restriction in its flow is the ultimate cause of all disease. Exercise stimulates and helps move this "energy" through blocked areas of the body.

## Strength

Strength is not just for showing off in the weight room—it is essential as we get older. People who exercise regularly are far less likely to fall and break bones. This is because the exercise has made them stronger as well as given them better balance. Also, the larger muscle mass cushions the bones better and protects them if you should fall.

## Body Fat

There's nothing more fundamental to losing body fat than exercise. Not, as many people think, because the exercise burns the fat off, but rather because muscle burns fat even while you sleep (60–70 percent of the energy your muscles burn, even while sleeping, is fat). The more muscle you have, the more calories you burn. Every pound of muscle that you have burns fat calories 24 hours a day. If you add four pounds of muscle to your body, every day you automatically burn an extra 200 calories or so, free of charge (plus another 200 calories from your exercise). Or to think of it another way, you get to burn off a scoop of Häagen-Dazs® ice cream every two days—while sleeping.

## Biochemical Changes

Exercise produces "happy" biochemicals called endorphins. Sometimes referred to as "the runner's high," these endorphins drive away stress and depression and stimulate the immune system. In addition, exercise increases levels of human growth hormone (HGH) in the body. Aerobic exercise can increase HGH levels by as much as 200 percent, while weight training can boost HGH an astounding 400–800 percent.

## DIFFERENT TYPES OF EXERCISE

It's not my purpose in this chapter to teach you how to exercise—there are many books, DVDs, and websites that teach you how to do that—but rather to explain to you why you need to exercise and why you need to commit to multiple forms of exercise. Believe it or not, running every day won't cut it, nor will going to the gym and working out with weights every day. You need it all: cardiovascular/aerobic exercise, strength training, weight-bearing exercise, stretching, breathing, and balance. Let's explore why.

## Cardiovascular/Aerobic Exercise

By definition, cardiovascular/aerobic exercise is brisk physical activity that requires the heart and lungs to work harder to meet the body's increased oxygen demand. Aerobic exercise promotes the circulation of oxygen through the blood. The key part of the definition here is the word *oxygen*. The defining aspect of aerobic exercise is that it is of sufficient intensity to force the heart and lungs to work harder, and yet of low enough intensity to facilitate adequate oxygen transfer to the muscle cells without a buildup of lactic acid (a waste product that causes muscle "burn"). In other words, aerobic exercise involves repetitive movement of large muscle groups (such as your arms, legs, and hips) with all of the needed energy supplied by the oxygen you breathe. When you're aerobically fit, your body takes in and utilizes oxygen more efficiently to sustain the repetitive muscle movement. The health benefits of cardio include:

- Improved heart and lung function, resulting in increased blood supply to muscles and improved ability to use oxygen

- Lower heart rate and blood pressure

- Increased high-density lipoprotein (HDL) cholesterol and decreased triglycerides

- Improved glucose tolerance and reduced insulin resistance

- Lowered blood sugar levels and reduced risk of diabetes

- Reduced body fat and improved weight control

- Enhanced immune function, including increased resistance to viral and bacterial infections and cancer

- Longer life expectancy

There is a world of aerobic exercise to choose from. Pick one or two that you enjoy and can easily pursue. For example, don't choose swimming if you live in the desert and the nearest pool is sixty miles away. Running, jogging, and fast walking are all good choices. Biking (either road or mountain) and swimming are also good. If you belong to a gym or have home equipment, there are treadmills, elliptical trainers, spin cycles, and rebounders, with more options being added all the time.

### Interval Training

Interval training is a specialized form of aerobic workout that alternates bouts of heavy work with periods of rest or light work. As such, it works both your body's aerobic and anaerobic systems. During the high-intensity part of the workout, your body draws upon glycogen (a form of sugar) stored in the muscles for energy. No oxygen is required to produce energy during this phase of the workout, thus it is considered anaerobic. Anaerobic exercise produces an oxygen debt, the byproduct of which is lactic acid, experienced as the burning sensation in your muscles. During the slower parts of the workout, your heart and lungs work aerobically (with oxygen) to convert stored carbohydrates into energy and pay back the accumulated oxygen debt and break down the lactic acid.

With repeated interval training, your body adapts to the alternating stresses of the training. Your body builds new capillaries so it can more efficiently move oxygen into muscles and lactic acid out. Muscles develop a higher tolerance to the buildup of lactic acid, and your heart muscle is strengthened.

## Strength Training

Strength training involves the use of weights or some other form of resistance to build muscle and increase strength. Its health benefits include:

- Increased muscle strength
- Increased tendon and ligament strength
- Reduced body fat and increased muscle mass
- Better balance
- Lower blood cholesterol
- Improved glucose tolerance and insulin sensitivity

Contrary to popular opinion, strength training is not just for young people. Studies have shown that people in their seventies and eighties can experience strength gains of as much as 180 percent in a few weeks. Just two

45-minute weight (strength) training sessions a week can improve bone density, muscle mass, strength, balance, and physical activity in older women (ages 50–70).[4] After one year of strength training, women were physiologically younger by 15–20 years than when they began. Other studies have demonstrated the same results for men who weight train.

What kinds of strength training options are available? As with aerobics, there is a world of choices: free weights, stacked weight machines, and Nautilus circuits are available in most gyms. Other options include resistance training on Soloflex and Bowflex machines and push/pull resistance with the Delta Trimax machine. Pilates equipment and the Total Gym use your own body weight as resistance. Choose one that works for you and that you can do easily and regularly.

Again, it's worth noting that weight training is the ultimate way to burn calories fast. A pound of muscle burns up to nine times the calories of a pound of fat. In other words, strength training increases your resting metabolic rate, which is the number of calories you burn while sleeping or sitting. The trick is that muscle is active tissue—it requires a lot of energy just to maintain itself. In fact, every pound of new muscle you add to your body will burn about 60 calories per day. Adding just 10 pounds of muscle to your body (something that won't happen by sitting in front of your computer) will burn off the calorie equivalent of 62 pounds of fat over the next year, even while you are sleeping, and it will continue to do so year after year.

## Weight-Bearing Exercise

Weight-bearing exercise is actually a subset of certain aerobic and strength training exercises. It is exercise in which you force your body to support weight (your own included) while exercising. Studies have shown that weight-bearing exercise can help slow down the rate of bone loss and osteoporosis, and therefore reduce fractures. How does it do this? Weight-bearing exercise directly stimulates bone formation. Then it strengthens muscles that in turn pull and tug on bones—this pulling action actually causes the bones to become denser and stronger. Weight-bearing activities at any age benefit bone health. Studies have shown that even people in their nineties can increase bone mass with weight-bearing exercise.

The best weight-bearing exercises are weight-lifting, jogging, hiking with a backpack, stair climbing, step aerobics, racquet sports, and other activities that require your muscles to work against gravity. Swimming and simple walking won't do the trick. One exceptionally useful form of weight-bearing exercise is rebounding (bouncing on a mini-trampoline). The act of rebounding makes use of gravitational forces (g-forces), just like astronauts training in a centrifuge. Rebounding can actually achieve momentary g-forces of 3.5, which means that the bones of a 150-pound person will momentarily have to bear 525 pounds of weight on each bounce—a good workout.

The benefits of weight-bearing exercise are site-specific, meaning that you strengthen only the bones used directly in the exercise. So it's a good idea to participate in a variety of weight-bearing exercises. To maintain the bone-building benefits, the exercise needs to be done on a regular basis.

## Stretching

Stretching is the stepchild of exercise, with more lip service paid to it than actual practice. Stretching, though, is crucial to good health. The health benefits include:

- Reduced muscle tension

- Injury prevention

- Increased range of movement in the joints

- Enhanced muscular coordination

- Increased circulation of the blood to various parts of the body

- Increased energy levels (resulting from increased circulation)

- Stress relief

- Improved posture

- Improved organ function

Think for a moment of the opposite of stretching: tightness and restriction. By definition, you are talking about constriction in muscles and soft tissue, meaning reduced blood flow, a reduced supply of nutrients to the area of tension, and reduced removal of metabolic wastes. Areas that are tense and constricted, then, are breeding grounds for illness and organ dysfunction. Traditional Chinese medicine states that all disease results from restrictions in the flow of energy (*chi* or *qi*) in the body and the resulting energy imbalances. So, you can see that stretching is not just an issue of feeling good—it is essential for maintaining optimum health.

What kinds of stretching are good? Yoga is probably the best stretching exercise there is, but Pilates works well too. If nothing else, do five to ten minutes of simple stretching after your daily exercise routine as part of your cool-down time. It is not by accident that at sixty years old, I can still do full splits.

## Resistance Breathing

Proper breathing is a topic worthy of its own chapter (in another book), but for now let's focus on the advantages of resistance breathing. The concept is simple: putting a device in your mouth that restricts (in a controlled manner) your inhalations and exhalations, which forces your lungs to work harder. This, in turn, strengthens the muscles that make your lungs work and increases their capacity. There are a number of such devices available on the Internet and in health magazines. This type of exercise can significantly improve the strength of your respiratory muscles and increase your lung capacity. Studies have shown that these devices can increase breathing endurance by close to 300 percent. Considering how fundamental oxygen is to health, it's not hard to see the short- and long-term health and performance advantages of doing so. This is not just for performance athletes—the older you are, the more important this is.

## Balance

One other key aspect of exercise is balance. Why? Because like all other physical abilities, balance diminishes with age unless we consciously exercise it. Is that a bad thing? Only if you fall down and break your hip or wrist.

Here's a simple balance exercise that you can do daily. It takes just a couple of minutes and will produce quick improvement.

- Stand, while holding onto the back edge of a chair set beside you for support.

- Bend the leg nearest to the chair at the knee 90 degrees so that your knees are still together and the foot of the bent leg is projected out behind you. Get used to balancing on the one leg while holding the chair.

- Then turn to the other side and do the same thing with the other leg.

- After a couple of days, once you can comfortably balance like this, try taking your hand off the chair and balancing on the one leg without support from the chair.

- As you get more comfortable doing this, try to stop using your arms for balance and pull your hands in, palms together in front of your chest (a prayer position). This will force the act of balance to the muscles of one leg.

- Again, after several days, once you can comfortably balance like this, try closing your eyes and holding the pose for 30 seconds.

If you really want to improve your balance, many yoga poses are specifically designed as balance poses, utilizing the arms, legs, hips, and the entire body. On a more modern note, there's a new breed of vibrating-platform exercise equipment that forces you to balance while working out. The net effect is that because the balancing aspect forces you to use an entirely separate set of muscles in addition to your normal workout muscles, it dramatically accelerates the benefits of exercise.

## NUTRITION AND EXERCISE

Exercise is as important to good health as proper nutrition. Then again, your need for proper nutrition is increased by exercise. You will need more quality protein to build the muscles you are exercising. Soy and whey are the "in vogue" supplements for body builders, but I much prefer the combination of rice protein and yellow pea protein. It is virtually of the same quality and bioavailability as those other sources, but has the advantage of being hypoallergenic and extremely easy to digest.

You also need quality carbohydrates, especially ultra-long-chain carbohydrates (ULCs) such as pre-sprouted barley. ULCs release energy over several hours and do not spike sugar levels. High-quality fats are also critical—omega-3s and GLA (gamma-linolenic acid) in particular.

When exercising, you utilize more oxygen, which produces extra free radicals, so you will need more antioxidants to clear them. Look for a full-spectrum antioxidant, rather than a single source wonder supplement (see Chapter 10). And you will want higher intake of minerals (particularly electrolytes such as potassium, magnesium, calcium, sodium, and all the trace minerals) and water-soluble vitamins (vitamin C and all of the B vitamins, for example), since you will be using them up and sweating them out at an accelerated rate. Instead of drinking high-sugar sports beverages, you might want to consider just adding liquid trace minerals to your water.

The one area that you gain nutritionally while exercising is in detoxification. Exercise is its own form of detoxification: it removes waste from the lymph, stimulates peristalsis to remove waste from the colon, and accelerates the removal of waste through sweat and urine.

## GENERAL RECOMMENDATIONS

You need to cross-train for maximum benefit: do cardio/aerobic exercise, strength training, weight-bearing exercise, stretching, resistance breathing, and balance exercises. Find books, exercise DVDs, a personal trainer at your gym, or classes that you like and follow the program as laid out for you.

- The best form of cardio/aerobic exercise is interval training, which can be done with almost any form of aerobic exercise and many forms of strength training by alternating fast and slow versions of the exercise.

- Working out on an elliptical trainer or a cross-country ski machine is much easier on your body than jogging or running. Anything that involves a lot of bouncing on a hard surface (such as jogging) is likely to damage your knees and spine over time.

- Stretching should be done every day. It's invaluable as part of your aerobic and weight-training sessions to prevent injuries, and it's also great exercise on its own.

- Yoga is spectacular exercise that, if done properly, can incorporate all aspects of exercise in one. Some of the poses can build strength in the legs, arms, chest, abdomen, and in every muscle in your body. Other poses, such as the sun salutation, can work as the cardiovascular/aerobic portion of your workout. Yoga can stretch every part of your body and many poses improve balance as well. And no other form of exercise helps you master breathing and optimize your lungs to the extent that yoga can.

- Besides feeling really good, regular deep massage can be a powerful tool for speeding recovery from exercise, removing toxins from muscle tissue, and improving the overall results of your exercise program. I particularly like a form of body work called BioSync because of its unique ability to break up collagen cross-linking and restore the natural length and flexibility in muscle tissue. Saunas and steam baths likewise speed the removal of toxins from muscle tissue and accelerate recovery times. Check out the new generation of far-infrared saunas.

Of course, be sure to check with your doctor before starting any exercise program. But keep in mind, anyone can exercise. If all you can do is hobble around the bed using a walker, you can start with one trip around the bed the first day, two the next, three the third, and so on. If you're confined to bed or a wheelchair, work your upper body. Extend your limits. Move or die.

That finishes our discussion of the core Baseline of Health Program. In the remaining chapters, we'll explore the issues that have elicited thousands of questions at www.jonbarron.org over the last ten years—namely, treatments for specific ailments. And what better place to begin than with the "cholesterol myth."

# PART FIVE
# *Specific Conditions*

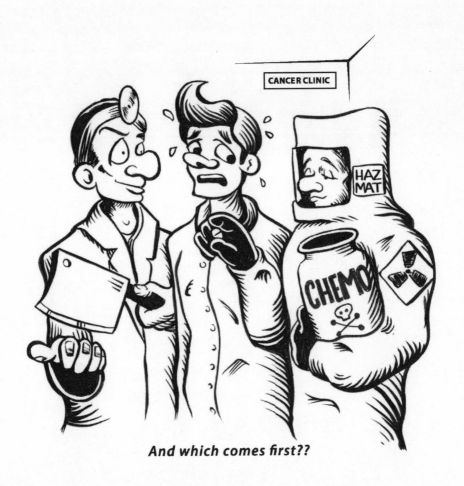

**And which comes first??**

# CHAPTER 18

# The Cholesterol Myth and Other Cardiovascular Stories

- **The Cholesterol Theory of Heart Disease**
- **Challenging the Theory**
- **An Alternative Theory**
- **Real Solutions for Cardiovascular Problems**
- **A Final Word on Cholesterol**
- **A New Key to Heart Attacks**

We live in a cholesterol obsessed world. Every day, we are bombarded with television and magazine advertisements that tell us we must lower our cholesterol (and why their company's drug can do it best). And every couple of years, a new announcement from the medical community tells us that we need to lower our national cholesterol targets—conveniently mandating that doctors encourage another 20 million or so more patients to get on a regimen of statin drugs for the rest of their lives. So, what's it all about? What is cholesterol, and should we really be so afraid of it?

Cholesterol is not a fat but rather a soft, waxy, "fat-like" substance that circulates in the bloodstream. It is not a villain. It is vital to life and is found in all cell membranes. It is necessary for the production of bile acids, steroid hormones, and vitamin D. Cholesterol is manufactured by the liver, but it is also present in all animal foods—abundant in organ meats, shellfish, and egg yolks, and contained in smaller amounts in all meats and poultry. Vegetable oils and shortenings contain no cholesterol.

Cholesterol cannot dissolve in the blood, so your liver combines it with special proteins called lipoproteins to "liquefy" it. The lipoproteins used by the liver are either very-low-density lipoproteins (VLDLs) or high-density lipoproteins (HDLs), which correspondingly produce LDL cholesterol and HDL cholesterol. HDL is called the "good" cholesterol because HDL particles prevent atherosclerosis by extracting cholesterol buildup from arterial walls and disposing of it through the liver. LDL cholesterol is called "bad" cholesterol because elevated LDL is associated with an increased risk of coronary heart disease. Thus, high levels of LDL and low levels of HDL (high LDL/HDL ratios) are considered by most doctors to be a risk factor for atherosclerosis, while low levels of LDL and high levels of HDL (low LDL/HDL ratios) are considered desirable.

It is important to note that the liver not only manufactures and secretes LDL cholesterol into the blood, it also removes it. To remove LDL, the liver relies on special proteins called LDL receptors that are normally present on the surface of liver cells. LDL receptors snatch LDL cholesterol particles from the blood and transport them inside the liver. A high number of active LDL receptors on the liver surfaces are associated with the rapid removal of LDL cholesterol from the blood and low blood LDL levels. A deficiency of LDL receptors is associated with high LDL cholesterol blood levels. Note: It is also crucial that the cholesterol which has been stored in the liver by the LDL receptors be regularly "flushed" by the liver to make room for "new" deposits, or the process comes to a standstill, thus causing levels to soar in the bloodstream. It's probably worth mentioning that the concept that you might have to flush cholesterol stored in the liver to make room for new cholesterol coming from the bloodstream, a foundational tenet in the alternative health community, has not yet made its way into the medical establishment's cholesterol theory of heart disease.

In point of fact, the liver is responsible for over 80 percent of your cholesterol level, while diet accounts for less than 20 percent. Yes, genetics plays a role in how efficiently your liver works and how many LDL receptors there are on the surface of your liver, but lifestyle and its effect on the liver plays a far bigger role.

## THE CHOLESTEROL THEORY OF HEART DISEASE

According to the cholesterol theory of heart disease (and despite all that you may have heard, it is only a theory), LDL cholesterol in the blood combines with other substances such as cellular waste products, calcium, and fibrin (a clotting protein) to form arterial plaque, which attaches itself to the inner lining of the arteries. Over time, cholesterol plaque causes thickening of the artery walls and narrowing of the arteries, a process called atherosclerosis. Arteries that supply blood and oxygen to the heart muscles are called coronary arteries. When coronary arteries are narrowed by atherosclerosis, they are incapable of supplying enough blood and oxygen to the heart muscle during exertion. Lack of oxygen to the heart muscle (ischemia) causes chest pain. Formation of a blood clot in a coronary artery can clause complete blockage of that artery, leading to death of heart muscle tissue—a heart attack. (Of course, an artery significantly narrowed by atherosclerosis is that much more easily blocked by a blood clot.) Atherosclerotic disease of the coronary arteries (coronary heart disease) is the most common cause of death in the United States, accounting for about 750,000 deaths annually.

## Causes of High Cholesterol

Again, according to the cholesterol theory of heart disease, both heredity and diet have a significant influence on a person's LDL, HDL, and total cholesterol levels. For example, familial hypercholesterolemia is a common inherited disorder whose victims have a diminished or nonexistent number of LDL receptors on the surface of liver cells. The resultant decreased activity of the LDL receptors limits the liver's ability to remove LDL cholesterol from blood. Thus, affected family members have abnormally high LDL cholesterol levels in the blood, and they also tend to develop atherosclerosis and heart attacks during early adulthood.

Diets that are high in saturated fats and cholesterol decrease the LDL receptor activity in the liver, thereby raising the levels of LDL cholesterol in the blood. Saturated fats are derived primarily from meat and dairy products and, according to most doctors, can raise blood cholesterol levels. Some vegetable oils made from coconut, palm, and cocoa are also high in saturated fats and are on the medical "no-no" list. On the other hand, most vegetable oils are high in unsaturated fats. Unlike saturated fats, unsaturated fats do not raise blood cholesterol (again, according to the theory) and can sometimes lower cholesterol. Olive and canola oil are high in monounsaturated fats, which may have a protective effect against coronary heart disease. And now doctors tell us to be sure to avoid hydrogenated and partially hydrogenated vegetable oils as the hydrogenation process produces trans-fats as a byproduct, and trans-fats raise LDL cholesterol. (At least on this one point, the cholesterol theory has finally caught up with alternative health theory.)

## Clinical Guidelines on Cholesterol Levels

In May 2001, the National Cholesterol Education Panel (NCEP) issued major new clinical practice guidelines on the prevention and treatment of high cholesterol levels in adults, lowering the target optimum level for LDL to less than 100. This was the first major update of the NCEP guidelines since 1993. The NCEP predicted that the new guidelines would increase the number of Americans "requiring" treatment for elevated cholesterol levels from 52 million to 65 million and would nearly triple the number of Americans who would need to take cholesterol-lowering drugs (from 13 million to 36 million). But for many doctors, 36 million people under experimental drug therapy are just not enough. Many "experts" are now pushing to set target limits for LDL to less than 80, which would mandate that tens of millions of additional Americans be on moderate to high doses of statin drugs for the rest of their lives, despite the fact that these drugs are known to cause significant liver damage.

Of course, there are the usual assortment of U.S. Food and Drug Administration (FDA)–approved double-blind studies to back these conclusions. In the past ten years, clinical trials have "conclusively" demonstrated that lowering LDL cholesterol reduces heart attacks and saves lives.[1] The benefits of lowering LDL cholesterol, according to these studies, include reducing the formation of new cholesterol plaques, eliminating existing plaques, preventing rupture of plaques, decreasing the risk of heart attacks, and lowering the chance of strokes.

## CHALLENGING THE THEORY

So, what's my problem? Quite simply, it's that cholesterol doesn't cause plaque to accumulate on arterial walls. If it did, then why doesn't anyone ever have clogged veins, only clogged arteries? Think about that for a moment. If high levels of LDL cholesterol promote the formation of plaque and its accumulation on arterial walls, then why doesn't it accumulate on the walls of veins? And the answer is because the problem is centered in the walls of the arteries, not in the cholesterol circulating in the bloodstream. That's the cholesterol myth.

To understand what I'm talking about, it's first necessary to understand the beneficial role that arterial plaque plays in the human body (yes, beneficial), because therein lies the key to understanding cholesterol. The role of plaque is as "repair cement" for arterial walls. If there is any damage to the arterial wall, your body will whip up some plaque from the cholesterol, calcium, and fibrin in the bloodstream to "patch" the damage before the arterial wall develops a leak, which would cause you to bleed internally. Cholesterol isn't part of the problem; it's part of the solution—to a different problem.

With that in mind, let's now look at some of the basic assumptions of the cholesterol theory of heart disease.

- Does eating a high-cholesterol diet automatically lead to heart disease? Absolutely not. Look at the results seen on the Atkins Diet, which include lowered cholesterol levels. This is pretty remarkable considering that this diet encourages the consumption of high-cholesterol foods, including large amounts of meat and dairy. Only synthetic trans-fats and refined carbohydrates need to be restricted on the program.

- Does eating a high–saturated fat diet automatically lead to heart disease? Again, no. Consider the traditional Eskimo diet, which is probably the diet with the highest saturated fat content in the world because of all the whale and seal blubber consumed. Eskimos on that diet have virtually no heart disease, that is, not until they shift to a modern Western diet. (Unfortunately, both the Atkins Diet and the Eskimo diet are associated with different problems in the long term. Eskimos on the traditional diet, for example, have an extremely high rate of osteoporosis because their diet promotes high acid levels in body tissue. The odds are we will see similar results down the road from those who live on the Atkins Diet for any period of time.)

- Does lowering cholesterol in the diet automatically reduce cholesterol levels in the bloodstream? Not necessarily—as evidenced by all the advertisements on television for statin drugs.

- Does lowering cholesterol in the bloodstream reduce the formation of new plaques? In many cases it does, but not necessarily for the reasons promoted. The primary reason may be that you've minimized the ability of the body to effect repairs. You haven't got rid of the problem—merely the ability of the problem to manifest in one particular set of symptoms.

- Do statin drugs reduce the incidence of heart attack and stroke? Yes, but as we will discuss shortly, probably not because of their ability to lower cholesterol and not without significant side effects.

## AN ALTERNATIVE THEORY

I would like to propose now an "arterial damage" theory of heart disease. Quite simply, it says that since your body produces arterial plaque in response to arterial damage, excessive plaque buildup and the concomitant hardening and narrowing of the arteries is a response to excessive damage to the arterial walls. And why only the arteries and not the veins? Because arterial walls contain significant amounts of muscle tissue that make the arterial wall particularly susceptible to damage, while veins contain much less muscle tissue and are thus less likely to suffer damage. What causes damage or inflammation to the arterial walls? As it turns out, several things.

- High homocysteine levels—Homocysteine is an amino acid produced as a normal byproduct of the breakdown of methionine (from proteins), which is an essential amino acid acquired mostly from eating meat. Homocysteine generates superoxide and hydrogen peroxide radicals, both of which have been linked to damage of the endothelial lining of arterial vessels. Studies have shown that too much homocysteine in the blood is related to a higher risk of coronary heart disease, stroke, and peripheral vascular disease.[2]

- Too much omega-6 fatty acid in the diet—The body converts linoleic acid, the primary fatty acid found in bottled vegetable oil, to arachidonic acid. The COX-2 enzyme then converts the arachidonic acid to the hormone-like prostaglandin E2 (PGE2) and to the cytokines interleukin-1 (IL-1), interleukin-6 (IL-6), and tumor necrosis factor alpha (TNFa), all of which promote inflammation in the body in general and in the arterial walls in particular. If you can't remember all of the biochemicals just mentioned, don't worry about it. All you have to remember is that excess consumption of most vegetable oils leads to inflammation of your arterial walls.

- High levels of grain-fed meats in the diet—Eating high levels of meats and animal fat from grain-fattened animals saturates the body with large amounts arachidonic acid—the same as with vegetable oils. As a point of interest, the high levels of arachidonic acid found in most meat are accumulated from the conversion of omega-6 fatty acids present in the grains used to fatten them. That means that only minimal levels of arachidonic acid are found in range-fed beef. If you can find it, range-fed beef is far healthier for you than the more common grain-fed variety.

- High acid diets—Diets high in meat, sugar, grains, and starch raise acid levels in body tissue, thereby making it hard for the body to clear the lactic acid that builds up in muscle tissue from normal muscle activity. This is a major factor and is a particular problem for arteries, since the arterial wall contains significant amounts of muscle tissue (again, veins do not) so they can contract to maintain blood pressure when changing body position (from lying down to suddenly standing up, for example). The problem is that when the acid doesn't clear from the arterial muscle tissue, it irritates, inflames, and scars the inside lining of the arterial wall adjacent to the muscle tissue.

- High levels of circulating immune complexes in the blood—Circulating immune complexes (CICs) are created when you eat complex proteins (usually from wheat, corn, and dairy) that cannot be digested thoroughly. They make their way into the bloodstream, where they are treated as allergens by the body and combined with antibodies, thus forming CICs. When the number of CICs climbs beyond the ability of the body to eliminate them, they are deposited in the body's soft tissues, including the muscle tissue in the arterial walls, thereby triggering attacks by the body's immune system, resulting in inflammation.

- Inflammation in general—C-reactive protein (CRP) is an inflammatory marker, a substance that the liver releases in response to inflammation somewhere in the body. Studies indicate that men with high levels of CRP have triple the risk of heart attack and double the risk of stroke compared to men with lower CRP levels.[3] In women, studies have shown that elevated levels of CRP may increase the risk of a heart attack by as much as seven times.[4] The statin medicines (such as Lipitor® and Zocor®) reduce levels of CRP, which may be more significant in accounting for the ability of these drugs to lower heart disease risk than the role they play in lowering cholesterol. But there are far healthier ways to lower systemic inflammation—proteolytic enzymes, as we discussed earlier, are a good example.

## REAL SOLUTIONS FOR CARDIOVASCULAR PROBLEMS

There's an ad on TV with a message something like, "Cholesterol comes from the tiramisu you had for dessert and from your Aunt Sue. If changing your diet isn't enough, be sure and ask your doctor about our drug." That ad totally misses the point. In fact, as I pointed out earlier, diet only accounts for about 20 percent of your cholesterol level. Certainly, genetics matters if it short-changed you on the number of liver LDL receptor sites you have. But that hardly limits your options to statin drugs. You always have the option of optimizing the functionality of the receptor sites that you do have in order to facilitate the movement of cholesterol into the liver, out through the bile duct, and then out through the colon. How?

- Avoid trans-fatty acids like the plague—Hydrogenated and partially hydrogenated oils (the trans-fatty acids) are the number one killer in the modern diet. Among other things, they cause the LDL receptor sites to overload.

- Optimize the liver—Do a periodic liver flush that includes the use of lipotropic herbs (herbs that promote the utilization of fats) such as dandelion root to flush accumulated fats and cholesterol from the liver and gallbladder. By flushing fats from the liver, you facilitate the movement of cholesterol from the surface LDL sites into the liver and then on out through the bile duct.

- Supplement with water-soluble fiber such as psyllium or oat bran—Water-soluble fiber lowers total cholesterol and LDL cholesterol by binding with bile acids and preventing their reabsorption into the body. This lowers cholesterol as cholesterol is a major component of bile acids, which are used by the body to aid in the digestion of fats. If soluble fiber is present in the intestinal tract, it binds with the bile acids after they have helped break down the fats in your diet and escorts them out of the body. Since they are not reabsorbed because of the presence of water-soluble fiber, the liver has to draw more cholesterol from the blood to make more bile acids to be used for further digestion. The net effect is to lower cholesterol levels in the blood.

- Lower homocysteine levels—While there is a considerable amount we do not know about homocysteine, we do know how to use nutritional supplements to reduce its levels. This is done using a combination of folic acid, vitamin $B_{12}$, and trimethylglycine (TMG), which facilitates a process called methylation, along with vitamin $B_6$, which facilitates trans-sulfuration. Such a combined approach can normalize homocysteine in 95 percent of people.

- Optimize omega-6 to omega-3 fatty acid ratios—Begin by eliminating your use of the bottled vegetable oils found in your supermarket, except for olive oil or walnut oil, and supplementing with fish oil, krill oil, perilla oil, or flaxseed oil, which are all high in omega-3s. Much of the problem with inflammatory disorders actually stems from a lopsided imbalance in dietary intake of the omega-6 and omega-3 fatty acids and the resulting cascade in pro-inflammatory activity. The ideal ratio is roughly 1 to 1; however, as we discussed previously, people in industrialized countries have replaced much of their dietary saturated fat (on the mistaken advice of their doctors and the media) with vegetable oil omega-6s. Ratios of 20 to 1 and 30 to 1 are now not uncommon. From a biochemical standpoint, this sets the stage for major arterial inflammation.

- Take antioxidants—A good antioxidant formula that contains oligomeric proanthocyanidins (OPCs), such as green tea, pine bark, and grape seed extract, can help repair damage to arterial walls (see Chapter 10).

- Use proteolytic enzymes—This is one of the most important things you can do. The regular use of proteolytic enzymes can help eliminate CICs from the body, reduce overall inflammation, dissolve accumulated plaque, and repair arterial scar tissue. Although the evidence is purely anecdotal at the moment, we have seen extraordinary results using detoxification levels of these enzymes (see Chapter 11).

## A FINAL WORD ON CHOLESTEROL

So, is there anything to worry about with high cholesterol levels? Yes, well, sort of. High cholesterol levels are indicative of other problems—a canary in the coal mine. Among other things, they can be a warning signal for liver problems, dietary imbalances, high acid levels, and chronic inflammation, which may be a factor in the onset of Alzheimer's disease and cancer in addition to heart disease. High cholesterol levels and high levels of saturated fat in the blood "thicken" the blood. If the arteries are wide open, this is not a big problem, but if the arterial walls have been narrowed or hardened, the thickened blood significantly increases the odds of a heart attack or stroke.

Of course, there are a number of natural ways to thin the blood: *Ginkgo biloba* is a blood thinner, as are garlic and proteolytic enzymes (particularly nattokinase). Coumadin is not the only—in fact, not even the best—answer. The trick, of course, is to take care of the problem, not the warning signal.

Artificially suppressing cholesterol levels with statin drugs is a bit like feeling good about your car because you've disconnected your warning lights. Not very bright.

To lower cholesterol levels without subjecting yourself to the side effects of statin drugs, try doing a liver flush and then supplementing with niacin (vitamin $B_3$) and policosanol. Policosanol is a natural supplement made from sugar cane that works by helping the liver control its production and breakdown of cholesterol, as well as being a powerful antioxidant that prevents LDL oxidation. Clinical studies show that policosanol is as effective as prescription drugs in lowering cholesterol levels, without their dangerous side effects, and it also reduces the inflammatory response in the arterial wall.[5] And speaking of the side effects of statin drugs, two stand out.

- They deplete your body's levels of coenzyme $Q_{10}$, a critical nutrient that plays a role in cellular energy production. The heart requires high levels of $coQ_{10}$ and it is also vital for nerve function and muscle integrity. Side effects of $coQ_{10}$ deficiency can include heart failure, neuropathy, inflammation of the tendons and ligaments, and muscle wasting (a condition that is so common with cholesterol drug use, it's even picked up its own name—statin myopathy). Any doctor who prescribes statin drugs without also insisting that you use a $coQ_{10}$ supplement is either ignorant or negligent.

- Statin use can cause an increase in liver enzymes, which can potentially cause permanent liver damage. Unfortunately, liver problems may develop without symptoms, so people who take statins need to have their liver function tested regularly.

## A NEW KEY TO HEART ATTACKS

Unfortunately, many of us know someone who has had a heart attack. In most instances, doctors have attributed the cause to smoking, eating habits, weight problems, high cholesterol, or high blood pressure. But a growing number of people—actually half of those who have heart attacks—are experiencing sudden heart attacks without the normal warning signs, shocking doctors and family members who thought they were healthy. Due to the nature of unexpected heart attacks, doctors so far have not been able to study the illness, understand its causes, or properly treat patients.

After years of scientific research, this is starting to change. Thanks to a

## JUST FOR FUN—QUESTIONS FOR YOUR DOCTOR

Remember, the cholesterol theory of heart disease is only a theory, a theory that is increasingly being discredited. The International Network of Cholesterol Skeptics (THINCS) is a steadily growing group of scientists, physicians, other academics, and science writers from various countries. Members of this group represent different views about the cause of atherosclerosis and cardiovascular disease. Although they do not agree on everything, the one thing they all stand against is the concept that animal fat and high cholesterol play a role in heart disease. You can check out their website at www.thincs.org. And for those of you who enjoy challenging your doctor, or if you just want to test how up-to-date their clinical knowledge is, ask them the following questions.

- If cholesterol is the main culprit in heart disease, why don't veins ever get narrowed and blocked?

- If high-cholesterol foods are responsible for raising cholesterol levels, then why do people on the high-cholesterol Atkins Diet experience such a significant drop in cholesterol levels?

- Why do Eskimos, who eat a traditional diet of almost pure saturated fat (whale and seal blubber), have almost a zero incidence of heart disease?

- If the liver is responsible for regulating up to 80 percent of my cholesterol levels, why would I want to take statin drugs for lowering cholesterol considering that the number one known side effect of statin drugs is liver damage?

major study conducted in Paris, we may have finally found the significant contributing factor: a fatty acid.[6] The study shocked the medical community, which expected to find genetics or stress at the root of the problem. But after thirty-five years of research, involving 5,240 middle-aged Parisian men with no known cardiovascular disease, doctors are now shifting their attention to non-esterified fatty acid (NEFA). Doctors found that when age, body mass index (weight), heart rate, systolic (or diastolic) blood pressure, tobacco consumption, parental history of myocardial infarction or sudden death, cholesterol, triglycerides, fasting plasma glucose (diabetic status), and insulin concentration were simultaneously entered into a matrix that looked at how and why each person died, they found that the fasting plasma NEFA concentration remained an independent risk factor for sudden death.

Circulating NEFA concentration in the blood is a factor that deserves added attention. It isn't just implicated in sudden heart attacks,[7] but there is also growing evidence that it's implicated in the onset of cancer too.[8] So, what exactly are non-esterified fatty acids? In short, NEFAs in the blood represent a buildup of excess omega-6 fats in the body. As we discussed in Chapter 7, this is caused by eating an overabundance of polyunsaturated fats such as corn, peanut, sunflower, and safflower oils—in other words, virtually every vegetable oil and processed food you buy in the supermarket. Although members of the medical community might be "shocked" by this information, it would barely elicit a knowing nod from anyone who has read this far.

How do NEFAs cause sudden heart attacks? Scientists are still trying to find a direct link, but some studies have shown that high levels of NEFAs can alter potassium channels, which means they inhibit the proper flow of potassium in and out of heart cells.[9] This is important since the heart is a pump controlled by the exchange of ions through the aforementioned channels, thereby generating electrical signals. Voltage dependence is regulated by the concentration of extracellular potassium. As external potassium is raised, the voltage range of the channel opening shifts to more positive voltages. Simply put, heart cells regulate the positive potassium charge with other ions and the result is a heartbeat. Upset the balance and you upset the heartbeat—and NEFAs upset the balance. Also, scientists found a correlation between NEFAs and high intracellular sodium and calcium levels, which also affect heart rhythms. And finally, studies have shown that an overabundance of NEFAs can interfere with endothelial nitric oxide production, which can lead to hypertension.[10]

Numerous studies have shown that a dietary supplement of omega-3 fatty acids can reduce the NEFA concentration in plasma and in cell membranes and suppress fast heart rhythms associated with heart attacks. Eating fish and taking omega-3s reduces the risk of sudden cardiac arrest. Another option, of course, is just cutting back on the amount of highly refined, high omega-6 vegetable oils.

## GENERAL RECOMMENDATIONS

Eating and cooking with processed oil is a part of the problem, but our dietary ratio of omega-6 to omega-3 fatty acids needs to change. What can we do to protect ourselves from NEFAs and balance our omega ratios? First of all, those of you who follow the guidelines of the Baseline of Health Program will be covered.

- Stop using all plastic fats. Eliminate all hydrogenated and super-refined vegetable oils. Again, there is a huge difference between highly refined and cold-pressed oils. They are not the same, and they behave very differently in the body.

- Stop cooking with high omega-6 oils, such as safflower, sunflower, and corn oil, and shift to olive and walnut oils (low temperature), coconut and grape seed oils (higher temperature), avocado and rice bran oils (highest temperature), and organic butter (in moderation).

- Eat omega-3-rich foods such as walnuts, flaxseeds, leaf lettuce, and cold-water fish. I would caution on the amount of fish since most fish is contaminated with mercury and PCBs. One solution is to eat wild salmon from Alaska. You can also take a molecularly distilled fish oil, flax oil, perilla oil, or krill oil supplement. When it comes to flax, I use ground flaxseed and prefer the seed to the oil because of its beneficial fiber and its higher lignan content, which has anticancer and cardiovascular-promoting benefits.

- Make sure you get enough B vitamins, including $B_{12}$, folic acid, and trimethylglycine (TMG), and pro-methylation supplements such as SAMe.

- Take the amino acid carnitine. Research shows that carnitine carries fatty acids into the mitochondria of your cells where they are quickly burned for fuel or cell energy. Some doctors recommend 400–500 mg of acetyl-L-carnitine, three times a day. This can naturally force the body to "burn up" the NEFAs in the bloodstream and use them to energize your body.

- For overall heart protection and maximum health benefits, shift from a high-glycemic, refined carbohydrate diet to a more Mediterranean-style diet.

When it comes to cardiovascular disease in general, remember that NEFAs are only one aspect of heart disease and that you should still eat healthy, exercise, supplement with the homocysteine-protectant supplements, and quit smoking. I also highly recommend systemic proteolytic enzymes, which can help eliminate CICs from the body, reduce overall inflammation, dissolve accumulated plaque, and repair arterial scar tissue. In addition, a good antioxidant formula helps repair arterial damage, and a regular liver detox helps keep fats and cholesterol from accumulating where they don't belong.

Many of our health problems have resulted from following the mistaken medical advice to shift away from the old natural standbys (olive oil, butter) to ultra-refined, low saturated fat, high omega-6 vegetable oils. Once again, we let medical doctors (who do not study nutrition) tell us what to eat to stay healthy, with disastrous results. How many millions of people have died because the medical community and government health agencies convinced them to consume vast amounts of omega-6 fatty acids? And now, whoops, they're changing their minds! Albert Einstein once said that insanity was doing what you've always done and believing that one day the results will be different. Why do we believe that one day the "health establishment" will actually get "health and nutrition" right? Maybe it's time to stop the insanity and just get back to the basics of good health.

Note: An eagerly awaited trial, sponsored by Merck and Schering-Plough and completed in 2006 (but not released until 2007), found that after several years on two types of cholesterol-lowering medications, patients reduced their cholesterol levels, but reaped no significant health benefits unless they already had heart disease. These results would be no surprise to anyone who just read this chapter. As a side note, in December 2007, a Congressional committee began investigating why Merck and Schering-Plough held back releasing the data for more than a year.

In the next chapter, we'll take a look at the state of cancer treatment here at the beginning of the twenty-first century.

# CHAPTER 19

# *Let's Talk About Cancer*

- **The State of Cancer Today**
- **The Cancer Industry**
- **Cancer and Its Causes**
- **Understanding the Failure of the "War on Cancer"**
- **The Game is Rigged**

*I*'m not going to prescribe or play doctor in this chapter, but rather explore the nature of cancer on a theoretical basis. Nevertheless, I think you will find that this exploration opens up a whole range of possible treatment options—once you understand the true nature of the disease.

## THE STATE OF CANCER TODAY

First, let's talk about the state of cancer in the United States today. If you believe what you read in the press, cancer treatment is making great strides: diagnosis and treatment are better than ever, more people are being saved than ever before, people are living longer after diagnosis, discovery of the cancer gene and the elusive "cure for cancer" are right around the corner, and things have never looked better for winning the "war on cancer."

On the other hand, if you look just below the surface, you find an entirely different story:

- We spend $209 billion a year on cancer treatment in the United States.[1]

- In the February 9, 1994, issue of the *Journal of the American Medical Association*, the "war on cancer" was declared a failure: "In all age groups, cancer incidence is increasing. . . . Few new effective treatments have been devised for the most common cancers."

- The incidence of cancer is soaring, up between 800 and 1,700 percent in the last 100 years (depending on whose numbers you look at). According to the American Cancer Society, one in every 2.5 Americans will get some form of invasive cancer in their lives, and half of those who get it will die from it.[2] Now, it is true that the rates for some forms of cancer—prostate, colon, and breast cancers—have dropped slightly in the last couple of years, but that drop is only relative to the extremely high levels that were reached in the last 100 years. Rates for other forms of cancer, such as lymph cancer and pancreatic cancer, have soared.

- More people are dying from cancer than ever before. In the early 1900s, cancer was a rare occurrence in the American population. Today, it is the number two killer in the United States, trailing only heart disease.

So, which story is true? They can't both be true, can they? Actually, they can—sort of. Benjamin Disraeli, one of England's great prime ministers, once said, "There are three kinds of lies in the world: lies, damn lies, and statistics." And that's exactly what we have here: statistical lies. Just do a little logical thinking and the truth begins to shine forth. So, let's take these claims one at a time and see what the truth is behind them.

## Lies, Damn Lies, and Statistics

### *"More people are surviving cancer than ever before."*

If mortality rates are virtually unchanged (as stated in the *Journal of the American Medical Association*), but 800 to 1,700 percent more people are getting cancer than ever before, then 8–17 times as many people will be saved with no improvement in treatment, would they not? Thus, the remarkable claims you see in the press. On the other hand, what you don't hear as often is that 8–17 times as many people are also dying from cancer—thus, the rise of cancer to its position as the number two killer in the United States. It's also worth keeping in mind that the population of the United States has increased 400 percent in the last hundred years (75 million to 300 million). That means you can divide both the survival and mortality rates by four to adjust for the increased population. If you do that, you more than wipe out all of the survival gains, but you're still left with increased mortality of three to five times. And that's how cancer has risen from virtual obscurity to become a devastating killer in the U.S., claiming several hundred thousand people a year.

So, which is the most important statistic? Quite simply, none of them. It's the fact that survival rates are virtually unchanged. What that means is that modern medicine isn't really making much of a difference. In fact, mortality rates are actually worse than they first appear. Consider that when a cancer patient undergoes chemotherapy and then succumbs to pneumonia because their immune system has collapsed from the treatment, it is recorded as death by pneumonia, not cancer. Now, add all of the people who have died from the side effects of chemotherapy and radiation, and you find that mortality rates are not just unchanged but have gone backward.

For several years now, the medical community has been talking about the great strides it's been making in treating breast cancer, and as evidence researchers points to declining incidence and mortality statistics. But, once again, we've been "Disraelied." A recent study found that virtually all of the reduction seen in breast cancer incidence and mortality is the result of a reduction in the use of hormone replacement therapy by the medical community.[3] In other words, the reductions have almost nothing to do with improved treatment but rather are the result of fewer doctors using a treatment that gives their patients terminal cancer. The medical community continues to brag about its "success" with breast cancer as though this new information never existed. It seems that *chutzpah* is now a medical term.

### *"People are living longer with cancer than ever before."*

If better testing is diagnosing cancer earlier than ever before, then, by definition, people would be living longer after diagnosis, even with no real change in the effectiveness in treatment or the actual survival rate, would they not? The truth is that people are not really living longer (not much, anyway)—they're just being given a longer death sentence. Now, those producing these statistics claim to have accounted for this quirk, but they haven't really. For one thing, they don't account for the number of people who die from the side effects of treatment.

## THE CANCER INDUSTRY

Are we being scammed and lied to? Are cures being deliberately suppressed, as some people claim? Although many in the alternative health community believe otherwise, I think the answer to both questions is no. There is no scam and no deliberate suppression. On the other hand, with $209 billion being spent every year on cancer in the United States, cancer has become, quite simply, a major industry. And therein lies the problem: you now have vested interests competing for a piece of this monstrous pie. This leads to a series of major problems.

First, no one has an interest in preventing cancer, since that doesn't produce any money. All interest is in finding "a cure for cancer." This is where the money is. And any cure found must be proprietary, otherwise no money can be made. This is another area in which the deck is stacked against alternative treatments. Since it now takes several hundred million dollars to approve a new drug or treatment in the U.S., any program that is not proprietary can never be approved, because no one can afford to take it through the testing process if they don't own the rights to it. When you hear drug companies complain about the high cost of drug approval, don't believe it. They love it because that's what keeps small players from disrupting their multi-billion dollar profit factory.

The system also ensures that any cure must come from within the medical community—to justify all of the money being raised and spent and, in fact, to justify the doctor's very existence as a doctor. I believe this is probably the biggest single problem because, in the end, ego trumps money.

Because the cancer industry is structured this way, it means that even though it's relatively easy to reduce the incidence of cancer by close to 90 percent (back to the levels experienced 100 years ago), no one in the medical community will tell you about it. And how exactly do you cut cancer incidence by 90 percent? Just remove the cancer-causing toxins from your body—toxins that didn't even exist 100 years ago but are now present in our bodies in substantial amounts. And start regenerating your body with the essential cancer-preventing nutrients that have been removed from the mass-produced, processed foods that make up the bulk of today's diet.

Even though there are natural treatments that are at least as effective as chemotherapy, radiation, and surgery (not hard to do, since these modalities are so ineffective and have such deleterious side effects), no one in the medical community will tell you about them. And even though the concept of a "cure for cancer" is basically bogus, you will still be asked to contribute billions of tax dollars to search for it.

I know a woman who had breast cancer and had run through all the usual medical treatments to no avail. She was dying and, in fact, had been sent home to die by her doctors. As a last resort, she went on the Baseline of Health Program and experienced a total recovery. To celebrate her recovery, she now runs regularly in "breast cancer" races to raise money for "medical" research—and she's absolutely oblivious to the contradiction.

## CANCER AND ITS CAUSES

Does anyone really believe that cancer somehow magically appears in isolated spots in your body for no particular reason? Do they also believe that removing or destroying that "isolated" cancer means that you're cured? Do the above statements sound silly, or even absurd, to you? Well, virtually all modern cancer research and treatments are based on these two premises. Think about it. The "cure" for cancer as practiced by the medical establishment is to surgically remove it, burn it out with focused beams of radiation, poison it with chemotherapy, or all of the above together. If we truly want to end the cancer scourge, we need to look elsewhere for answers. In fact, we need to consider an entirely different paradigm.

I submit to you that cancer is fundamentally a disease of the immune system. What do I mean by that? In your body, as part of the normal metabolic process, you produce anywhere from a few hundred to as many as 10,000 cancerous cells each day. Everybody does. So why doesn't everybody get cancer? Because, as we discussed in Chapter 14, your immune system has the ability to recognize each of those aberrant cells and remove them from your body. That's what a healthy immune system does.

Then why do some people get cancer? Because one of three things happens (and, more often than not, all three together):

1. You expose yourself to toxins and outside influences (such as heavy metals, radiation, rancid fats, viruses, bacteria, parasites, etc.) that dramatically increase the number of cancerous cells your body produces so that not even a healthy immune system can handle the load.

2. You compromise your immune system to the point that it can no longer handle all of the cancerous cells your body produces, thus allowing some of them to take root and establish themselves.

3. Circulation (in the broad sense) is impeded, leading to both 1 and 2 above.

### Exposure to Toxins and Other Outside Influences

The influence of some of these factors is known beyond a doubt, while others are more hypothetical (but with strong circumstantial support).

- Exposure to radiation is a known cause of cancer. Incidentally, just two computerized tomography (CT) scans during your life exposes you to as much radiation as if you stood just two miles from ground zero at Hiroshima.[4]

- Exposure to radon gas seeping up from the ground and into our houses is also a known carcinogen. Radon gas is the number two cause of lung cancer in the U.S., second only to smoking cigarettes, according to the EPA,[5] surgeon general, and the American Lung Association. Millions of homes and buildings contain high levels of radon gas.

- Living in cities with polluted air dramatically increases your chances of getting lung cancer, although, to be sure, some cities such as Los Angeles have made significant strides in improving their air quality over the last twenty years.

- There is now strong circumstantial evidence that viruses and bacteria are a major factor in producing cancer.

- Prolonged exposure to cigarette smoke is a known carcinogen.

- Chlorine in our water is a known carcinogen. In fact, there are over 2,000 known carcinogens in our water supply.

- Excessive estrogen is the only known cause of uterine cancer and plays a major role in several other kinds of cancer, including breast and prostate cancers.

- Improper elimination and the improper balance of bacteria in the colon are known to be cancer causers. Colon cancer is now the second leading cancer among men and women combined.

- Excessive buildup of free radicals is a risk factor for cancer. Related to this is the consumption of rancid fats and trans-fatty acids.

- Excessive sugar intake feeds cancer. Most cancer cells rely on glycolosis (the conversion of glucose to pyruvate) to power themselves.

- Repeated acid reflux will eventually stress the lining of the esophagus enough so that esophageal cancer results.

Does it sound overwhelming? It's only overwhelming if you're looking for a "magic bullet" cure, and then you would need dozens of bullets—one for each type of cancer. Once you understand that simple protocols such as the Baseline of Health Program will eliminate virtually all of these factors from your body in one fell swoop, then the whole concept of preventing and reversing cancer becomes much less intimidating.

## Compromised Immune System

How do we compromise our immune systems? As it turns out, almost every which way you can imagine.

- How good can your immune system be (even taking all the supplements in the world) if your colon is packed with old fecal matter? A substantial portion of your immune system then has to combat the effects of self-toxicity. Clean up your intestinal tract and you free up your immune system.

- Beneficial bacteria manufacture potent immune boosters such as transfer factor and lactoferrin right in your intestinal tract—if the bacteria are there and functioning. In other words, the proper balance of beneficial bacteria in your intestinal tract can substantially boost your immune system by increasing internal production of a number of powerful immune factors. Without those factors, your immune system is marginalized.

- Taking proteolytic enzymes between meals relieves stress on the immune system by helping to eliminate circulating immune complexes (CICs) from the body. Given today's enzymatically challenged diet, this is essential to prevent a total breakdown of your immune system.

- Proper diet and nourishment boost your immune system. Each immune cell in your body is manufactured from the food you eat. A nutritionally deficient diet means functionally deficient immune cells. You can't build the same immune cell out of pepperoni pizza, beer, and Ding Dongs® that you can out of whole, living foods. Supplementation with the proper vitamins, minerals, and phytonutrient complexes will significantly enhance the production of your body's immune cells.

- Deficiencies of the key fatty acids are a sure invitation to cancer. In fact, some of the fatty acids actually work as immune system modulators that help keep it properly programmed so it doesn't attack itself.

- Antioxidants boost the immune system in multiple ways. One example is curcumin: published studies prove that curcumin can increase the white blood cell count by 50 percent in just twelve days.[6]

- Cleaning out the liver improves its ability to produce immune factors and remove bacteria from the blood. An impaired liver is like a death sentence to your immune system.

- Cleaning out the blood and preserving your blood's pH (acid/alkaline balance) also helps to improve immune function. In fact, low pH (acidic) in body tissues is almost a guarantee for the onset of cancer.

- Invading pathogens can eventually overwhelm the immune system, rendering it incapable of performing its normal protective functions.

- Your mental attitude matters. There is a strong statistical correlation between depression and cancer.

- Lack of exercise reduces immune function and causes the lymph to stagnate, further compromising the immune system, not to mention promoting lymph cancer.

- The ingredients in a single can of cola can depress parts of your immune system by as much as 50 percent for as long as six hours. So what does that mean if you drink four to five cans of cola a day, or more?

Again, what at first appears to be overwhelming becomes quite manageable when we view it as part of the whole. The Baseline of Health Program addresses each one of these concerns.

## Impeded Circulation

I'm using the term *circulation* in the broadest sense, as it applies to all of the body's circulatory systems: blood, lymph, and energy.

If there is any restriction of blood circulation (caused by anything from narrowing of the arteries to tension in the surrounding muscle tissue) several problems arise. Sufficient oxygen can no longer reach key areas of the body. Oxygen is a cancer destroyer. Sufficient nutrients can no longer reach that area of the body, thus starving it, weakening it, and making it vulnerable to mutation. And the waste material produced by the cells can no longer be efficiently removed. The buildup of toxic waste in the cells eventually leads to cancer. And more and more studies are now identifying inflammation itself as a major factor in the onset of cancer.[7]

Your lymph is your body's sewer system, removing dead cells, waste, toxic matter, heavy metals, bacteria, etc., from body tissues. If for any reason your lymph is stagnant, you end up poisoning yourself. Cancer is a likely outcome.

Fundamentally, our bodies are pure energy systems. As you look more and more closely at the subatomic structure of all matter, the physical world begins to disappear. All that's left is a series of forces and probabilities that create the illusion of matter as we know it. Certainly, we have to deal with this illusion (the physical world) as we see it and experience it, but we also have to deal with the consequences of the world of energy, which remains unseen but is nevertheless the true reality behind all physical matter. A major factor in the onset of cancer is when these energies in our body become unbalanced or diminished in any way. Cancer cells are almost exclusively low-energy cells.

## UNDERSTANDING THE FAILURE OF THE "WAR ON CANCER"

Once we understand what cancer actually is, it's easy to understand why medical treatments for cancer have had such dismal results. Medical treatments, for the most part, are based on eliminating the "symptoms" (or manifestation) of the cancer in your body. They do absolutely nothing to eliminate the actual "cause" of the cancer—to remove the factor that initiated the growth of the cancer in the first place. Think about this for a moment. Does chemotherapy, radiation treatment, or surgery do anything for any of the causes of cancer that we discussed? No—all they do is "attempt" to remove the manifestation of the cancer that results from these causes. Is it any wonder they have had such a poor track record? Even worse, we can see that radiation and chemotherapy significantly compound the problem because they are actually known carcinogens.

### Chemotherapy

Chemotherapy drugs are some of the most powerful carcinogens known. The prime cancer treatment we use today actually fills your body with some of the most powerful cancer-causing drugs in existence. The absurdity of it is mind-boggling. Even if you temporarily destroy the current cancer in your body by poisoning it with these drugs, haven't you significantly increased your chances of getting cancer down the road?

Researchers tracked 2,169 people treated as children and adolescents at St. Jude Children's Research Hospital, in Memphis, Tennessee, for acute lymphoblastic leukemia.[8] Their cancer had gone into complete remission and their health was monitored for an average of nineteen years. The researchers found that the childhood leukemia survivors were 13.5 times more likely than the general population to develop the most serious types of cancer. In addition, the study found that the incidence of new cancers increased steadily for these cancer survivors during the thirty years after their leukemia treatment.

Medical treatments do nothing to improve immune function. In fact, chemotherapy and radiation destroy immune function in your body. This is the most absurd aspect of the modern medical approach in dealing with cancer—it destroys the very system in your body that can actually eliminate and prevent the recurrence of that cancer and then does nothing to repair that damage. At the very least, this is highly irresponsible. I have seen numerous people who have chosen to use immune-boosting formulas while undergoing chemotherapy and have actually seen their immune function increase (even double) during the course of treatment.

Most damning of all, these treatments are deadly in and of themselves. Chemotherapy drugs are not only carcinogenic, they are incredibly toxic. The fundamental premise behind their use is actually frightening: "We're going to give you some of the most powerful poisons we know of in the hope that we can kill the cancer faster than we kill you. Of course, if we're wrong, you'll die from the treatment and not your cancer. And at the very least, since it is so poisonous, you're going to feel really sick, much worse than you've ever felt in your life. Your hair may fall out; you'll vomit repeatedly. But, of course, it's worth it if it works. And it is your only option."

What about the long-term consequences? Does your body just shrug off the effects of chemotherapy and move on? Of course not. And the consequences are not just to the body, but to the mind too. New studies show that chemotherapy promotes a lingering intellectual deficit.[9] It was found that while more people survive cancer, there has been an increase in cognitive impairment, even years after treatment. Chemotherapy, and specifically tamoxifen, seems to impact the brain negatively, creating cognitive deficit, even though researchers are unsure exactly how. The real question is why the researchers were so surprised. Chemotherapy is an indiscriminant treatment: it assaults the body with highly toxic poisons and attacks and damages every cell in the body, which is why it has so many side effects.

Orthodox chemotherapy is toxic, immunosuppressant, and carcinogenic, so why do the majority of doctors and oncologists still push chemotherapy? First, what is considered an "effective" cancer treatment is a matter of definition. The U.S. Food and Drug Administration (FDA) defines an "effective" drug as one that achieves a 50 percent or more reduction in tumor size for twenty-eight days. But in the real world this definition is completely arbitrary and virtually meaningless. In the vast majority of cases, there is absolutely no correlation between shrinking tumors for twenty-eight days and the cure of the cancer or extension of life. So, when a doctor says "effective" to a cancer patient, it does not necessarily mean it cures cancer or will help you live longer, only that it temporarily shrinks the tumor.

Second, most doctors just don't know what else to do. They face patients who they feel have hopeless conditions and justify the continual loss of life brought about by these drugs because it's the only alternative they know (along with surgery and radiation). They refer to this stage not as therapy but as experimentation, which is better than telling a patient there is no hope. As for oncologists, they have devoted countless hours to the understanding of poisonous, deadly compounds and how to administer these drugs. This is all they know too. They want to help cancer patients, but they don't have other options in their arsenal, certainly not options that come from outside the medical fraternity.

Third, as commonly seen in all major industries, as long as drug companies and the cancer industry see profits in these treatments, there will be little motivation to change. Dr. George D. Lundberg, former editor of the *Journal of the American Medical Association*, pulled no punches when he said of chemotherapy: "[It's] a marvelous opportunity for rampant deceit. So much money is there to be made that ethical principles can be overrun sometimes in a stampede to get at physicians and prescribers."[10]

And in a small percentage of cases, chemotherapy absolutely does help, which is not to say that other approaches wouldn't work as well or even better. But it is, in fact, this minimal success rate that fuels the continued use of the therapy. Based on these occasional short-term successes, doctors will often pressure patients to opt for the therapy even when it has little chance of success in their particular cases.

But above and beyond everything else, it's important to understand that chemotherapy does nothing to address the underlying cause of the cancer. No doctor has ever told their patient they got cancer because they were suffering from a chemotherapy deficiency!

## Surgery

More and more women are now opting for voluntary breast removal (bilateral prophylactic mastectomy) after testing positive for what is being called "the breast cancer gene."[11] This is obviously not a simple issue with a "one size fits all" conclusion. It's also important to note there is a huge piece being left out of the equation, a piece that could significantly affect outcomes.

Women who have a mutation in one of the known breast cancer genes, *BRCA1*, and a strong family history of the disease, can have up to an 80 percent risk of developing breast cancer during their lifetime. On the other hand, the gene mutation without a strong family history results in only a 10 percent chance of developing breast cancer. That's an 800 percent variation in outcome, depending on family history. It's also worth noting that the odds of getting breast cancer if you have the mutated gene and no family history are actually just about the same as if you didn't have the bad gene at all.[12]

This brings us to the missing piece of the equation—family history. What does "family history" actually mean? Most people assume it means genetics, but not necessarily. It also means that you and your family live much of your lives in the same environment, eating the same diet and following similar lifestyles. For example, according to recent studies, if you grow up on a farm, you, your siblings, and your parents have a 200–400 percent increased risk of breast cancer.[13] There are also numerous studies that equate high dairy consumption with increased rates of breast cancer, most likely associated with high levels of estrogens and growth hormones found in commercial dairy products.[14] If that's what your family served at the dinner table, that's what you all ate together, and it's also likely to be what you and your new family will be eating when you move out. Heavy metals such as cadmium may also play a role in increasing breast cancer rates.[15] So, if you grew up in an environment high in cadmium, then you and your family would face the same increased risk.

You get the idea: often what people term "family history" is, in fact, nothing more than shared environmental and dietary history—and you can change that environment and history:

- Pesticides can be detoxified out of the body

- Estrogen dominance can be balanced out with natural progesterone cream

- Heavy metals can be chelated out of the body

Even with a bad gene and a family history, you might be able to lower your odds of getting breast cancer back to 10 percent or less. When faced with that number, prophylactic removal of breasts doesn't sound like such a good idea. And again, it's important to remember that surgical removal does not get rid of the underlying cause of cancer, just one place that it might manifest. The bad gene is not the actual cause of the cancer—it merely makes you more susceptible. If it were the actual cause, then you wouldn't have an 800 percent variation in the numbers of women who have the bad gene and get cancer. Something else is affecting that 800 percent variation. If you opt for this surgery, you may not get breast cancer, but you haven't changed your odds of getting uterine cancer, liver cancer, lymph cancer, etc.

## Most Current Research is a Waste of Time and Money

Most current cancer research is "magic bullet" nonsense. Take the search for the cancer gene. Are there genes that give one a predisposition for getting cancer? Absolutely. This is exactly what the Baseline of Health Program talks about when it refers to your Personal Health Line at the time of birth. But looking for a cancer cure by finding the cancer gene will do nothing to eliminate all of the other factors responsible for cancer. And we already know how small a role the "cancer gene" plays in the onset of cancer: there has been an 8-fold to 17-fold increase in the incidence of cancer in the last hundred years, but not even one-millionth of 1 percent of that increase can be related to genes. Genes evolve over hundreds of thousands (if not millions) of years, which means that the so-called cancer gene has had no impact on the huge increase we've seen since 1900. Virtually 90 percent of the cancer that we see today cannot possibly have anything to do with genes. So, at best, genes are responsible for only a small percentage of the minimal cancer rates we had in the early 1900s, and finding the "cancer gene" will affect only that tiny percentage of cancer. Genes may create tendencies, but in most cases they are not the underlying cause. Bottom line: look not for a cure in the cancer gene.

There is, however, a ray of hope in the world of medical research. In the last few years, medical research has started committing resources to the development of methods to harness and enhance the body's natural tendency to defend itself against malignant tumors. Immunotherapy represents a new and powerful weapon in the arsenal of anticancer treatments. Sometimes referred to as "biological response modifiers" or as "biological therapies," these new treatments—such as interferons and other cytokines, monoclonal antibodies, and vaccine therapies—have generated renewed interest and research activity in immunology.

## THE GAME IS RIGGED

The concept of working with the body to completely remove cancer from the body is old news to the alternative health community, but it is a revolutionary concept for medical science and holds great promise for the future—when they finally work it out. Fortunately, you don't have to wait for medical science to experience many of the benefits of these kinds of therapies. They have been available for decades in the world of alternative health. So, why have they been ignored?

According to the medical establishment, there are no effective alternative treatments for cancer. Your only options are chemotherapy, radiation, and surgery. In fact, in half the states in this country, it is illegal for a medical doctor to prescribe anything other than these options as a treatment for cancer. The sad thing is that it absolutely is not true—there are effective alternatives. But don't they test promising alternative therapies, and in each and every case find them ineffective? And the answer is: yes, they test them, but they unconsciously skew the tests so that alternative therapies cannot pass.

The problem is that, in almost all cases, alternative therapies are administered as part of a comprehensive program. Now that we've discussed the nature of the disease, it's easy to see why a comprehensive program is the only thing that makes sense. Nevertheless, when the medical community decides to test the validity of a particular treatment, they insist on separating out the pieces from the whole and testing each piece in isolation.

This would be akin to using the wrong approach in testing a prospective football quarterback (American football, that is). The "alternative approach" (the correct option) would be to put him on the field with an entire team and see how he plays. The "medical approach" would be quite different. "How can we really tell if he's any good if there are other players on the field?" ask the doctors. "Great receivers could catch lousy passes and we'd never know. A great offensive line could make him look good by blocking so well that he had all the time in the world to find his receivers. The only way to truly tell if he's any good is to put him on the field alone against an entire all-pro defensive team and see how he does." And, of course, the moment the ball is hiked, he's swarmed under and tackled, failing the test.

But then how do drugs pass this kind of testing? Quite simply, drugs, by design, are "magic bullets." In effect, they put the quarterback out on the field alone, but armed with an assault rife. Of course, as soon as the ball is hiked, he shoots the entire defensive team and walks across the goal line for a touchdown, passing the test. Unfortunately, although he scores, there are side effects—the other team is dead and the game is over—but he did score.

Alternative therapy, like football, is a team game. On occasion, you may get good results using just one component or another, but overall you will get the best results when you run the program as a whole. To isolate components of a program from the whole is to treat them as drugs. That's not what they are, and they will fail that test by definition. But that's not the only way that medical testing procedures are rigged against alternative therapies.

Another way of looking at it is that traditional medical treatments are subtractive, whereas alternative therapies are additive. Chemotherapy, for example, is an all-or-nothing proposition in application. If you use chemotherapy, you wipe out your immune system, which pretty much ends the possibility of using your immune system to overcome the cancer. That means medical treatments have to work consistently in a high enough percentage of cases or they are dismissed as invalid. That makes sense when testing subtractive therapies like drugs, but it makes no sense for testing alternative therapies, which are additive. Nevertheless, that is the criterion used to evaluate alternative therapies. And even here, the medical establishment plays with a rigged roulette wheel. Doctors routinely prescribe chemotherapy for advanced lung cancer cases where the success rate is less than 1 percent, far below the 30 percent marker set for placebos. Any alternative therapy with a 1 percent success rate would be laughed into oblivion by the establishment.

Testing alternative therapies as though they were subtractive drugs dooms many of them to false failure. An alternative treatment that would be dismissed as ineffective because testing showed it to be only 10 percent effective in isolation might nevertheless be an invaluable part of a comprehensive program that contained seven of these 10 percent–effective components— giving you a 70 percent chance of overcoming your cancer if used in combination. Or a component might have no effectiveness by itself but serve to amplify the effectiveness of another component. Remove the first component and the second component comes up short in testing. Nevertheless, the medical establishment deliberately chooses not to test alternative therapies in this way, thus condemning all the individual components of a program with the "quackery" label. So, the only way you hear about effective alternatives is by word of mouth or anecdotal evidence. Fortunately, the effectiveness of some of these programs is so strong that it is impossible to suppress their success, which is why more and more people are turning to effective alternatives. Are all the alternatives effective? Of course not. Are there quacks out there? Absolutely. Unfortunately, because the establishment suppresses all information regarding alternatives, it makes it that much harder to separate the wheat from the chaff. So, until better information is available, it's buyer beware. Then again, as we've already seen, that caution is at least as valid when it comes to the treatments your doctor offers you.

And lest I forget, one of the biggest arguments against alternative therapies is that they are a waste of money. Please! We spend $209 billion a year in the United States alone on a medical "war on cancer" that has been declared a failure by its very generals. Spending $100 a month on supplements is a drop in the bucket compared to that expenditure. To claim that alternative therapies pick your pocket is, at the very least, hypocritical.

## GENERAL RECOMMENDATIONS

### Preventing vs. Reversing

It is much easier to prevent cancer than to reverse it. The reason is simple: isolated cancer cells are not very strong and have no built-in support mechanisms, but once they take root and begin to multiply, they build awesome support systems and acquire a life of their own. In the case of tumors, for example, this includes the development of fully functional, complex vascular systems capable of providing tremendous amounts of nutrition and sustenance (unfortunately, at the expense of your body's vital organs). Also, once they take root, cancer cells are able to manifest their most important attribute—immortality. Unlike normal cells in your body, which have a limited life span (one of the main reasons we age and die), cancer cells generally do not age and die. Functionally, they can live forever, and this gives them a major competitive advantage over healthy cells in your body.

Nevertheless, your body is capable of reversing an established cancer—doctors see it all the time and call it a "spontaneous remission"—but it is far easier to prevent cancer. What do you do to prevent or reverse cancer? This is the big question, isn't it? But unfortunately I cannot prescribe or recommend any particular treatments in this book. That would be against the law. However, it is not inappropriate to give you some guidelines.

## Chemotherapy, Radiation, and Surgery

First, surgery might play a role in treatment if a tumor is so large, for example, that it impinges on another organ, thereby threatening near-term death. In that case, surgery might make sense to give you the time to pursue alternatives. On the other hand, I would be very leery of any chemotherapy or radiation treatments and would need to see very convincing statistical evidence that those particular treatments were indeed effective for my particular type of cancer, at my particular age. The success rate for chemotherapy is highly age-dependent. It is much more likely to be effective with the young who have strong immune systems, dropping to about 50/50 by age 50. And by 50/50, I don't mean that it's effective 50 percent of the time, but rather that it's a 50/50 call as to whether doing chemotherapy or nothing at all is the better option in terms of survivability. And by age 55, you're statistically better off doing nothing rather than subjecting yourself to chemotherapy. Remember, chemotherapy and radiation are "subtractive" treatments, a single role-of-the-dice crap shoot—you either win the big pot or end up bankrupt. And, in gambling, the odds are always with the house. If you opt for chemotherapy or radiation, it is absolutely imperative that you do something to improve your odds. You need to repair your immune system concurrent with your treatment. Check with your doctor about using natural immune enhancers during your therapy as they have consistently produced spectacular results in similar circumstances.

## Alternative Therapies

It's now time to take a look at the "additive" therapies—the ones that remove the toxins from your body and build your body's natural defenses against cancer. They are additive in the sense that they can all build off each other. Do everything, do it all at once, do it intensively, and repeat it. And once you have the cancer on the run, keep doing it until there is no sign of cancer for at least six months (so it doesn't sneak back in).

By everything, I mean the Baseline of Health Program, which is specifically designed to clean out and nourish virtually every major system in your body. It is by no means a cancer treatment but rather a system for optimizing the health of all the major body systems. For that reason, it serves as the core of any program you use to deal with catastrophic illness, including cancer. Following the Baseline of Health Program is the best method available for preventing cancer from taking root in your body, and it also offers the best base from which to launch any program intended to reverse cancer once it has taken root. It can play a significant role in removing from your body the toxins that promote the growth of aberrant cells and in rebuilding and optimizing your immune system.

When using the Baseline of Health Program as part of a regimen for reversing cancer, you need to do it completely (no exceptions), intensively, and repeatedly. Be sure to change your diet. In November 2007, the World Cancer Research Fund and the American Institute for Cancer Research published their report on diet, exercise, and cancer. Their primary conclusion was that about 40 percent of all cancers are linked to food, lack of exercise, and body weight. Specifically, excess body fat and red meat are linked to an increased risk of common cancers.[16] The liver cleanse and detoxification are crucial, and don't forget supplementing with omega-3 fatty acids, juice fasting, mental exercises, and physical activity—these are all key elements of the program.

In addition, specific anticancer protocols to check out in the library or on the Internet include:

- The Budwig diet.

- Specialized antioxidants like curcumin, green tea, selenium, and L-carnosine.

- Acemannan concentrates from aloe help build the immune system.

- Ellagitannin extracts from red raspberries and pomegranates are proven powerful anticarcinogens, as is graviola.

- Using high doses (12 tablespoons a day) of stabilized rice bran.

- AHCC (Active Hexose Correlated Compounds).

- Modified citrus pectin.

- Anvirzel and its low-cost alternative, oleander soup.

- Consider eliminating all forms of propyl alcohol (internal and external) from your life since there are indications these may play a role in fostering the growth of cancer-promoting parasites in the body.

- Ozone therapy has been shown to be effective in burning cancers out of the body. It's administered using rectal insufflation.

- Rife technology is available in several machines that have expanded on the work of Royal Rife. The basic premise is that cancers can be eliminated by frequencies tuned to the individual electromagnetic signature of that particular disease. The medical establishment and self-appointed "quack-busters" try to discredit these machines. Nevertheless, they work if you find the right machine, perhaps not as consistently as some proponents would have you believe, but the technology can be a powerful addition to any cancer therapy.

• Track down a scalar-energy charging-chamber or consume large amounts of scalar-enhanced products to help raise cellular energy levels.

## A Cure for Cancer?

Let's be clear—this is not a cure for cancer. Anyone who says they have a "cure" for cancer is misinformed. A "cure" is a simple impossibility, even within the medical community. When I see advertisements for hospital-based cancer programs where patients talk about being "cancer free" for five or seven years, I scoff. The simple truth is that no one is cancer free, ever—an important point to keep in mind.

First of all, not everyone gets well, no matter what program they use. That's the nature of life. Sometimes it's simply because there are so many variables. For example, if your house is concentrating radon gas seeping up from the ground below and you never checked for it and didn't know, then you could be doing every therapy program in the world and your odds of overcoming lung cancer would be significantly lessened. Then again, if you live in the middle of farm country and are continually exposed to pesticides, that too lessens your odds, no matter what you do. Sometimes, you just don't know. Even in those cases, your odds are still *significantly* better on a program designed to detoxify your body rather than on a program that adds more toxins to it.

Also, it's important to remember that every day of your life your body produces anywhere from a few hundred to as many as 10,000 cancerous cells as part of its normal metabolic processes. That's why I say you're never completely cancer free. The only question is: can your body deal with those cells and prevent them from taking root and multiplying? That's it, pure and simple. Any program that reinforces your body in that agenda is good and will improve your odds dramatically. Any program that undermines it is "questionable." The choice is yours.

Note: A June 2008 study in *Proceedings of the National Acdemy of Sciences* found that by making dietary and lifestyle changes, people were able to alter cancer genes and radically reduce their cancer risk. During the course of the study, on average, 453 cancer-promoting genes were "switched off" in test subjects, while 48 cancer-fighting genes were "switched on"—again, purely by changing diet, lifestyle, and supplementation. Bottom line: the Baseline of Health Program can even alter the outcome of genetically induced cancer.

Cancer has certainly been the plague of the last half of the twentieth century, but at the beginning of the twenty-first century, new plagues are emerging. In the next chapter, we will explore "The Plagues of Our Time."

# CHAPTER 20

# *The Plagues of Our Time*
## *Diabetes, Osteoporosis, Alzheimer's Disease, and Multiple Sclerosis (MS)*

- **Diabetes: The Echo Effect**
- **Osteoporosis: Stop the Insanity**
- **Alzheimer's Disease: A New Collective Nightmare**
- **Multiple Sclerosis (MS): Letting the Body Heal Itself**

For many years now, cancer and heart disease have been the focus of our fears—the dreaded killers of our generation. Now, new terrors are emerging, and like the giant mutant ants from the 1954 science fiction movie *Them!*, they are not natural terrors. They are monsters of our own creation, largely the result of inapt choices. In just the last 10–20 years, diabetes, osteoporosis, Alzheimer's disease, and multiple sclerosis (MS) have emerged from relative obscurity to become front page news. We now receive several thousand questions a year on these four diseases alone at the Baseline of Health Foundation. Make no mistake; these are the plagues of our time.

## DIABETES: THE ECHO EFFECT

Type 2 diabetes is not like any other disease. Most diseases, such as cancer and MS, are linear: you get the disease and it progresses in a straight line, from point A to point B. It may have regressions and remissions in which it backs up on its linear path for a bit, but then it picks up steam and once again proceeds down the same track to its ultimate conclusion. Diabetes does not do that. It follows multiple, mutually reinforcing paths—an echo effect, if you will, with each echo (or effect) reinforcing and amplifying all the others. This distinction is of vital importance because it mandates multiple points of intervention if you wish to reverse diabetes and not just slow its progression.

## Understanding Insulin

Despite long intervals between meals and the erratic intake of high-glycemic carbohydrates, blood sugar levels normally remain within a narrow range. In most people, this range is from about 70–110 mg per dl. A blood sugar reading of 100 equates to about a fifth of an ounce [5 grams] of sugar total in the bloodstream of an average 165-pound [75-kg] male. The body's mechanisms for restoring a normal blood glucose level when it steps outside its range (either low or high) are extremely efficient and effective. High blood sugar levels are regulated by the hormone insulin, which is produced by beta cells in the islets of Langerhans in the pancreas. These cells are extremely sensitive to variations in blood glucose levels and, under normal circumstances, respond with extraordinary speed to any variation.

When you eat high-glycemic foods, you suddenly increase the amount of sugar in your blood. This increase triggers the beta cells to release insulin, which travels in the blood to cells throughout the body, where it facilitates the uptake of sugar in the individual cells so the sugar can be quickly converted to energy. If you eat too much sugar (beyond what the cells can use for energy), insulin tells the body to store the excess sugar as glycogen in the liver (and also, to a lesser degree, in muscle tissue). When the glucose levels come down to acceptable levels, this triggers the beta cells to stop the production and release of insulin, which allows the process to stabilize. When blood glucose levels drop too low, however, the hormone glucagon is released from alpha cells in the pancreas, which triggers the release of the sugar stored in the liver as glycogen, once again bringing blood sugar levels back to normal. Release of insulin is strongly inhibited by the stress hormone noradrenaline (norepinephrine), which is why blood sugar levels increase so dramatically during stress.

## The Initial Sound: Insulin Resistance

On the surface of the cells of your body sit insulin receptors, minute "lock and key" chemical gateways, like little doors that open and close, that regulate the inflow of blood sugar. After many years of exposure to a high-glycemic diet, these cells become damaged by so much insulin that their "doors" begin to malfunction and shut down. As a result, the fat cells, muscle cells, and liver cells of the body become resistant to insulin so that normal amounts of insulin are no longer adequate to produce a response. The cells require ever greater quantities of insulin to open the resistant receptors and achieve even a minimal response. Insulin resistance in fat cells results in the breakdown of stored triglycerides, which elevates free fatty acids in the blood. Insulin resistance in muscle cells reduces glucose uptake, which keeps sugar levels high in the blood, and insulin resistance in liver cells reduces glucose storage, which also raises blood glucose levels.

With more and more cell doors jammed shut, your body needs to produce ever more insulin to "push" the glucose into the cells. More insulin causes even more doors to close and, as this vicious cycle continues, a condition called "insulin resistance" sets in. This is a primary cause-and-effect response by your body. If normal insulin levels are not enough to make the cells behave properly, the beta cells in your pancreas continue to sense high levels of glucose in the blood and they go into overdrive to pump out ever greater quantities of insulin in an attempt to bring blood sugar levels back to normal. In most cases, this extra insulin is enough to bring things back under control—for a time—but with two significant side effects:

- It puts undue stress on the beta cells in the pancreas. They can only operate in overdrive for so long before they burn out. At that point, not only can they no longer produce sufficient levels of insulin even under prodding, but they eventually lose all ability to produce insulin under any conditions.

- The increased insulin comes with a whole host of its own side effects.

## The First Echo: Damage from High Sugar Levels

Too much sugar in the blood leads to increased thirst in the body's attempt to get rid of the extra sugar. This leads to increased urination and starts putting an extra burden on your kidneys. Too much sugar causes the small blood vessels throughout the body to narrow as your body tries to reduce the damage caused to organs by minimizing the ability of the excess sugar to reach them. The higher the blood sugar level, the more the small blood vessels narrow. The blood vessels thus carry less blood, and circulation is impaired. Poor circulation in turn results in complications such as kidney disease, poor wound healing, and foot and eye problems. This sugar imbalance also alters fat metabolism, increasing the risk that cholesterol-laden plaque will build up in the large blood vessels. Finally, sugar also sticks to proteins, causing their structural and functional properties to be changed. It is a primary

reason that wounds don't heal since they have trouble making quality collagen, the connective tissue that is the major structural protein in the body.

In addition, stress results in the adrenal glands pumping adrenaline into
the bloodstream, which increases free fatty acids in the blood and shuts off
the release of insulin. In obesity, less insulin is able to reach the insulin-
responsive muscles and, in the end, there is not enough insulin to meet the
demand. Diabetic neuropathy (damage to nerves caused by diabetes) affects
the peripheral nerves, such as those in the feet, hands, and legs. Symptoms
include numbness, tingling, and pain.

## The Second Echo: Excess Insulin Damage

Excess sugar is not the only problem associated with diabetes. Excess insulin
is also a killer. Insulin is the master hormone of your metabolism. When it
is out of balance and your insulin levels are consistently elevated, a long list
of deadly complications are created:

- Heart disease
- Hardening of the arteries and damage to artery walls (elevated insulin lev-
els are directly implicated in the damage done to arterial walls that leads
to atherosclerosis)
- Increased cholesterol and triglyceride levels
- Elevated blood pressure
- Vitamin and mineral deficiencies
- Kidney disease
- Fat-burning mechanism is turned off, leading to the accumulation and
storage of fat (weight gain and obesity)

## The Third Echo: Destruction of the Beta Cells

This is the big echo, in which the other effects get ramped up to catastrophic levels. When blood sugar levels rise even slightly above 100 for as little as
two hours, beta cell failure is detectable. People who maintain blood sugar
levels of as little as 110 can lose as much as 40 percent of their beta cell capacity in as little as two years.[1] In other words, the very cells of your body
responsible for keeping blood sugar under control are destroyed by the excess
blood sugar they are unable to control, which echoes back on the beta cells
in the pancreas, destroying even more of them and thus causing blood sugar

levels to rise even further. This then reverberates through the body once again, echoing back once more on the pancreas, killing even more beta cells—on and on until there are no beta cells left to destroy.

## The Fourth Echo: Breakdown of the Body

At a certain point in the process, when your body can no longer produce any insulin and resists even the insulin you take through injection, you begin to experience the ravages of diabetes:

- Neuropathy
- Amputation
- Kidney failure
- Heart disease
- Blindness
- Death

## Limitations of the Medical Approach to Diabetes

Although the situation may sound grim, it's not hopeless. It does, however, present the limitations of the medical approach and shows why the Baseline of Health Program, which deals with the whole body, is likely to produce significantly better results. Standard medical treatment (i.e., drugs) offers several flawed approaches to treating diabetes.

Drugs like metformin seek to inhibit the absorption of high-glycemic carbohydrates in the intestinal tract and enhance insulin sensitivity in the body, thereby reducing the need for extra insulin. The major problem with metformin is its effect on the gastrointestinal system, ranging from a mild loss of appetite to nausea, vomiting, abdominal discomfort, cramps, flatulence, and diarrhea. Many patients find these symptoms impossible to cope with and discontinue the medication. Lactic acidosis, a serious condition in which the cells of the body do not get enough oxygen to survive, is a rare but dangerous side effect of metformin. It is caused by a buildup of lactic acid in the blood. Most of the cases have been in people whose kidneys were not working well (an inevitable problem with diabetes).

Drugs like glyburide work by stimulating the pancreas to release more insulin. Glyburide is so effective that you need to carry glucose pills with you in case you produce so much insulin that your blood sugar drops too low and you fall into a diabetic coma. Although this rarely happens, it is indicative of the larger problems with glyburide. It raises insulin levels so high that your body faces all of the problems of high insulin levels discussed above. It does not repair beta cells but just forces them to work harder, thus speeding up the day when they break down and become totally dysfunctional. Also, extra insulin covers you when the beta cells in your pancreas have burned out and can no longer produce sufficient insulin (by themselves or when stimulated by drugs such as glyburide)—until, that is, your body's insulin resistance is so high that no amount of insulin is adequate for the task at hand. At that point, your body goes into rapid decay.

## Alternative Therapies for Stopping the Echoes

Any viable alternative therapy needs to address the problems that medicines do not. It also needs to work *with* the body so it can be effective over the long term. And an effective alternative needs to stop all of the echoes, so that nothing bounces back to retrigger the problems. With that in mind, in addition to changing your diet (no more sodas and high-glycemic snack foods), you may want to explore the following protocol.

- Inhibit absorption of high-glycemic foods, without creating unwelcome responses in the intestinal tract (such as those experienced using metformin). This can be accomplished with herbs, including nopal cactus and *Gymnema sylvestre.*

- Naturally reverse insulin resistance, so less insulin is required, using konjac mannan (glucomannan from the Asian plant konjac), Cinnulin PF (a proprietary cinnamon extract developed by the U.S. Department of Agriculture), chromium GTF, and omega-3 fatty acids.

- Repair beta cells in the islets of Langerhans in the pancreas to optimize insulin production reserves as opposed to forcing the cells to dramatically overproduce as with glyburide, which leads to inevitable burnout. Useful supplements include *Gymnema sylvestre* and alpha-lipoic or R-lipoic acid.

- Lower blood sugar levels through proper diet and herbal supplementation with fenugreek extract, bitter melon (*Momordica charantia*), corosolic acid, and mulberry.

- Reduce stress. Remember, adrenaline suppresses the release of insulin.

- Protect organs and proteins from damage caused by higher than normal levels of sugar through a mixture of antioxidants and nutraceuticals, such as L-carnosine, acetyl-L-carnitine, dimethylaminoethanol (DMAE), coenzyme $Q_{10}$ (co$Q_{10}$), alpha-lipoic or R-lipoic acid, and benfotiamine (fat-soluble vitamin $B_1$).

• Protect organs from damage caused by higher than normal insulin levels by cleaning the blood with a blood-cleansing formula, proteolytic enzymes, and omega-3 fatty acids.

Does this protocol work? In 2006, I tested a trial formula containing nopal cactus, konjac mannan, *Gymnema sylvestre*, fenugreek extract, Cinnulin PF, *Momordica charantia*, and corosolic acid through an independent clinical trial. This herbal mix performed better than the prescription drug metformin. It produced an average 54-point drop in fasting blood sugar levels in six weeks; the lowest drop out of the fifty people tested was 42 points and the highest 106.

The bottom line for preventing and reversing diabetes is to do everything, and do it all at once. Since diabetes is not a straight-line, progressive disease, you need to stop every "echo" so no aspect of the disease can reverberate and start the whole process moving downhill again. You need to stop it all, all at the same time, or it will all start again.

## OSTEOPOROSIS: STOP THE INSANITY

There's an old saying, "Insanity is doing the same thing over and over and thinking that some day the result will be different." Now, you can argue that's also the definition of persistence, but when it comes to osteoporosis, it truly is the definition of insanity. Amazingly, 99 percent of the medical community and the media promote a solution for osteoporosis that not only does not work, but also has been proven to actually exacerbate the problem. And that's not the worst part: even more insane is the fact that although research has shown that taking more calcium and drinking more milk actually contributes to osteoporosis and makes it worse, our doctors don't just tell us to continue doing these things, they tell us that it's not working because we're not doing enough.

Osteoporosis is a generalized skeletal disorder characterized by thinning of the bone and deterioration in its architecture, causing susceptibility to fracture. The key phrase here is "susceptibility to fracture." There are two types of osteoporosis. Type I osteoporosis (post-menopausal osteoporosis) generally develops in women after menopause, when the amount of estrogen in the body decreases. This process leads to an increase in the resorption of bone (the loss of bone substance). Type I osteoporosis is far more common in women than in men, and typically develops between the ages of fifty and seventy. The decrease in the overall strength of the bone leads primarily to wrist and spine fractures. Type II osteoporosis (senile osteoporosis) typically happens after the age of seventy and affects women twice as frequently as men. Type II osteoporosis involves a thinning of both the hard outer bone and the spongy bone inside. This process leads to hip and spinal fractures. Approximately 20 percent of women and 40 percent of men with osteoporosis have a secondary cause such as hyperthyroidism or lymphoma.

Osteoporosis has been recognized as a major public health problem for only the last twenty years. (In the old days, it was just called "widow's stoop.") The increasing incidence of fragility fractures, such as spinal, hip, and wrist fractures, first became apparent from epidemiological studies in the early and mid-1980s. Today, approximately 10 million Americans (8 million women and 2 million men) have osteoporosis. Another 34 million show signs of low bone mass indicative of future osteoporosis.[2]

At the present time, the majority of hip fractures (the major danger from osteoporosis) occur in Europe and North America. In fifty years, however, it is estimated that 75 percent of all hip fractures will occur in developing countries,[3] with the number of hip fractures rising three-fold to 6.3 million a year. The rate of increase for osteoporosis is faster than the growth in population, and it is growing in parts of the world that have never shown much evidence of it previously.

## The Medical Mantra: Hormones and More Calcium

At one time, the medical mantra was that it's all hormonal—"it's a woman's disease"—which meant hormone replacement therapy (HRT) was the answer. But as more study results came in, that theory became unsustainable, at least by itself. It couldn't explain the dramatic increase in the incidence of osteoporosis in the United States and throughout the world, and it couldn't explain the ever-increasing number of men who were becoming afflicted. So, a new theory had to be developed—the bone mineral density theory. According to this theory, people weren't getting enough calcium in their diets so they weren't able to build enough bone mineral density to serve as a reserve as they got older; thus, they couldn't compensate for the natural bone loss that occurred as they aged. The obvious solution, according to the medical community, was calcium supplementation. So, according to the latest wisdom, we should:

- Drink more milk

- Take calcium supplements

- Use HRT to rebalance hormonal levels

- Drink fluoridated water since fluoride builds bone mass[4]

- Use Fosamax®, the latest wonder drug to prevent the destruction of bone

If you go to a doctor and ask about osteoporosis, 99 percent of them will recommend some combination of the above, even though we now know that the protocol doesn't work and, in fact, contributes to osteoporosis.

Why doesn't it work? A number of people in the alternative health community have argued for years that excessive calcium doesn't help the problem; it contributes to it. Magnesium is far and away the more important mineral (but still a secondary piece of the puzzle) when it comes to bone loss. To understand what's going on here, let's begin by quickly discussing how the body builds bones.

First, your bones are living tissue, not dead cement. By living tissue, I mean that bone is comprised of living cells (osteoclasts and osteoblasts) that are continually removing and replacing the mineral deposits that we normally think of as bone. The brilliance of this system might not at first be obvious. After all, what possible advantage could there be to getting rid of good bones? Isn't that osteoporosis? But it's only osteoporosis when we mess up the balance, when we lose more bone than we build. If building and replacing bone wasn't a dynamic process, how could you mend broken bones or replace aging fragile bones? And if the process went only one way (just building bone), your body would eventually become one solid mass of bone as your bones continued to grow and grow. When you are healthy, it is this dynamic process of removing old bone minerals and replacing them with new bone minerals that keeps your skeletal system healthy, as long as that process is in equilibrium. As with almost all diseases, it is deviation from the natural state of balance that causes problems, when we start losing bone minerals faster than we replace them. That's osteoporosis.

So, what causes us to go out of balance? Again, if you believe most of what you read and hear, it's hormonal imbalance and insufficient calcium in the diet so that we cannot grow new bone fast enough—thus the need for calcium supplements, high dairy intake, and HRT. But the facts don't bear this out: the incidence of hip fractures (a good indicator of osteoporosis) in countries that have the highest dairy consumption (Norway, Sweden, and the U.S.) is fifty times higher than in countries like New Guinea and South Africa that have extremely low consumption of dairy products (and animal products in general).[5] High calcium intake does not prevent osteoporosis, not even among people who use coral calcium supplements.[6]

## A Balanced Lifestyle

The simple truth is that if we live a balanced lifestyle, we actually need very little calcium (of the right sort) to maintain healthy bones. The problem we have is not that we get too little calcium but rather that we have made choices that dramatically accelerate the rate of bone loss, to the point that we can never consume enough calcium to overcome the deficit. What accelerates bone loss to such a degree and what can be done about it?

- Lack of sufficient weight-bearing exercise accelerates bone loss. Thus, increasing exercise helps reverse it.

- Insufficient boron and vitamin $D_3$ contribute to bone loss.

- Insufficient magnesium in the diet is more of a factor than insufficient calcium. One study showed that, after nine months, women on magnesium supplements increased bone density by 11 percent.[7]

- Increasing the amount of gamma-linolenic acid (GLA) and eicosapentaenoic acid (EPA) in the diet helps increase bone density.

- Avoiding fluoride in your drinking water is vital. Fluoride collects in the bones and, although it "technically" increases bone mass and density, the evidence is strong that fluoride intake can dramatically reduce the quality of your bones and double the incidence of hip fractures.[8] Bottom line: although your bones may be denser if you have fluoride in your water, they are far more brittle.

- Balancing out hormones. Does that mean that I'm recommending hormone replacement therapy? Hardly. HRT, as it is practiced, increases your risk of cancer and offers only a temporary reprieve from osteoporosis.

What most people don't realize is that bone loss accelerates rapidly in women once they stop using estrogen, causing a "catch-up" effect. By age eighty, women who had taken HRT for ten years and then stopped for ten years will lose 27 percent of their initial bone density, while those who were never treated will lose about 30 percent. The only way you would get continued benefit is to take HRT for the rest of your life, which would likely be shorter because of the increased risk of developing breast and endometrial cancers. HRT doesn't build bone—it only slows the rate of loss for a short period of time and at great risk. Natural progesterone cream, on the other hand, increases bone strength and density by stimulating osteoblasts, your bone-building cells, and does not carry the same risks.

- Fosamax is problematic because it works by totally destroying the equilibrium of the bone-building process by killing osteoclasts, the cells that remove old bone so your osteoblasts can build new bone in its place. Yes, if you kill off the osteoclasts, your bones are going to get denser because instead of replacing old bone, the new bone will "cram" itself into whatever space it can find. Unfortunately, this also means that your bones are going to get weaker because you're not eliminating the older, damaged bone. Fosamax builds a house of cards that must ultimately collapse.

- But all of the above factors pale in comparison to the problem of a high-acid diet. This is the reason the incidence of osteoporosis has soared and why more men are now suffering. A high-acid diet (meat, fish, poultry, eggs, dairy, cooked grains, and refined sugars) leaches calcium from your body by forcing it to use calcium from your bones to buffer the high acid content so that your blood pH remains constant and you don't die. The problem with dairy is that because of its high phosphorus content, it actually takes more calcium to buffer it than you receive from the dairy, thus the high incidence of osteoporosis in countries that consume a lot of dairy. I am not saying that dairy is the biggest culprit—most of the other acid foods are worse, particularly high-sugar, phosphoric acid–laden colas—I just single out dairy because it's always identified as building strong bones, when the opposite is true.

So, what is one to do? Well, first reread Chapter 7 on diet, which lays out the ground rules for helping your body build bone. Minimizing the intake of animal foods (to less than three ounces a day) and the elimination (or at least minimization) of refined grains and sugars are both helpful. At that point, the amount of highly absorbable calcium that you get in your diet (from foods such as romaine lettuce, broccoli, sesame seeds, and bok choy) will be more than adequate for most people to build strong bones.

Think about cows for a moment. How do cows grow such large, strong bones considering that they don't drink milk and they don't take calcium supplements? They eat grass—low in calcium, but high in magnesium (magnesium is the basis of chlorophyll in plants). Consider the fact that the traditional Eskimo diet contains over 2,000 mg of calcium a day, but because their diet is so acidic (virtually 100 percent of the food is from animal sources), it produces the highest hip fracture rate in the world.[9] The bottom line is that calcium supplementation will not save you from the consequences of a high-acid-forming diet. And if you absolutely can't change to a more alkaline diet, then taking supplemental calcium (not milk) to buffer the excess acid probably makes sense. It won't repair any damage, but it will protect against some of the destruction you are inflicting on yourself.

## ALZHEIMER'S DISEASE: A NEW COLLECTIVE NIGHTMARE

Alzheimer's disease is set to become our next big medical terror. In the early 1900s, it was infectious diseases. From 1950 to around 1975, it was heart disease. And from the mid-1970s to now, it has been cancer. But rising rapidly in our consciousness, Alzheimer's looks ready to take its place as our new collective bogey man.

So, what is Alzheimer's? First, let's separate dementia and Alzheimer's, as they are not the same thing. Dementia refers to a progressive decline in cognitive function beyond what might be expected from normal aging. Alzheimer's is only one possible cause; strokes, for example, may damage parts of the brain and lead to dementia. Common prescription drugs such as sleep aids, antianxiety drugs, antidepressants, allergy drugs, and even cold remedies can cause dementia as a side effect. Medical authorities say that side effects from prescription drugs are responsible for only a minority cases, but even according to these conservative sources, such side effects may still represent 15–30 percent of all dementia diagnoses.[10] Alzheimer's, on the other hand, is defined by two distinct brain abnormalities: amyloid plaques and neurofibrillary tangles.

An estimated 4.5 million Americans have Alzheimer's disease, a number that has more than doubled since 1980.[11] Worldwide, it is estimated that there are currently 18 million people with Alzheimer's disease.[12] This figure is projected to nearly double by 2025 to 34 million people and reach 52 million by 2050. The cost of Alzheimer's in the United States alone was estimated to be $67.3 billion in 1991, climbing to at least $100 billion based on 1994 data, with projections of at least $160 billion a year by 2010.[13]

Scientists do not yet fully understand what causes Alzheimer's disease. Truth be told, there probably is not one single cause, but several factors that affect each person differently. The greatest known risk factor for Alzheimer's is increasing age. Most individuals with the disease are sixty-five or older. The likelihood of developing Alzheimer's doubles about every five years after age sixty-five; after age eighty-five, the risk reaches nearly 50 percent.[14]

Risk genes increase the likelihood of developing the disease, but do not guarantee it will happen. Scientists have so far identified one Alzheimer's risk gene called apolipoprotein E-e4 (APOE-e4). They have also found rare genes that directly cause Alzheimer's but in only a few hundred extended families worldwide.

There appears to be a strong link between serious head injury and future risk of Alzheimer's. Modest head trauma, however, seems to produce no increased risk. Some of the strongest evidence links brain health to heart health. Your brain is nourished by one of the body's richest networks of blood vessels. Every heartbeat pumps about 20 to 25 percent of your blood to your head, where brain cells use at least 20 percent of the food and oxygen your blood carries. Reduce that flow, and you damage your brain.

One study linked sufferers of diabetes to a 65 percent higher risk of developing Alzheimer's disease.[15] A more recent study puts the risk at almost double.[16] New research also indicates that inflammatory stress leading to metabolic changes in brain proteins may be a significant factor.[17] And, finally, there is the much debated aluminum connection. Much of the ambiguity may be because researchers are looking at the wrong culprit. There are indications that aluminum by itself may not be a significant trigger for Alzheimer's, but aluminum and fluoride together may be.[18]

## Avoiding Alzheimer's

So, because there probably is not a single cause but rather several factors, the search for "the cure" for Alzheimer's is likely to be fruitless, in addition to being extremely expensive (but with massive amounts of research money available, it will continue nonetheless). Everything we know about Alzheimer's disease says that it is not primarily related to genetics but rather to deteriorating conditions connected with the aging process. Most of those conditions can be ameliorated, or even reversed, through the use of diet and lifestyle changes and the use of supplements.

What can we do to improve our odds of being among the 50 percent who are unafflicted at age eighty-five? Quite a lot actually, and even better, nothing other than what you should already be doing to maintain optimum health. If you're following the Baseline of Health Program, you're already covered. Here are some specifics as they apply to Alzheimer's.

### Heart Health

The connection of Alzheimer's with cardiovascular disease would appear to have two primary components: reduced flow of oxygen and nutrients to the brain resulting from restricted arteries, and inflammation of areas of the brain caused by many of the same factors that cause inflammation of arterial tissue, which leads to the hardening of the arteries and the buildup of arterial plaque. Dietary changes, such as avoiding heavy consumption of saturated fats and trans-fatty acids, makes sense. Also, reduce consumption of high omega-6 vegetable oils and supplement with omega-3 fatty acids. Lower homocysteine levels by using a supplement that includes vitamin $B_{12}$, folic acid, and trimethylglycine (TMG). Also, regular use of methylation supplements, such as S-adenosyl-L-methionine (SAMe), is useful.

### Inflammation

Systemic inflammation is starting to emerge as one of the biggest risk factors you face as you age. It is now implicated in everything from heart disease to cancer to Alzheimer's. Reducing that inflammation is not difficult. Omega-3 fatty acids play a key role here, so supplementation is crucial. A good systemic proteolytic enzyme formula can also work wonders.

### Diabetes

The primary culprit when it comes to diabetes, however, appears to be glycation, the uncontrolled reaction of sugars with proteins. It's similar to what happens to sugars when you heat them and they caramelize—glycation is what happens when excess sugars caramelize the proteins in your body. (The carmelized proteins are called AGEs, or advanced glycosylation end-products.) It's a major factor in the aging process, and it's particularly devastating to diabetics. Thanks largely to the destructive effect of sugar and aldehydes, the protein in our bodies tends to undergo destructive changes as we age. This destruction is a prime factor, not only in the aging process itself, but also in the familiar signs of aging such as wrinkling skin, cataracts, and the destruction of our nervous system, particularly our brains. So, how does this work in our brains? Quite simply, AGEs contribute to amyloidosis, the process by which beta amyloid plaques are formed in the brain.[19] For therapeutic options that can help reduce advanced glycosylation end-products and the concomitant increase in beta amyloid plaques in the brain, see the recommendations for diabetes earlier in this chapter.

### Heavy Metals

Not just aluminum and fluoride but excess levels of all heavy metals, including lead, can cause deterioration of brain function. Regular use of a heavy metal–chelating formula makes a great deal of sense.

### Exercise

Regular exercise, not just physical but also mental, is critical. Regular aerobic exercise (interval training, in particular) improves oxygen flow to the brain. Even regular dancing has been shown to help. Weight-bearing exercise can increase human growth hormone production by as much as 800 percent, which is important because HGH can promote the repair of damaged brain cells. And stretching opens up circulation to every area of the body.

Thinking exercises that challenge your mind make a huge difference. Playing bridge, chess, or a musical instrument all help. In fact, studies have shown that people who do just four crossword puzzles a week have a 47 percent reduced risk of Alzheimer's disease.[20] What's a five-letter word beginning with *S* and ending with *T* that describes people who understood what I just said?

## MULTIPLE SCLEROSIS (MS): LETTING THE BODY HEAL ITSELF

Multiple sclerosis is one of those diseases that responds extraordinarily well to the Baseline of Health Program, but as we have already seen, it is hardly unique. It is merely representative of how effective the program can be in dealing with a whole range of catastrophic illnesses. But it is an especially good example because the results have been so dramatic. The vast majority of the MS patients who have gone on the whole program have experienced a dramatic, long-term improvement in symptoms—not a cure, but a significant improvement in symptoms.

MS is an autoimmune disease in which the body's immune system attacks myelin, a key substance that serves as a nerve insulator and helps in the transmission of nerve signals. From a medical standpoint, what we understand about multiple sclerosis is mostly hunches and guesswork. Nevertheless, it does appear that MS (as with most idiopathic autoimmune disorders) is the result of an overall system imbalance triggered by things within our ability to alter and that the final causative factor in the chain of events is inflammation.

Whatever the initiating cause of MS, there is considerable evidence that a misprogrammed immune system is involved. The theory is that a virus, bacteria, or environmental toxin excites an immune response, which destroys the invader and builds a memory of it so that the immune system can respond more quickly the next time it sees that invader. There is reason to believe that in MS, the immune system gets confused and identifies peptides in the myelin as identical to the peptides found in the original invader. This "mistaken identity" causes the immune system to attack the perceived invader (the myelin), thereby inflaming and damaging the myelin surrounding the nerve cells.

Once again, we find commonality with so many other catastrophic illnesses. Look at the increasing incidence of thyroid diseases such as Graves' disease. What triggers the immune system to attack the thyroid? Why does medicine only deal with the final effect and not the possible causes if the disease is triggered by out-of-balance hormones and environmental factors? Why does the same program, the Baseline of Health Program, work so well when dealing with such different diseases as MS and Graves' disease?

It's no secret that hormones significantly impact autoimmune disorders and any disorder related to systemic inflammation. For example, MS is more common in women than men, as are most thyroid disorders such as Graves' disease, and the progress of these diseases follows the rise and fall of hormones during the monthly cycle.[21] It has also been known for years that pregnant woman with MS get better in the last trimester of their pregnancy.[22] In the third trimester, the hormone estriol (the gentle estrogen) is at high levels. It appears that a key role of estriol is to inhibit the "escape" of white blood cells from blood vessels into the central nervous system, where they can then attack myelin. In testing with MS patients, after the first three months of estriol treatment, brain scans showed the number of lesions in a group with relapsing-remitting MS decreased by 82 percent, and the volume of those lesions decreased by 79 percent (both compared with pre-treatment scans).[23] The decrease persisted for the rest of the first treatment period. When the women stopped taking the estriol over the next six months, the number of lesions gradually increased again, all the way back to pre-treatment levels. In another study, administering estriol until treatment levels reached levels consistent with those in late pregnancy completely ameliorated the disease.[24] And in recent studies, researchers found that testosterone therapy for those who have MS may help improve cognitive function and slow brain atrophy.[25] It's believed that testosterone helps protect nerve cells from damage caused by the kind of autoimmune attack that occurs in people with MS.

The primary medical treatment offered is the immunomodulator interferon beta-1a. For many people, it can reduce symptoms for up to four years, but over time, as the body forms neutralizing antibodies, its effectiveness diminishes.[26] It also comes with a host of side effects, including fatigue, chills, fever, muscle aches, and sweating. Symptoms of depression are also possible.

But a look at the possible causative factors in MS makes clear that interferon beta-1a intervenes at only the very last steps of a progressive deterioration and does nothing to eliminate the underlying causes—a common problem with the medical approach to virtually all of the autoimmune disorders. Factors that we need to account for if we truly want to reverse MS include bacteria and viruses; chemical toxins, pesticides, and heavy metals; diet; hormones; plaque buildup; scarring; protein damage; minimizing both the production of advanced glycosylation end-products and the body's glycemic response; immune system imbalance; and inflammation.

## A Multifactorial Approach to MS

Although not specifically designed for MS, the Baseline of Health Program addresses each of the above factors just as a matter of course, simply by following the program. It does so, not because it is MS-specific but rather because it is designed to improve the health of the entire body, to simply allow the body to do what it was designed to do—work properly and stay healthy. And that's why it is just as effective when dealing with most other forms of catastrophic illness. This is significant, or should be, to anyone with an open mind.

## GENERAL RECOMMENDATIONS

The subtitle of this book is "A Step-By-Step Guide to Optimum Health and Relief from Catastrophic Illness." By simply following the principles of the program, you naturally protect yourself from virtually all of the major illnesses of our time. Am I claiming that the Baseline of Health Program cures MS or any other catastrophic illness? Not at all—after all, only medical doctors make such claims. All I'm saying, and the facts bear it out, is that your body is designed to keep these diseases at bay, if you let it do its job. Problems arise when the body either becomes too toxic or lacks the proper nutrients to do what it was designed to do.

Consider MS, as an example: for thirty years of your life you don't have the disease, and then you do. What changed that caused it to appear? If you can reverse those changes, then doesn't it make sense that the symptoms of the disease would disappear also, as long as you keep those changes away? That's what we're talking about here—not curing anything, just bringing your body back to the state it was in before symptoms manifested. After that, your body just does what it was designed to do.

We're almost done now—just one topic left. What topic do you think elicits more questions than any other at www.jonbarron.org? The answer, of course, is aging. Once considered the inevitable curse of life, people have now begun to believe it's their right to fight it. And the truly amazing thing is, you can!

# CHAPTER 21

## Aging—It's Not Just for the Old

- **The Purpose of Aging and Death**
- **The Things We Do to Ourselves**
- **Micro-Level Factors**
- **Macro-Level Factors**

*P*robably no other area in alternative health is more subject to over-promising and under-delivering than antiaging medicine, especially with the Baby Boomer generation now approaching retirement age. We're talking about every "magic bullet" under the sun, from face rejuvenation creams to human growth hormone supplements. Ah, if only it were that simple! Aging is not the result of any single factor, but is the cumulative result of a number of factors, including:

- Cell senescence (the aging of cells)
- Diminished telomerase activity (an enzyme involved in DNA replication)
- Protein degradation
- Advanced glycosylation end-products (AGEs)
- Excess sugar in the blood
- Progressive systemic inflammation
- Dehydration
- Accumulated toxic buildup in organ tissues
- Reduced circulation
- Reduced cellular energy production and impeded energy flows in the body
- Changes in hormone levels and hormone balance

- Excessive body weight
- Body wear and tear

The above list is hardly complete. We could also add stress, the accumulation of free radicals in the body, and the cumulative results of poor nutrition, for example. The key here is not to identify every single factor (an impossible task), but to understand that if you want to slow the aging process, you have to look at more than a "magic bullet" approach involving one or two supplements. The only way to maximize health and life span is to use a whole-body, systemic approach. In other words, you need to do everything at once. The good news is that there are definitely steps that you can implement to help retard the aging process and keep you more youthful, more energized, and healthier for longer than you ever thought possible.

Before we address these factors of aging and present a program for slowing down and even reversing some of them, we need to separate the factors into three categories in order to decipher clues as to how to handle them. The three primary categories that affect how we age are:

- The things that we do to ourselves, which are easily correctable (relatively speaking).
- The micro-level factors programmed into our cells, which until a few years ago seemed impossible to change.
- The macro-level factors programmed into our bodies as we age, such as hormonal changes, many of which can be modified.

## THE PURPOSE OF AGING AND DEATH

Although it may not seem so from an egocentric point of view, aging and death are good things for the species. The concept is simple—adaptation and evolution. In order to ensure the survival of the species, nature selects those traits most useful for survival in a particular environment and passes them on to the next generation. The species evolves over time so it becomes more and more capable of surviving in its environment. But why do "we" have to die after passing on our genetic information? From a genetic point of view, if the older generation did not die off, it wouldn't allow the species to advance because the older generations would continue to procreate and advance the "older" gene pool generation after generation. It's only by eliminating the older gene pool that the species evolves.

In order to accomplish its purpose, nature has programmed our bodies with certain time bombs. For example, at the micro level, our cells can replicate only so many times before the cells become non-functional and die off. And at the macro level, genes program certain changes into our bodies so that once our "biological" usefulness has been fulfilled, aging is accelerated. Menopause is a prime example.

The benefits of this process of the old dying off and being replaced by the new is not just reserved for the next generation. Although it may not seem so, it does provide immediate benefits for us too. We can see it at work in our bones, for example. Our bones grow and renew as older bone dies off and is replaced by new, less fragile bone. If all we had was our original bone, we wouldn't be able to repair broken bones.

You may have seen the movie based on this premise called *Death Becomes Her*, in which characters played by Goldie Hawn and Meryl Streep become immortal. They cannot die, and the cells in their bodies cannot die, but without death and replacement, there is no mechanism for repairing damage. By the end of the film, although they are both alive, their bodies have suffered ghoulish but comical damage. This whole mechanism of death and replacement works—if it weren't such a personal issue when we ourselves die, we'd all be pleased with the process. It's worth noting that the only "immortal" cells in our bodies are aberrant cancer cells.

## Tampering with Nature?

A number of people have suggested that trying to change this process is contrary to the laws of nature and shouldn't be attempted. However, I don't think so, and I would like to submit to you an opposing "genetic" point of view. If the purpose of the whole process is to advance the species, then as humans we have a new element added to the equation because we rely on our brains, on intelligence, for our advantage in the world. Other species advance primarily by improving their gene pool as it relates to physical adaptation, but humans advance not just according to physical traits but also according to what we know and how we think. Knowledge and experience are becoming far more important for the survival of mankind than for any other species. Books and computers can capture the knowledge of an individual, but not their experience. And the longer we can hold onto that experience, the greater our species' chances of survival.

I believe that nature supports this premise. As our knowledge grows, we are now learning that we can indeed manipulate and alter some of the limiting factors that nature built into the "early prototypes" of our bodies. In a sense, at the point knowledge has become fundamental to our survival, nature is allowing us to view and alter some of these previously hidden secrets.

Another point to consider is that some scientists believe that we are not actually "living longer," but that we are merely living closer to our built-in limit of around 150. If so, then all we are really doing is helping people live the length of life their bodies were designed to live, which would make the "tampering with nature" question moot. In either case, let's discuss some of those things we've learned.

## THE THINGS WE DO TO OURSELVES

The damage we do to ourselves is the easiest to correct. In fact, virtually everything we've talked about in previous chapters addresses this issue, which means that most of what you have already read about optimizing your health is exactly what you need to be doing to prolong life. Just to reiterate, here is a quick summary of some of the key points.

### Compromized Immune System

One of the major causes of death is the collapse of the immune system as we age. This makes us susceptible to everything from pneumonia to cancer. Some of this is inevitable, of course, but it is amazing how much of it can be prevented, and even reversed, by following the principles of the Baseline of Health Program.

### Inflammation

Chronic inflammation is a major aging factor and a primary contributor to premature death. It is implicated in everything from lung problems to chronic heart disease and even cancer. There are a number of things we can do that help reduce inflammation far better and more safely than taking an aspirin every day. Probably the two most important are regular intake of systemic proteolytic enzymes and bringing the ratio of omega-6 to omega-3 fatty acids closer to the 1:1 ratio where it needs to be.

### Toxins

Every day, we are exposed to over 100,000 "new" chemicals that have been released into the environment over the last century. Many of them are chemical estrogens, potent in amounts as small as a billionth of a gram. Cleansing those toxins out of our bodies with colon, liver, heavy metal, blood, and kidney detoxification is essential for maximizing health and increasing life span. In addition, modern industry has released untold tons of free heavy metals, including mercury, cadmium, lead, and aluminum, into the environment—all of which is eventually making its way into our bodies.

## Poor Circulation

When we talked about cancer, we explored how any restriction in blood circulation reduces the amount of oxygen and nutrients that reaches our cells and increases the buildup of toxic waste in those same cells. We also explored how poor circulation in our lymph system accelerates the aging process and promotes the onset of age-related diseases such as cancer. And finally, we discussed how a major factor in the aging/disease process is when the energies in our body become unbalanced or diminished in any way, or if they cannot circulate freely to all parts of the body.

## Free Radicals

Free radicals play a major role in the aging process as well as in the onset of cancer, heart disease, stroke, arthritis, possibly allergies, and a host of other ailments. The link between free radicals and the "aging diseases" is one of the most important recent scientific discoveries. The use of a full-spectrum antioxidant supplement at a maintenance level may provide the ultimate defense against the premature aging effects of free radicals. At therapeutic levels, antioxidants can play a significant role in reversing many of the effects of aging and disease. In the world of antiaging, antioxidants are the "celebrities" of the moment, with a new one blazing across the media every few months. It's hard to have missed the stories about noni, mangosteen, gogi, açaí, pomegranate, and resveratrol over the last couple of years.

## Lack of Exercise

Exercise fundamentally changes every system and function in your body. And the older you get, the more important it is, and the more pronounced the benefits are. The operative concepts, however, when it comes to exercise are balance and common sense. If you overdo it, the benefits start to reverse, and you risk ligament and cartilage injury and even damage to the immune system. Over-exercise is counterproductive and eventually breaks the body.

Moderate exercise, on the other hand, can double the strength of a person in their nineties in just a few weeks.

## Poor Diet and Nutrition

The key thought to remember is that you can't build the same life expectancy into your body with pepperoni pizza, beer, and Ding Dongs® that you can with healthy, living foods.

## Negative Thoughts

What you think absolutely matters—not just mentally, but physically. Stress and depression are major aging factors.

## Smoking

Smoking not only shortens your life, it makes you look older in the process. This is not just an issue of vanity—your skin is a window to your overall health. This is easily seen in heavy smokers. The dried up, heavily wrinkled, gray skin seen on the outside of the body is highly reflective of the damage that is also being done out of sight in the lungs and cardiovascular system. If your skin doesn't have a rosy, youthful glow, then you might want to start making changes in your lifestyle according to the Baseline of Health Program.

## Excessive Calories and Sugars

Of all of the things that you can do to increase longevity, only one has been proven to actually extend life across the board: caloric restriction. Caloric restriction is the only means of retarding aging that is both extensively researched and proven. This is not the same as dieting or starvation. Rather, it entails the reduction of caloric intake while maintaining the optimal intake of essential nutrients, especially vitamins and minerals.

Caloric restriction appears to produce the following effects: it lowers body temperature, raises dehydroepiandrosterone (DHEA) levels, and lowers plasma insulin levels. Interestingly enough, lowering plasma insulin levels itself also tends to lower body temperature and increase levels of DHEA (the youth hormone), indicating that insulin may be a prime factor in the aging process. This was supported by studies showing that the sugar-regulating drug metformin might be just as effective as caloric restriction in reversing aging and revitalizing the elderly.[1]

Does that mean we should all be taking metformin? Not necessarily. First, although, as far as drugs go, metformin is relatively benign, it is not totally without side effects (it occasionally causes death from lactic acidosis, for example). But it is quite likely that a minor change in lifestyle and the use of natural supplements can offer the same benefits with no negative side effects and at less cost. For example:

- Cut way back on your intake of high-glycemic foods.

- Use natural glucoregulatory herbs with your meals. As we discussed in relation to diabetes, these include herbs such as nopal cactus, konjac mannan, *Gymnema sylvestre*, fenugreek extract, banaba leaf extract (corosolic acid), bitter melon (*Momordica charantia*), blueberry leaf extract, and cinnamon extract (Cinnulin PF). The use of these herbs will significantly slow down the rate at which your body absorbs simple carbohydrates, thereby minimizing the insulin response. In essence, these herbs mimic the activity of metformin without the side effects.

- Go on a regular fasting program. Start with just one day a week on fresh juice and superfoods such as chlorella, spirulina, wheatgrass, and presprouted barley. Then supplement that with a three-day fast once a month, and a one-week fast twice a year. Short-term fasting produces many of the benefits of long-term caloric restriction, and it's a lot easier to do.

It's never too late to start. Studies have shown that caloric restriction is just as effective in extending life span late in life as it is earlier. In fact, many of the major benefits can be gained in as little as four weeks on the program.

## MICRO-LEVEL FACTORS

Unlike the things we do to ourselves that accelerate aging and are easily correctable (relatively speaking), the micro-level factors that promote aging are programmed into our very cells. Until a few years ago, these factors seemed impossible to influence, but this is changing. Of all of the things that make us "old," two things stand out because, until now, they have been so untouchable—the Hayflick Limit and the glycation of proteins.

### The Hayflick Limit

The Hayflick Limit, named after the person who discovered it almost forty years ago, refers to the fact that all cells have only a limited capacity to continue to divide through the course of our lives. The numbers are different for each type of cell in the body, but by early adulthood, half of those divisions have been used up. By mid-life, perhaps only 20–40 percent of those divisions are left. At that point, old age starts taking over. In effect, the Hayflick Limit determines life span at the cellular level. With each division, a cell becomes less likely to divide again, until finally it stops dividing altogether and becomes senescent. Cell senescence is the final step before cell death. Senescent cells are still alive and metabolically active, but they're no longer capable of dividing. More importantly, senescent cells exhibit all of the characteristics that so bother us about old age, such as the difference between the supple skin of a child and the wrinkled skin of the elderly.

As cells approach the Hayflick Limit, they divide less frequently and become aberrant. They take on wildly irregular forms, no longer line up in parallel arrays, assume a granular appearance, and deviate from their normal size and shape. This distorted appearance, called the senescent phenotype, is accompanied by a state of declining functionality that, until recently, was thought to be irreversible.

## The Glycation of Proteins

Glycation is the uncontrolled reaction of sugars with proteins, similar to what happens when you heat sugars and they caramelize. In effect, glycation is what happens when excess sugars caramelize the proteins in your body. It's a major factor in the aging process, and it's particularly devastating to diabetics. Your body is mostly made up of proteins. In fact, proteins are the substances most responsible for the daily functioning of your body. That's why anything that causes protein deterioration has such a dramatic impact on the body's function and appearance. Thanks largely to the destructive effects of sugar and aldehydes, the protein in our bodies tends to undergo destructive changes as we age. This destruction is a prime factor not only in the aging process itself but also in the familiar signs of aging, such as wrinkling skin, cataracts, and the destruction of our nervous system, particularly the brain.

## Supplements to Reverse Cellular Aging

As it turns out, not only can we reverse the aging process at the cellular level now, and actually do it quite simply and quickly, but we can also reverse aging at the system level and the organ level. And for that matter, we can reverse it in terms of how we look and feel, and by that I mean our skin and hair and energy levels. This also affects our life span as well. There are a number of nutraceuticals that can play a role, but three stand out: L-carnosine, dimethy-laminoethanol (DMAE), and acetyl-L-carnitine. Based on everything we know, supplementing with a combination of these nutrients is one of the most effective and safest steps we can take to help turn back the clock at the cellular level.

## L-Carnosine

L-Carnosine is a naturally occurring combination of two amino acids, ala-nine and histidine, that was discovered in Russia in the early 1900s. Because much of the research was done in Russia, it was largely unavailable in the United States until just a few years ago. Now, though, there have been a number of studies and experiments in other parts of the world verifying everything done in Russia, and more. Most notably, there was a series of astonishing experiments done in Australia that proved that carnosine rejuve-nates cells as they approach senescence. Cells cultured with carnosine lived longer and retained their youthful appearance and growth patterns.

It was discovered that carnosine can actually reverse the signs of aging in senescent cells. When the scientists transferred senescent cells to a culture medium containing carnosine, those cells exhibited a rejuvenated appearance and often an enhanced capacity to divide. When they transferred the cells back to a medium lacking carnosine, the signs of senescence quickly reap-peared. In other words, the carnosine medium restored the juvenile cell phe-notype within days, whereas the standard culture medium brought back the senescent cell phenotype. In addition, the carnosine medium increased cell life span, even for old cells. When the researchers took old cells that had already gone through 55 divisions and transferred them to the carnosine medium, they survived up to 70 divisions, compared to only 57–61 divisions for the cells that were not transferred. This represents an increase in the number of cell divisions for each cell of almost 25 percent. But in terms of cell life, the increase was an astounding 300 percent. The cells transferred to the carnosine medium attained a life span of 413 days, compared to just 126–139 days for the control cells.[2]

Increased Life Expectancy—What does carnosine mean for actual life expectancy? A more recent Russian study on mice has shown that those given carnosine are twice as likely to reach their maximum life span as untreated mice. The carnosine also significantly reduced the outward "signs of old age" and made the mice look younger: 44 percent of the carnosine-treated mice had young, glossy coats in old age as opposed to only 5 percent in the untreated mice. Another important difference between the treated and the untreated mice was in their behavior: only 9 percent of the untreated mice behaved youthfully in old age versus 58 percent of the carnosine-treated mice.[3]

Auto-Regulator—Carnosine has the remarkable ability to throttle down bodily processes that are in a state of excess and to ramp up those that are under-expressed. For example, carnosine thins the blood of people whose blood tends to clot too much and increases the clotting tendency in those with a low clotting index.[4] Another example is that carnosine suppresses excess immune responses in those who have "hyper" immune systems, whereas it stimulates the immune response in those with weakened immune systems, such as the aged.[5] And carnosine even seems to have the ability to normalize brain wave functions.[6]

Controlling Protein Glycation—Carnosine protects cellular proteins from damage in at least two ways. First, it bonds with the carbonyl (or aldehyde) groups that, if left alone, attack and bind with proteins.[7] Second, it works as an antioxidant to prevent the formation of oxidized sugars, also called advanced glycosylation end-products (AGEs).[8] The less AGEs in your body, the younger you are. Both of these processes have important implications for antiaging therapy.

Alzheimer's Disease Prevention—Carnosine has also been proven to reduce, or completely prevent, cell damage caused by beta amyloid, one of the prime protein risk factors for Alzheimer's disease. The presence of beta amyloid leads to damage of the nerves and arteries of the brain. Carnosine blocks and inactivates beta amyloid, in effect, protecting neural tissues against dementia.[9] The key is that carnosine not only prevents damaging cross-links from forming in proteins, it eliminates cross-links that have previously formed, thus restoring normal membrane function in cells. This is true not only in the brain, but in all the organs of the body.

There is, however, one "gap" in carnosine's usefulness—lipofuscin. Lipofuscin is a pigment commonly found in aging brains and in other tissues such as the skin. By itself, it is not dangerous but merely a byproduct of harmful reactions, such as free-radical damage and protein/aldehyde damage, that have already taken place. In the case of aldehydes, for example, when you supplement with carnosine, it quickly binds with the aldehydes, preventing them from damaging the proteins. The byproduct of this reaction is lipofuscin. So, once again you have inactive lipofuscin compounds, but this time as the result of preventing protein damage. In a sense, with carnosine you trade protein damage for lipofuscin. This, however, can lead to another problem. If enough lipofuscin accumulates over time (a process accelerated when you supplement with carnosine), it can interfere with proper cellular and organ functions. It's important, therefore, to continually remove the lipofuscin so it doesn't build up, and that's were DMAE comes in.

### Dimethylaminoethanol (DMAE)

DMAE is the perfect companion to carnosine in an antiaging formulation, because it reinforces carnosine's antiaging properties and provides a series of complementary benefits of its own, particularly in the brain. DMAE is a naturally occurring nutrient, with oily fish such as wild salmon and sardines among its primary sources, that enhances acetylcholine synthesis. Adequate levels of acetylcholine are important for proper memory function. Normally found in small amounts in our brains, DMAE has been shown to remarkably enhance brain function when used as a supplement.

Many people may have heard of the antiaging results that Romanian scientist Ana Aslin achieved using something called GH3 (procaine). GH3 breaks down in the body to form DMAE and para-aminobenzoic acid (PABA). In other words, DMAE is the key active component in Ana Aslin's antiaging formula.

The important point to remember, though, is that one of DMAE's prime actions is that it flushes accumulated lipofuscin from your body—from the neurons in your brain, from your skin, and from all other organs. It also complements carnosine in that DMAE has been shown to inhibit and reverse the cross-linking of proteins and extend life span. In a French double-blind study, individuals who were given 1,200 mg per day of DMAE for five days showed significant improvements in alertness and neuromotor control, with decreased anxiety. Studies have also shown that DMAE can help improve memory, concentration, and the ability to focus.[10]

Clinical studies of DMAE have used up to 1,600 mg per day with no reports of significant side effects. In some cases, people may experience slight headaches, muscle tension, or insomnia if they take too much too quickly. These effects are easily eliminated if intake is reduced and then gradually increased. Although there is no direct connection, many manufacturers recommend that women who are pregnant or breastfeeding, anyone who suffers from convulsions, epilepsy, or seizure disorders, and people with manic-depressive illness should avoid using DMAE. This is probably more of a legal issue than a medical one. Surprisingly (or maybe not so surprisingly if you think about it), for a substance found readily in nature, it is heavily regulated in some countries, such as Canada, where a prescription is required.

### Acetyl-L-Carnitine

Like DMAE, acetyl-L-carnitine (ALC) is a perfect complement to L-carnosine. Although your body can synthesize L-carnitine in the liver, it depends on outside sources (meat being a primary one) to fulfill its requirements. This can present a problem for vegetarians since L-carnitine performs several key functions in the human body. For one, it can improve the functioning of the immune system by enhancing the ability of macrophages to function as phagocytes. And it can improve the functioning of muscle tissue and has been shown to increase running speed when given prior to exercise.[11] It also plays a major role in cellular energy production by shuttling fatty acids from the main cell body into the mitochondria (the cell's energy factories) so that the fats can be oxidized for energy. Without carnitine, fatty acids cannot easily enter the mitochondria.

Acetyl-L-carnitine is a specialized form of L-carnitine that is often deficient, even in meat eaters. It performs virtually all of the same functions as L-carnitine, only better. In terms of cellular energy production, in addition to shuttling fatty acids into cell mitochondria, ALC provides acetyl groups from which acetyl-coenzyme A (a key metabolic intermediate) can be regenerated. This is important because acetyl-coenzyme A facilitates the transport of metabolic energy and boosts mitochondrial activity. Also, the addition of the acetyl group makes ALC water soluble, which enables it to diffuse across the inner wall of the mitochondria and to cross all cell membranes more easily. In particular, ALC readily crosses the blood-brain barrier, where it provides a number of specialized neurological functions. Studies have shown that acetyl-L-carnitine can inhibit the deterioration in mental function associated with Alzheimer's disease and slow its progression.[12] Part of this is a result of its ability to shield neurons from the toxicity of beta amyloid protein. As a result, ALC improves alertness in Alzheimer's patients.

Through its action on dopamine (a chemical messenger used between nerve cells) and dopamine receptors, ALC seems to play a major role in preventing and/or minimizing the symptoms of Parkinson's disease. ALC retards the decline in the number of dopamine receptors that occurs as part of the normal aging process and (more rapidly) with the onset of Parkinson's disease.[13] In fact, many researchers believe that Parkinson's may be caused by a deficiency of dopamine. ALC also inhibits tremors and may even play a role in helping with MS by inhibiting (and possibly reversing) the degeneration of myelin sheaths.[14]

Overall, ALC helps slow down the aging process of the brain:

- Retards the inevitable decline in glucocorticoid receptors that occurs with aging.

- Slows the age-related deterioration of the hippocampus.

- Retards the inevitable decline in nerve growth factor receptors that occurs as we age.

- Stimulates and maintains the growth of new neurons within the brain and helps to prevent the death of existing neurons.

- Protects the NMDA (N-methyl-D-aspartic acid) receptors in the brain from age-related decline. NMDA receptors play a critical role in "synaptic plasticity," a key cellular mechanism involved in the brain's learning and memory functions.[15]

- Inhibits the excessive release of adrenaline and the depletion of luteinizing hormone–releasing hormone and testosterone that occurs in response to stress.

- Enhances the function of cytochrome oxidase, an essential enzyme of the electron transport system. This is important because reduced cytochrome oxidase activity is characteristic of neurodegeneration.[16]

The mind-boosting effect of acetyl-L-carnitine is often noticed within a few hours, even within an hour, of supplementing. Most people report feeling mentally sharper, having more focus, and being more alert. And ALC, like DMAE, helps flush lipofuscin from the body, especially from the brain.

## MACRO-LEVEL FACTORS

Now, let's touch on the hormonal changes programmed into our bodies, changes that affect aging at the macro level. Hormones are your body's chemical messenger system, telling your body what to do and when. In regard to aging, they tell your body how to age and when, and changes in any hormone can affect aging.

- Changes in estrogen and progesterone levels relate to the onset of menopause in women (andropause in men), the change most women associate with aging.

- Changes in testosterone affect our outlook on life (our "drive"), the disappearance of muscle mass, and the shrinkage of our bodies associated with old age.

- Growth hormone affects everything from muscle/fat ratios to the graying of hair.

- When melatonin levels drop as we age, it affects things as diverse as how well we sleep to how strong our immune system is—even how resistant we are to cancer.

Reestablishment of a youthful hormonal balance can be achieved by neutralizing the effects of xenoestrogens on the body and by supplementing with bioidentical hormones in small amounts, or by supplementing with herbs or secretagogues that assist your own body in increasing production of the necessary hormones (see Chapter 13).

## GENERAL RECOMMENDATIONS

Other than the addition of L-carnosine, DMAE, and acetyl-L-carnitine, everything that you need to do to slow down the aging process has already been covered in the Baseline of Health Program. In other words, at the same time you're optimizing health and protecting yourself from catastrophic illness, you're slowing down the aging process and maximizing your life potential with no additional effort. With that in mind, let's focus on the three "new" nutraceuticals in question.

L-Carnosine—While it is true that some people who supplement with carnosine are going to notice everything from younger-looking skin to more energy, you shouldn't focus on short-term benefits. If any short-term benefits are noticed, you should consider them an added bonus. The reason you want to supplement with carnosine is to protect against the long-term ravages of aging. Some experts recommend using only 50–100 mg of carnosine a day; others say that if you don't take 1,000–1,500 mg a day it won't work because your body metabolizes the first 500 mg or so. All of these experts are ignoring the simple fact that different people need different amounts. For example:

- The older you get, the more you need.
- If you eat a mostly vegetarian diet, you need more.
- If you're diabetic or just have trouble with blood sugar, you need more.

If you're young and healthy and include meat in your diet, then 250–500 mg a day makes sense. As you get older, and if you're starting to show signs of aging or glycation (such as cataracts), then consider increasing the dosage up to 1,200 mg a day, maybe even as high as 1,500 mg a day. Carnosine levels in our bodies directly correlate with both the length and quality of our lives. And since carnosine levels decline with age, supplementation with carnosine represents one of the most powerful things you can do to hold back the ravages of old age.

DMAE—Typically, dosages of 100–500 mg of DMAE a day are taken in two to three doses with meals. While the best dosage has not yet been discovered, it is known that doses of less than 100 mg per day do not have much effect. At 400 mg per day, however, alertness and mental powers are improved. Overdosing can cause insomnia, headaches, or muscle tension, which disappear when dosage is lowered. No serious adverse effects have been reported. However, it is thought that DMAE may make epilepsy and bipolar depression worse in those who are undermethylated (see Chapter 10), so people with these health problems should avoid DMAE.

Acetyl-L-Carnitine—The typical daily dosage of ALC for long-term use is 100–400 mg once a day (preferably in the morning) or spread throughout the day. At dosages over 500 mg, you may experience over-stimulation or slight nausea. However, many people use up to 1,000–1,500 mg a day with no problems.

Look, getting older may be beyond your control, but how you age is not. Following the principles of the Baseline of Health Program can help you prevent and reverse catastrophic illness as well as the signs and symptoms of aging.

Whew! All done! All that's left is put it all together with some specific recommendations to get you started on the road to taking back control of your health.

# CONCLUSION

# Building Your Baseline of Health Day by Day

*T*he secret to health—the secret to all of the success that the great "miracle doctors" share—is that they look to raise every inch of a person's Personal Health Line. If you do that, the odds of good health (even of recovery from many terminal diseases) are remarkably favorable. If you want great health, maximized physical performance, or relief from illness that has not responded to allopathic medicine, stop looking for magic bullets and start working with your entire body. Variations of this program have proven so effective that thousands of people have experienced remarkable healings by using it. The results may very well astound you . . . and your doctor. (If you are on any medication or have a major illness, be sure to work with your physician.)

This program is the synthesis of all the best that is taught by today's miracle doctors. It is designed to empower your own body to throw off illness and keep the illness from returning. And for those of you who are already healthy, it is designed to keep you that way—to maximize your body's defense and repair mechanisms so you never get sick in the first place. It can even help maximize athletic performance, as I verified working with a number of riders on the Kelly Benefit Strategies/Medifast Pro Cycling Team during the 2007 season.

That said, I need to mention that over the years, I've given close to 2,000 talks on the Baseline of Health Program, which focuses on working with the entire body. After each talk, I am invariably surrounded by people who tell me how impressed they are with the idea of not looking for magic bullets and dealing with the entire body, and how much sense it makes to them. They absolutely understand the concept and why it's necessary to do everything in the program. And then, as surely as night follows day, they ask "the question"—"But I have condition X, so what herb or supplement should I take?" I understand. We've all been conditioned by years of modern medicine to look for magic bullets.

Given that fact, I'm going to do the unforgivable and break the Baseline of Health Program into pieces. Don't get me wrong; it's absolutely far and away better to do the entire program. Picking and choosing pieces is like shooting craps—sometimes you get lucky, but in the end the odds favor the house. And the sicker you are, the more necessary it is that you don't diddle about: do the program all at once, several times in a row, in rapid succession, and make no compromises. But if you're like most people, in fair to middling health, or even a high-performance athlete who follows this program, you can take it in pieces. And yes, some of the pieces of the program are more essential than others.

## THE BASELINE OF HEALTH PROGRAM

| SUPPLEMENT/ACTION | SCHEDULE | | | |
| | DAILY FOR EVERYONE | DAILY FOR MEN AND WOMEN OVER 30 | PERIODIC | SPECIAL OCCASIONS |
| --- | --- | --- | --- | --- |
| Digestive enzymes | • | | | |
| Food-grown multivitamin/mineral | • | | | |
| Proteolytic enzymes | • | | | |
| Liquid trace minerals | • | | | |
| Superfoods | • | | | |
| Psyllium or flax fiber | • | | | |
| Sugar metabolizer | • | | | |
| Antioxidants | • | | | |
| Omega-3 fatty acids | • | | | |
| Probiotics | • | | | |
| Vitamin D | • | | | |
| Full-spectrum vitamin E | • | | | |
| L-carnosine | • | | | |
| Coenzyme $Q_{10}$ | • | | | |
| Immune boosters | • | | | |

| | SCHEDULE | | | |
|---|---|---|---|---|
| SUPPLEMENT/ACTION | DAILY FOR EVERYONE | DAILY FOR MEN AND WOMEN OVER 30 | PERIODIC | SPECIAL OCCASIONS |
| Pathogen destroyers | • | | | • |
| Brain enhancers | • | | | • |
| Women's progesterone cream | | • | | |
| Women's testosterone formula | | • | | |
| Men's progesterone cream | | • | | |
| Men's testosterone formula | | • | | |
| Growth hormone secretagogue | | • | | |
| Estriol cream for women | | | | • |
| Other hormones (melatonin, pregnenolone, 7-Keto DHEA) | | • | | • |
| Colon detoxification | | | • | |
| Liver detoxification | | | • | |
| Heavy metal detoxification | | | • | |
| Blood cleanse | | | • | |
| Kidney flush | | | • | |
| Colon corrective formula | | | | • |
| Stress reduction | | | | • |
| Energy boosters | | | | • |
| Joint enhancers | | | | • |
| Lifestyle changes (exercise, relaxation, hydration, juice fasting, diet) | • | | | |

## DAILY FOR EVERYONE

The first three items in this list are essentially my sine qua non of health. If I do these regularly along with proper eating, periodic juice fasting, detoxification, and exercise, my health is going to be pretty darn good.

- At one time, I considered a broad-based vitamin/mineral supplement the cornerstone of the Baseline of Health Program, but now I personally use more digestive enzymes than any other single supplement. If I could only take one supplement, it would probably be a high-quality digestive enzyme formula with every meal. (See Chapter 11.)

- Nevertheless, a broad-based vitamin/mineral supplement is still a major component of the program because it's virtually impossible to get everything you need nutritionally from the modern diet. Vitamin isolates have a role in punching up certain nutrient levels, but I recommend taking a biodynamically grown, living-food, multivitamin/mineral complex (see Chapter 9).

- A liquid trace-mineral supplement is a core supplement as well, preferably one that contains electrically charged micelle colloidal particles that help break surface tension and make the trace minerals more bioavailable (see Chapter 9).

The rest of the items in this list are somewhat "optional." To put it another way, the more you do wrong in your daily life—eat badly, don't exercise, etc.—the more of the following items become mandatory for basic health maintenance. If you're looking for optimum health, then the more you do, the better, regardless of how well you're living. For what it's worth, I do virtually all of them. (Men and women obviously use formulas that are specific to them.)

- The more I use proteolytic enzymes between meals, the more attached I become to their benefits. I now consider their regular use almost essential for optimum health (see Chapter 11).

- Superfoods should become a regular part of your diet, if not daily, then at least two to three times a week. Look for superfood mixes that combine ingredients such as hypoallergenic rice and pea protein, ultra-long-chain carbohydrates, green foods (chlorella, spirulina, barley grass, wheat grass), good fats, and antioxidants. Either mix them in juice or blend them in fruit smoothies. (See Chapter 9.)

- Water-soluble fiber in the form of freshly ground golden flaxseed, psyllium seed husks, or stabilized rice bran solubles should be used to supplement most diets (see Chapter 7).

- If you eat any grains or moderately high-glycemic carbohydrates, use a fiber-based metabolic sugar enhancer to block receptor sites and slow the glycemic response. Look for fibers such as konjac mannan, nopal cactus, fenugreek, and *Gymnema sylvestre*. (See Chapters 7 and 20.)

- A full-spectrum antioxidant is essential to control free-radical damage, prevent disease, slow down the degradation of organs, and extend life (see Chapter 10).

- The best sources of omega-3 fatty acids are fish oil, krill oil, and high-lignan cold-pressed, organic flax oil. Each has features that make it unique and invaluable. I use all three, mixing them to get a total of 3 grams each day. (See Chapter 7.)

- Use a good probiotic to keep beneficial bacteria populations in the gut at optimum levels (see Chapter 4).

- Vitamin D deficiency is emerging as a major source of age-related conditions. Taking 1,000 IU a day of $D_3$ is not too much, particularly if you don't spend much time in the sun. And even if you spend time in the sun, it's still worth supplementing as you get older. In fact, 2,000 IU to as much as 5,000 IU a day is not out of the question as you age. (See Chapter 21.)

- High-quality vitamin E supplementation promotes health, especially of the cardiovascular system. Make sure you use a full-spectrum supplement that emphasizes gamma-tocopherol vitamin E and all of the tocotrienols (see Chapters 9 and 10).

- L-carnosine is an expensive supplement, but it's also one of the reasons that I don't look sixty years old. As we discussed in the last chapter, dosage is age-related, diet-related, and related to whether or not you have sugar problems. At my age, I use 1,500 mg a day in combination with DMAE and acetyl-L-carnitine. (See Chapter 21.)

- For cardiovascular health, I use ubiquinone or coenzyme $Q_{10}$, 50 mg a day (see Chapter 18).

- I rotate through immune boosters such as echinacea formulas, AHCC (Active Hexose Correlated Compounds), and colostrum. I also use pathogen destroyers, such as garlic, olive leaf extract, and oil of oregano, semi-regularly (a couple of times a week) and as needed when I feel illness coming on. (See Chapter 14.)

- I find that brain enhancers, such as the herbs *Ginkgo biloba* and *Bacopa monniera*, definitely improve my short-term concentration and maximize the outlook for long-term cognitive function (see Chapter 10).

## Lifestyle Changes

Even though lifestyle changes do not involve supplements, they are a fundamental part of the Baseline of Health Program. If you are not already doing so, incorporate these changes into your daily life as soon as possible. They are not optional.

Exercise—Even if you are ill (especially if you are ill), you must exercise. If all you can do is hobble around the bed with a walker, do it. Do one lap around the bed the first day, and two laps the next. Ultimately, you should be doing some weight-bearing exercise, some cardio, some stretching, and some breathing exercises. Cycle through them on a day-by-day basis, but do something every day. (See Chapter 17.)

Relaxation—Meditate or pray deeply, morning and evening. Other options are to watch your breath or use biofeedback devices. In other words, use whatever technique that helps you relax. At the end of each session, practice healing visualizations and affirmations. Use a nerve tonic or beverage as needed. (See Chapter 16.)

Hydration—Some say that you get all the water you need in the foods you eat, but that's just not true. You need to drink a minimum of 64 ounces of pure water every day. Soda and coffee do not count; if you think they do, try washing your clothes in them. (See Chapter 8.)

Juice Fasting—I'm a proponent of juice fasting. One of the best investments you can make in your health is a good juicer. Both fresh vegetable and fresh fruit juices are great, but I would recommend emphasizing vegetable juices as they are more alkalinizing and contain less sugar. My basic recommended protocol is:

- Fast one day a week on juice supplemented with one or more superfoods.

- Every month, do a three-day juice/superfood fast.

- Twice a year, as part of a bi-annual liver detoxification, do a five to six day juice/superfood fast.

Here's an important thought for you to keep in mind: if all you do is fast just one day a week, in seven years you will have fasted for a total of an entire year. Just one day a week can have a major impact over time. What do you think a year of fasting every seven years would do to optimize your health, let alone slow down any weight gain you might otherwise have experienced? Finally, if you are seriously ill, start a juice fast immediately; drink up to a gallon of diluted fresh juice a day (an 8-ounce glass every hour you're awake). (See Chapter 6.)

Diet—If you can't be perfect in your dietary habits, at least be better than you are now. If you have a really bad day (filled with chili dogs, beer, and cupcakes), do a one-day juice fast the next day. Your body has a remarkable ability to repair itself, if you give it a chance. And again, if you are seriously ill, you have no choice. You must totally clean up your act until you are well: no cooked foods, no processed foods, and lots of raw organic fruits and vegetables, especially fresh juices. Once you're feeling better, don't jump right back into your bad habits. Continue on your health program for at least six months after symptoms clear. It's crucial to make sure any last hidden remnants of disease have been eliminated before easing up on the program. (See Chapter 7.)

## DAILY FOR MEN AND WOMEN OVER THIRTY

By the time you're thirty, because of exposure to chemical estrogens, your hormonal system is out of whack. You need to consider supplementation with all natural progesterone cream and testosterone-balancing formulas. The only caution on progesterone formulas is to not overdo it. The idea is to mimic nature, not blow it away. If the progesterone cream doesn't do the trick, women might want to consider estriol cream, which is mild and cancer protective and may be all you need. If not, talk to your doctor about bio-identical estrogen.

Also, if you're over thirty, a good growth hormone secretagogue makes sense. If nothing else, 2,000 mg a day of an arginine/ornithine supplement will help. However, if you have herpes, don't use the arginine as it can stimulate the virus. As for the other hormones—melatonin, pregnenolone, and 7-Keto DHEA—use them as needed. Incidentally, "daily" here means on-again/off-again as described in Chapter 13.

## PERIODIC

There are those (and I'm one of them) who say that any health program should begin with a thorough detoxification. It will maximize the benefits of any supplements you take. I also understand that many people are either afraid of detoxes or find them too inconvenient. Keep in mind that whether you start with them or not, at some point they are an indispensable part of the Baseline of Health Program. My recommendation for most people is:

- A colon cleanse combined with a good heavy metal detoxification—two to four times a year.

- A blood/liver detoxification, immediately preceded by a stone-softening program that also works as a kidney flush—two to four times a year. To make things easy, I do the detoxes on a seasonal basis:
  - Spring—Colon/heavy metal detox
  - Summer—Liver/blood/kidney detox
  - Fall—Repeat the colon/heavy metal detox
  - Winter—Right after the holidays are over is the perfect time for a repeat of the liver/blood/kidney detox. Incidentally, every January, we now do a group post-holiday detox, with people from all over the world doing the detox at the same time and supporting each other. (See Chapters 3 and 6.)

For more information on detoxing than could fit in the book, including day-by-day, step-by-step walk-through instructions, check the Detox Center at www.jonbarron.org.

Note: If seriously ill, the detoxification programs need to be done immediately, back to back. Then take one week off and repeat, and repeat again as long as necessary. If you are on any medications, be sure to check with your doctor first.

## SPECIAL OCCASIONS

If needed, take a colon activator daily to avoid retaining fecal matter. Also, the worse you eat and/or the more contact you have with toxins, the more often you need to cleanse and detoxify. Other "as needed" formulas include stress reducers, energy enhancers, and joint support formulas.

## GENERAL RECOMMENDATIONS

That's the Baseline of Health Program in a nutshell. Before I close, let me make one final comment. Although, I have taken my shots at modern med-

# JONBARRON.ORG

As I stated way back in the Preface, the core of the Baseline of Health Program hasn't changed over the last ten years, but there has indeed been tremendous change in the environment surrounding the program, including the availability of "new" ingredients and "new understandings" of some old favorite ingredients, new areas of interest as they hit the news, changing focus on specific health issues, and the increasing interface of modern medicine with alternative health. And by the time you read this, many of those things will have changed yet again.

Make no mistake, this book will serve as a solid core reference for years to come, but if you want to stay up to date on all of the latest information, I invite you to visit www.jonbarron.org. There are over 1,000 pages of reference material, hours of audio files including recordings of radio appearances, video files including some of my television interviews, and a daily blog that explores the most current health issues. Consider signing up for the free semi-monthly newsletter, where I explore the hottest health issues in detail.

icine, I'm actually very supportive of doctors (if I get a hernia, I'm at the doctor's office in a heartbeat) and am extremely optimistic about some of the things I see coming in the future. We've certainly got a long way to go, but I believe that many of the mainstream treatments that we consider barbaric today will go the way of the dinosaur and that many pharmaceuticals will be replaced with high-level metabolic moderators and immune enhancers. Cancer research is already turning in this direction. I also see a bright future for gene therapy and stem cell research (despite the opportunity for great abuse) in helping alleviate many of the illnesses we face today. Finally, there's bio-mechanical medicine, which is starting to give hope to the blind and movement to the paraplegic. I believe this is all coming in the future.

That said, no amount of medical advancement will make:

- Unhealthy fast food into health enhancing nutrition

- A plugged colon incidental

- An overtaxed liver beneficial to your health

- A body filled with hundreds of toxic chemicals and heavy metals healthy

Besides, even if advancements are coming in the future, they don't help in the here and now. Ultimately, if you want optimum health or want to overcome illness, you have no choice. You cannot wait for some "magic bullet" that is unlikely to come in the near future—you must take charge of your own health, and you must do it now. Don't count on the medical system to take care of you; no amount of tinkering and funding can stop the inevitable train wreck barreling toward us. How can any health-care system survive up to half of the population living for 20–30 years with severe diabetes, let alone the other half suffering from cancer, heart disease, osteoporosis, Alzheimer's disease, and MS? There isn't enough money in the world to cover it. The only way that health care can survive—the only way you can survive—is if you take back control of your health and start doing those things that allow your body to stay healthy. Or to put it another way, the only way to save health care is to stop using it. Start living the baseline of health.

I wish you good health and long life.

# References

## Introduction

1. Heffler, S., S. Smith, S. Keehan, et al. "Health Tracking Trends: U.S. Health Spending Projections for 2004–2014." *Health Affairs* (February 23, 2005). Available online at: http://content.healthaffairs.org/cgi/content/full/hlthaff.w5.74/DC1. Employee Benefit Research Institute. "National Health Care Expenditures 1995." *EBRI Databook on Employee Benefits*, 4th ed. Employee Benefit Research Institute, March 1997.

2. Cutler, D.M., A.B. Rosen, and S. Vijan. "The Value of Medical Spending in the United States, 1960–2000." *New Engl J Med* 355 (2006): 920–927.

3. Zwillich, Todd, and Laura Gilcrest. "U.S. Healthcare Earns Sorry Score." United Press International (UPI) (September 20, 2006).

4. Cutler, D.M., A.B. Rosen, and S. Vijan. "The Value of Medical Spending in the United States, 1960–2000." *New Engl J Med* 355 (2006): 920–927.

5. Hoyert, D.L., M.P. Heron, S.L. Murphy, et al. "Deaths: Final Data for 2003". Centers for Disease Control and Prevention (CDC), Division of Vital Statistics, National Vital Statistics Reports, April 19, 2006.

6. Centers for Disease Control and Prevention (CDC). "Leading Causes of Death, 1900–1988."

7. National Digestive Diseases Information Clearinghouse. "Digestive Diseases Statistics for the U.S." NIH Publication No. 06-3873, December 2005.

8. "Past and Projected Female and Male Life Expectancy at Birth, United States, 1900–2050." U.S. Department of Commerce, Bureau of the Census.

9. Centers for Disease Control and Prevention (CDC), National Center for Chronic Disease Prevention and Health Promotion. "Incidence of Diagnosed Diabetes per 1000 Population Aged 18–79 Years, by Age, United States, 1997–2004." National Diabetes Surveillance System.

10. Lewis, Ricki, Ph.D., U.S. Food and Drug Administration. "The Rise of Antibiotic-Resistant Infections." *FDA Consumer* (September 1995).

11. Carlsen, E., A. Giwercman, N. Keiding, et al. "Evidence for Decreasing Quality of Semen During Past 50 Years." *Br Med J* 305 (1992): 609–613.

12. Kaplowitz, P.B., S.E. Oberfield, and the Drug and Therapeutics and Executive Committees of the Lawson Wilkins Pediatric Endocrine Society. "Reexamination of the Age Limit for Defining When Puberty is Precocious in Girls in the United States: Implications for Evaluation and Treatment." *Pediatrics* 104:4 (1999): 936–941. Herman-Giddens, M.E., E.J. Slora, R.C. Wasserman, et al. "Secondary Sexual Characteristics and Menses in Young Girls Seen in Office Practice: A Study from the Pediatric Research in Office Settings Network." *Pediatrics* 99:4 (1997): 505–512.

13. Christianson, A., C. Howson, B. Modell, March of Dimes. "The March of Dimes Global Report on Birth Defects: The Hidden Toll of Dying and Disabled Children." March of Dimes Report 31-2008-05, 2006.

14. Wild, S., G. Roglic, A. Green, et al. "World Health Organization, Global Prevalence of Diabetes: Estimates for the Year 2000 and Projections for 2030." *Diabetes Care* 27 (2004): 1047–1053.

15. National Institute of Diabetes and Digestive and Kidney Diseases. "Digestive Diseases in the United States: Epidemiology and Impact Diverticulosis and Diverticulitis." NIH Publication No. 02-1163. NIDDK (January 2002).

16. Centers for Disease Control and Prevention (CDC) Media Relations. "Asthma Rates in U.S. Increase." CDC (April 24, 1998).

17. Commission for Environmental Cooperation. *Children's Health and the Environment in North America, 2005–2006.* Montreal, Quebec, Canada: Commission for Environmental Cooperation, 2006, p. 4.

18. American Cancer Society. "All Women at Risk For Developing Breast Cancer." *The Breast Cancer Fact Sheet* (September 28, 2005), 3.

19. American Cancer Society. "National Action Plan for Childhood Cancer." ACS Publication 02-5M-No. 2406 (August 16, 2002).

20. Brown, M.L., J. Lipscomb, C. Snyder. "The Burden of Illness of Cancer: Economic Cost and Quality of Life." *Annu Rev Public Health* 22 (2001): 91–113. NIH Cost of Illness Report to the U.S. Congress, 2005. "National Health Care Expenditures Projections: 2003–2013." National Institutes of Health, 2005.

21. Lazarou, J., B.H. Pomeranz, P.N. Corey. "Incidence of Adverse Drug Reactions in Hospitalized Patients: A Meta-analysis of Prospective Studies." *JAMA* 279 (1998): 1200–1205.

22. Lazarou, J., J.H. Gurwitz, et al. "Why Learn about Adverse Drug Reactions (ADR)?" *Am J Med* 109:2 (2000): 87–94.

23. Lazarou, J., B.H. Pomeranz, P.N. Corey. "Incidence of Adverse Drug Reactions in Hospitalized Patients: A Meta-analysis of Prospective Studies." *JAMA* 279 (1998): 1200–1205.

24. Kohn, L.T., J.M. Corrigan, M.S. Donaldson, Institute of Medicine. "To Err Is Human: Building a Safer Health System." Executive Summary, Institute of Medicine, 1999.

25. Siegel-Itzkovich, J. "Doctors' Strike in Israel May Be Good for Health." *Br Med J* 320 (2000): 1561.

26. Phillips, D., N. Christenfeld, L. Glynn. "Increase in U.S. Medication-Error Deaths Between 1983 and 1993." *Lancet* 351 (1998): 643–644.

## Chapter 1: The Thieves of Health

1. McTaggert, Lynne. "Spin Doctors of Cancer." *What Doctors Don't Tell You* 7:3 (July 1996).

2. Office for National Statistics. "Breast Cancer." October 4, 2005.

3. Leaf, C. "Why We're Losing the War on Cancer and How to Win It." *Fortune* 149:6 (March 22, 2004): 76–82, 84–86, 88.

4. Culbert, Michael. *Medical Armageddon*. San Diego: C and C Communications, 1994.

5. Stevenson L.W. "Beta-Blockers for Stable Heart Failure." *N Engl J Med* 346 (May 2002): 1346–1347.

6. Cooper W.O., S. Hernandez-Diaz, P.G. Arbogast, et al. "Major Congenital Malformations after First-Trimester Exposure to ACE Inhibitors." *N Engl J Med* 354 (2006): 2443–2451. Friedman, J.M. "ACE Inhibitors and Congenital Anomalies." *N Engl J Med* 354 (2006): 2498–2500.

7. Boden, W.E., R.A. O'Rourke, K.K. Teo, et al. "Optimal Medical Therapy With or Without PCI for Stable Coronary Disease." *New Engl J Med* 356:15 (2007): 1503–1516.

8. Families USA. "Report: Cost Overdose: Growth in Drug Spending for the Elderly." July 15, 2000. (Data for the Families USA report were prepared by the PRIME Institute of the University of Minnesota).

9. Millenson, Michael L. "Demanding Medical Evidence: Doctors and Accountability in the Information Age." Robert Wood Johnson Foundation, Issue 2 (September 1998).

10. Kaufman, M. "Study Cites Marked Drop in FDA's Warning Letters." *Washington Post* (June 27, 2006): A19.

11. Union of Concerned Scientists. "FDA Scientists Pressured to Exclude, Alter Findings; Scientists Fear Retaliation for Voicing Safety Concerns." July 20, 2006. Available online at: www.ucsusa.org/news/press_release/fda-scientists-pressured. html.

12. Alonso-Zaldivar, Ricardo. "FDA Pledges Conflict Reforms." *Los Angeles Times* (July 25, 2006): A12.

13. Ibid.

14. Greider, Katharine. *The Big Fix: How the Pharmaceutical Industry Rips Off American Consumers*. New York: Public Affairs Reports, 2003.

15. Kaufman, M. "Study Cites Marked Drop in FDA's Warning Letters." *Washington Post* (June 27, 2006): A19.

16. Greider, Katharine. *The Big Fix: How the Pharmaceutical Industry Rips Off American Consumers*. New York: Public Affairs Reports, 2003.

17. Gibson, M.J., N. Brangan, D. Gross, et al. "How Much are Medicare Beneficiaries Paying Out-of-pocket for Prescription Drugs?" Washington, DC: AARP Public Policy Institute, September 1999.

18. Gandhi, T.K., S.N. Weingart, J. Borus, et al. "Adverse Drug Events in Ambulatory Care." *N Engl J Med* 348:16 (2003): 1556–1564.

## Chapter 3: Intestinal Cleansing

1. Adams, P.F., G.E. Hendershot, M.A. Marano. "Current Estimates from the National Health Interview Survey, 1996." National Center for Health Statistics. *Vital Health Stat* 10 (1999): 200.

2. Kozak, L.J., M.F. Owings, M.J. Hall. "National Hospital Discharge Survey: 2002 Annual Summary with Detailed Diagnosis and Procedure Data." National Center for Health Statistics. *Vital Health Stat* 13 (2005): 158. Burt, C.W., S.M.

Schappert. "Ambulatory Care Visits to Physician Offices, Hospital Outpatient Departments, and Emergency Departments: United States, 1999–2000." National Center for Health Statistics. *Vital Health Stat* 13 (2004): 157.

3. Sandler, R.S., J.E. Everhart, M. Donowitz, et al. "The Burden of Selected Digestive Diseases in the United States." *Gastroenterology* 122 (2002): 1500–1511.

4. International Foundation for Gastrointestinal Disorders. "About Constipation." November 25, 2006. Available online at: www.aboutconstipation.org/.

## Chapter 5: Your Mouth Is Killing You

1. Geerts, S.O., M. Nys, M.P. De, et al. "Systemic Release of Endotoxins Induced by Gentle Mastication: Association with Periodontitis Severity." *J Periodontol* 73 (2002): 73–78.

2. Andriamanalijaona, R., H. Benateau, P.E. Barre, et al. "Effect of Interleukin-1beta on Transforming Growth Factor-beta and Bone Morphogenetic Protein-2 Expression in Human Periodontal Ligament and Alveolar Bone Cells in Culture: Modulation by Avocado and Soybean Unsaponifiables." *J Periodontol* 77:7 (July 2006): 1156–1166.

3. Kut, C., A. Assoumou, M. Dridi, et al. "Morphometric Analysis of Human Gingival Elastic Fibres Degradation by Human Leukocyte Elastase Protective Effect of Avocado and Soybean Unsaponifiables (ASU)." *Pathol Biol (Paris)* 46:7 (September 1998): 571–576.

4. "Fluoride: Trading Tooth Decay for Cellular Death?" Available online at: www.mercola.com/2001/jul/25/tooth_decay.htm.

5. Walton, J., C. Tuniz, D. Fink, et al. "Uptake of Trace Amounts of Aluminum Into the Brain from Drinking Water." *Neurotoxicology* 16:1 (Spring 1995): 187–190.

6. Varner, J.A., K.F. Jensen, W. Horvath, et al. "Chronic Administration of Aluminum-Fluoride or Sodium-Fluoride to Rats in Drinking Water: Alterations in Neuronal and Cerebrovascular Integrity." *Brain Research* 784 (1998): 284–298.

7. Boyd, N.D., H. Benediktsson, M.J. Vimy, et al. "Mercury from Dental 'Silver' Tooth Fillings Impairs Sheep Kidney Function." *Am J Physiol* 261 (1991): R1010–R1014.

## Chapter 6: Cleansing Your Liver, Kidneys, and Blood

1. Environmental Defense. "Toxic Nation: A Report on Pollution in Canadians." November 2005. Available online at: www.jonbarron.org/pdf/b40fjwm0.pdf.

2. National Kidney and Urologic Diseases Information Clearinghouse. "Kidney and Urologic Diseases Statistics for the United States." Available online at: http://kidney. niddk.nih.gov/kudiseases/pubs/kustats/index.htm.

3. American Heart Association. "Heart Disease and Stroke Statistics, 2007 Update at a Glance." Available online at: www.americanheart.org/downloadable/heart/1166711577754HS_StatsInsideText.pdf.

4. Boden, W.E., R.A. O'Rourke, K.K. Teo, et al. "Optimal Medical Therapy With or Without PCI for Stable Coronary Disease." *N Engl J Med* 356:15 (April 2007): 1503–1516.

5. Omura, Y., Y. Shimotsuura, A. Fukuoka, et al. "Significant Mercury Deposits in Internal Organs Following the Removal of Dental Amalgam, and Development of Pre-cancer on the Gingiva and the Sides of the Tongue and Their Represented Organs as a Result of Inadvertent Exposure to Strong Curing Light (Used to Solidify Synthetic Dental Filling Material) and Effective Treatment: A Clinical Case Report, Along with Organ Representation Areas for Each Tooth." *Acupunct Electrother Res* 21:2 (1996): 133–160.

6. Omura, Y., S.L. Beckman. "Role of Mercury (Hg) in Resistant Infections and Effective Treatment of *Chlamydia trachomatis* and Herpes Family Viral Infections (and Potential Treatment for Cancer) by Removing Localized Hg Deposits with Chinese Parsley and Delivering Effective Antibiotics Using Various Drug Uptake Enhancement Methods." *Acupunct Electrother Res* 20:3–4 (1995): 195–229.

7. Klinghardt, D. "Amalgam/Mercury Detox as a Treatment for Chronic Viral, Bacterial, and Fungal Illnesses." *Explore* 8:3 (1997).

8. Barron, Jon. "Clinically Proven Oral Chelation." Baseline of Health Foundation. Available online at: www.jonbarron.org/newsletters/05/10-24-2005.php.

## Chapter 7: Diet—The Slow Killer

1. Yang, Y.J., et al. "Comparison of Fatty Acid Profiles in the Serum of Patients with Prostate Cancer and Benign Prostatic Hyperplasia." *Clin Biochem* 32 (August 1999): 405–409.

2. De Stefani, E., H. Deneo-Pellegrini, P. Boffetta, et al. "a-Linolenic Acid and Risk of Prostate Cancer: A Case-Control Study in Uruguay." *Cancer Epidemiol Biomarkers Prev* 9 (March 2000): 335–338.

3. Wild chimps love fresh baby monkey meat.

4. Brody, Jane E. "Studies Suggest a Harmful Shift in Today's Menu." *New York Times* (May 15, 1979): C1.

5. Cho, E., W.Y. Chen, D.J. Hunter, et al. "Red Meat Intake and Risk of Breast Cancer Among Premenopausal Women." *Arch Intern Med* 166 (2006): 2253–2259.

6. Violand, B.N., M.R. Schlittler, C.Q. Lawson, et al. "Isolation of *Escherichia coli* Synthesized Recombinant Eukaryotic Proteins that Contain Epsilon-N-acetylly-sine." *Protein Sci* 3:7 (1994): 1089–1097.

7. Beasley, Joseph, and Jerry Swift. "The Kellogg Report." Institute of Health Policy and Practice, 1989.

8. Grant, William. "Milk and Other Dietary Influences on Coronary Heart Disease." *Altern Med Rev* 3:4 (1998): 281–294.

9. Mettlin, C.J., E.R. Schoenfeld, and N. Natarajan. "Patterns of Milk Consumption and Risk of Cancer." *Nutr Cancer* 13 (1990): 89.

10. Galan, P., F. Cherouvrier, P. Preziosi, et al. "Effect of the Increasing Consumption of Dairy Products Upon Iron Absorption." *Eur J Clin Nutr* 45 (1991): 553–559.

11. Holick, M.F., Q. Shao, W.W. Liu, et al. "The Vitamin D Content of Fortified Milk and Infant Formula." *New Engl J Med* 326 (April 1992): 1178–1181.

12. Ramanujan, Krishna. "Insects Develop Resistance to Engineered Crops When Single- and Double-gene Altered Plants are in Proximity, Cornell Researchers Say." Cornell University News Service, June 17, 2005. Available online at: www.news.cornell.edu/stories/June05/Bt.kr.html.

13. Chaudhry, M. Rafiq. "Impact of Genetically Engineered Cotton in the World." Presented at the Second Meeting of the Asian Cotton Research and Development Network, November 2002,. Available online at: www.icac.org/cotton_info/speeches/ Chaudhry/2002/asiaI_presentation2002.pdf.

14. Gibbs, Gary. *The Food that Would Last Forever.* Garden City Park, NY: Avery Publishing Group, 1993.

15. Ibid.

16. Ibid.

17. Blanc, B.H., and H.U. Hertel. "Comparative Study about Food Prepared Conventionally and in the Microwave-Oven." *Raum Zeit* 3:2 (1992): 43.

18. Ibid.

19. Vallejo, F., F.A. Tomas-Barberan, C. Garcia-Viguera. "Phenolic Compound Contents in Edible Parts of Broccoli Inflorescences After Domestic Cooking." *J Sci Food Agricult* 83:14 (2003): 1511–1516.

## Chapter 8: Dying of Thirst

1. Batmanghelidj, F. *Your Body's Many Cries for Water.* Falls Church, VA: Global Health Solutions, 1995.

2. McTaggart, Lynne. *What Doctors Don't Tell You* 3:9 (January 1993).

3. Riggs, B.L., S.F. Hodgson, W.M. O'Fallon, et al. "Effect of Fluoride Treatment on the Fracture Rate in Postmenopausal Women with Osteoporosis." *N Engl J Med* 322:12 (1990): 802–809.

4. Danielson, C., J.L. Lyon, M. Egger, et al. "Hip Fractures and Fluoridation in Utah's Elderly Population." *JAMA* 268 (1992): 6.

5. Sowers, M.R., M.K. Clark, M.L. Jannausch, et al. "A Prospective Study of Bone Mineral Content and Fracture in Communities with Differential Fluoride Exposure." *Am J Epidemiol* 133 (1991): 649–660.

6. Varner, J.A., K.F. Jensen, W. Horvath, et al. "Chronic Administration of Aluminum-Fluoride or Sodium-Fluoride to Rats in Drinking Water: Alterations in Neuronal and Cerebrovascular Integrity." *Brain Research* 784 (1998): 284–298.

## Chapter 9: Vitamins, Minerals, and Phytochemicals

1. Ungoed-Thomas, Jon. "Official: Organic Really is Better." *The Sunday Times* (October 28, 2007). Available online at: www.timesonline.co.uk/tol/news/uk/health/ article2753446.ece.

2. Dagnelie, P.C., W.A. van Staveren, H. van den Berg. "Vitamin B-12 from Algae Appears Not to Be Bioavailable." *Am J Clin Nutr* 53 (1991): 695–697.

## Chapter 10: Antioxidants and Free Radicals

1. *Vitamin-Mineral Manufacturing Guide: Nutrient Empowerment, Vol. 1.* Lakeport, CA: Nutrition Resource, 1986.

2. Moon, S.O., W. Kim, et al. "Resveratrol Suppresses Tumor Necrosis Factor-alpha-Induced Fractalkine Expression in Endothelial Cells." *Mol Pharmacol* 70 (2006): 112–119.

3. Baur, J.A., K.J. Pearson, et al. "Resveratrol Improves Health and Survival of Mice on a High-calorie Diet." *Nature* 444 (November 2006): 337–342.

4. Godeau, R.L., C. Gavignet-Jeannin, et al. "The Effect of Procyanidolic Oligomers on Vascular Permeability: A Study Using Quantitative Morphology." *Pathol Biol (Paris)* 38:6 (June 1990): 608–616.

5. Chen, H., L. Teng, J.N. Li, et al. "Antiviral Activities of Methylated Nordihydroguaiaretic Acids." *J Med Chem* 41:16 (July 1998): 3001–3007.

6. Ayrton, A.D., et al. "Antimutagenicity of Ellagic Acid Towards the Food Mutagen IQ: Investigation into Possible Mechanisms of Action." *Food Chem Toxicol* 30:4 (1992): 289295. Castonguay, A., et al. "Antitumorigenic and Antipromoting Activities of Ellagic Acid, Ellagitannins and Oligomeric Anthocyanin and Procyanidin." *Int J Oncol* 10 (1997): 367–373. Constantinou, A., et al. "The Dietary Anticancer Agent Ellagic Acid is a Potent Inhibitor of DNA Topoisomerases in Vitro." *Nutr Cancer* 23:2 (1995):121–130.

7. Aviram, M., L. Dornfeld, M. Rosenblat, et al. "Pomegranate Juice Consumption Reduces Oxidative Stress, Atherogenic Modifications to LDL, and Platelet Aggregation: Studies in Humans and in Atherosclerotic Apolipoprotein E-Deficient Mice." *Am J Clin Nutr* 71:5 (2000): 1062–1076.

8. Gan, L., S.H. Zhang, Q. Liu, et al. "A Polysaccharide-Protein Complex from *Lycium barbarum* Upregulates Cytokine Expression in Human Peripheral Blood Mononuclear Cells." *Eur J Pharmacol* 471:3 (June 2003): 217–222.

9. Luo, Q., J. Yan, S. Zhang. "Isolation and Purification of *Lycium barbarum* Polysaccharides and Its Anti-fatigue Effect." *Wei Sheng Yan Jiu* 29:2 (March 2000): 115–117.

10. Zhang, X. "Experimental Research on the Role of *Lycium barbarum* Polysaccharide in Anti-peroxidation." *Zhongguo Zhong Yao Za Zhi* 18:2 (February 1993): 110–112, 128.

## Chapter 11: Enzymes = Life

1. Howell, Edward. *Enzyme Nutrition*. Wayne, NJ: Avery, 1985.

2. Felson, D.T., and Y. Zhang. "An Update on the Epidemiology of Knee and Hip Osteoarthritis with a View to Prevention." *Arth Rheum* 41 (1998): 1343–1355. Yelin, E. "The Economics of Osteoarthritis." In Brandt, K.D., M. Doherty, and L.S. Lohmander (eds.). *Osteoarthritis*. New York: Oxford University Press, 1998, pp. 23–30. Klein, G., et al. "Efficacy and Tolerance of an Oral Enzyme Combination in Painful Osteoarthritis of the Hip. A Double-blind, Randomised Study Comparing Oral Enzymes with Non-steroidal Anti-inflammatory Drugs." *Clin Exp Rheumatol* 24:1 (2006): 25–30.

3. Bendz, B., and P. Sandset. "Deep-vein Thrombosis in Long-haul Flights." *The Lancet* 358:9284 (2001): 837–838.

4. Miller, P.C., S.P. Bailey, et al. "The Effects of Protease Supplementation on Skeletal Muscle Function and DOMS Following Downhill Running." *J Sports Sci* 22:4 (2004): 365–372.

## Chapter 13: Balancing Hormone Levels in the Body

1. Kaplowitz, P.B., S.E. Oberfield, and the Drug and Therapeutics and Executive Committees of the Lawson Wilkins Pediatric Endocrine Society. "Reexamination of the Age Limit for Defining When Puberty is Precocious in Girls in the United States: Implications for Evaluation and Treatment." *Pediatrics* 104:4 (October 1999): 936–941. Herman-Giddens, M.E., E.J. Slora, R.C. Wasserman, et al. "Secondary Sexual Characteristics and Menses in Young Girls Seen in Office Practice: A Study from the Pediatric Research in Office Settings Network." *Pediatrics* 99:4 (1997): 505–512.

2. Cumming, D.C., S.R. Wall. "Non–Sex Hormone-Binding Globulin-bound Testosterone as a Marker for Hyperandrogenism." *J Clin Endocrinol Metab* 61 (1985): 873–876.

3. Panzer, C., S. Wise, G. Fantini, et al. "Impact of Oral Contraceptives on Sex Hormone–Binding Globulin and Androgen Levels: A Retrospective Study in Women with Sexual Dysfunction." *J Sex Med* 3 (2006): 104–113.

4. Schottner, M., D. Gansser, G. Spiteller. "Lignans from the Roots of *Urtica dioica* and Their Metabolites Bind to Human Sex Hormone–Binding Globulin (SHBG)." *Planta Med* 63:6 (1997): 529–532.

## Chapter 14: Optimizing Your Immune System

1. Associated Press. "Scientists May have Found Appendix's Purpose." (October 5, 2007). Available online at: www.msnbc.msn.com/id/21153898/.

2. Lews, Linda, M.D. FDA Memorandum, November 9, 2007. Available online at: www.fda.gov/ohrms/dockets/ac/07/briefing/2007-4325b_02_01_Tamiflu%20Background_Summary.pdf.

3. Barrett, B. "Medicinal Properties of Echinacea: A Critical Review." *Phytomedicine* 10:1 (2003): 66–86.

4. Wagner, H., A. Proksch. "An Immunostimulating Active Constituent from *Echinacea purpurea*." *Z Phytother* 2 (1981): 166–171.

5. Nanba, H. "Antitumor Activity of Orally Administered D-fraction from Maitake Mushroom (*Grifola frondosa*)." *J Naturopath Med* 4:1 (1993): 10–15.

6. Ishikawa, K. "Anti-HIV Activity in Cytopathic Effect of Proteoglucan Extracted from Maitake Mushroom." National Institutes of Health (January 23, 1991).

7. Furneri, P.M., A. Piperno, A. Sajia, et al. "Antimycoplasmal Activity of Hydroxytyrosol." *Antimicrob Agents Chemother* 48:12 (December 2004): 4892–4894. Renis, H.E. "Inactivation of Myxoviruses by Calcium Elenolate." *Antimicrob Agents Chemother* 8:2 (August 1975): 194–199.

8. United States Department of Agriculture. "Citricidal Effective Against Three Animal Viruses: Foot and Mouth Disease (FMD), African Swine Fever (ASF), Swine Vesicular Disease (SVD)."

9. Kienholz, V.M., B. Kemkes. "The Anti-bacterial Action of Ethereal Oils Obtained from Horseradish Root (*Cochlearia armoracia* L.)." (In German.) *Arzneimittelforschung* 10 (1961): 917–918.

10. Zhou, J., H.K.W. Law, C.Y. Cheung, et al. "Differential Expression of Chemokines and Their Receptors in Adult and Neonatal Macrophages Infected with Human or Avian Influenza Viruses." *J Infect Dis* 194 (2006): 61–70.

11. Kuttan, S.R., and G. Kutta. "Immunomodulatory Activity of Curcumin." *Immunol Invest* (1999) 28: 291–303.

## Chapter 15: It's All About Energy

1. "Hoaxes of the Ages." *U.S. News and World Report* (July 24, 2000).

2. Boyers, D.G., W.A. Tiller. "Corona Discharge Photography." *J Appl Physics* 44 (1973): 3102–3112.

3. "Transcranial Magnetic Stimulation." Harvard Health Publications, Harvard Medical School. Available online at: www.health.harvard.edu/press_releases/transcranial_ magnetic_stimulation.htm.

4. Ozdemir, S., O. Hulusi Dede, G. Koseoglu. "Electromagnetic Water Treatment and Water Quality Effect on Germination, Rooting and Plant Growth on Flowers." *Asian J Water Environ Pollution* 2:2 (2005).

5. Barrett, Stephen, M.D. "Homeopathy: The Ultimate Fake." QuackWatch. org. Available online at: www.quackwatch.org/01QuackeryRelatedTopics/homeo.html.

## Chapter 16: The Thought That Kills

1. Frasure-Smith, N., F. Lespérance, M. Talajic. "Depression and 18-Month Prognosis After Myocardial Infarction." *Circulation* 91 (1995): 999–1005.

2. Carney, R., K. Freedland, M. Rich, et al. "Ventricular Tachycardia and Psychiatric Depression in Patients with Coronary Artery Disease." *Am J Med* 95:1 (1993): 23–28.

3. Berkman, L., L. Leo-Summers, R. Horwitz. "Emotional Support and Survival after Myocardial Infarction: A Prospective, Population-based Study of the Elderly." *Ann Intern Med* 117 (1992): 1003–1009.

4. Morris, P.L., R.G. Robinson, P. Andrzejewski, et al. "Association of Depression with 10-year Post-stroke Mortality." *Am J Psychiat* 150 (1993): 124–129.

5. Talbot, Margaret. "The Placebo Prescription." *New York Times Magazine* (January 9, 2000).

6. "Less Banter in Surgery?" *New York Times* (February 7, 1984). Available online at: http://query.nytimes.com/gst/fullpage.html?sec=health&res=9C06E6D7143 BF934A35751C0A962948260.

7. Kein, Gerald. "Can You Anesthetize the Sub-Conscious Mind?" Omni Hypnosis Training Center, www.omnihypnosis.com/canyou.htm.

8. Bennett, H.L., H.S. Davis, and J.A. Giannini. "Non-Verbal Response to Intraoperative Conversation." *Br J Anaesthesia* 57:2 (1985): 174–179.

9. Kein, Gerald. "Can You Anesthetize the Sub-Conscious Mind?" Omni Hypnosis Training Center, www.omnihypnosis.com/canyou.htm.

10. A.A. Mason. "A Case of Congenital Ichthyosiform." *Br Med J* (1952): 422–423.

11. Klopfer, B. "Psychological Variables in Human Cancer." *J Projective Tech* 21:4 (December 1957): 331–340.

12. Edward, Rhiannon. "U.S. Drug Company Knew that 'Prozac Could Lead to Violence'." December 31, 2004. Available online at: http://news.scotsman.com/health. cfm?id=1477962004.

13. Kennedy Salaman, Maureen. "Medicating of America." *Health Freedom News* (June 2006). Available online at: www.thenhf.com/health_freedom_news_56.htm.

14. Fischer, E., B. Heller, M. Nachon, et al. "Therapy of Depression by Phenylalanine." *Arzneimittelforschung* 25 (1975): 132–133.

15. Kimura, K., M. Ozeki, L. Juneja, et al. "L-Theanine Reduces Psychological and Physiological Stress Responses." *Biol Psychol* 74:1 (2007): 39–45. Lu, K., M. Gray, C. Oliver, et al. "The Acute Effects of L-theanine in Comparison with Alprazolam on Anticipatory Anxiety in Humans." *Hum Psychopharmacol* 19:7 (2004): 457–465.

16. Schubert, H., and P. Halama. "Depressive Episode Primarily Unresponsive to Therapy in Elderly Patients: Efficacy of *Ginkgo biloba* Extract (EGB 761) in Combination with Antidepressants." *Geriatr Forsch* 3 (1993): 45–53.

17. Pittler, M.H., E. Ernst. "Efficacy of Kava Extract for Treating Anxiety: Systematic Review and Meta-Analysis." *J Clin Psychopharmacol* 20:1 (2000): 84–89.

18. Bhattacharya, S.K., A. Bhattacharya, K. Sairam, et al. "Anxiolytic-Antidepressant Activity of *Withania somnifera* Glycowithanolides: An Experimental Study." *Phytomedicine* 7:6 (2000): 463–469.

19. Ribeiro, M.D. "Effect of *Erythrina velutina* and *Erythrina mulungu* in Rats Submitted to Animal Models of Anxiety and Depression." *Brazil J Med Biol Res* 39:2 (2006): 263–270.

20. Estroff Marano, Hara. "Bedfellows: Insomnia and Depression." *Psychology Today* (July/August 2003).

21. Saul, Stephanie. "Sleep Drugs Found Only Mildly Effective, but Wildly Popular." *The New York Times* (October 23, 2007). Available online at: www.nytimes.com/2007/10/23/health/23drug.html?_r=1&pagewanted=print&oref=slogin.

## Chapter 17: Exercise—Move or Die

1. "UPI Poll: Most Have Exercise Regime." United Press (February 23, 2007).

2. Ogden, C.L., M.D. Carroll, L.R. Curtin, et al. "Prevalence of Overweight and Obesity in the United States, 1999–2004." *JAMA* 295 (2006): 1549–1555.

3. Thune, I., T. Brenn, et al. "Physical Activity and the Risk of Breast Cancer." *New Engl J Med* 336 (May 1997): 1269–1275.

4. Friedrich, M.J. "Women, Exercise, and Aging." *JAMA* 285 (2001): 1429.

## Chapter 18: The Cholesterol Myth and Other Cardiovascular Stories

1. "Randomised Trial of Cholesterol Lowering in 4,444 Patients with Coronary Heart Disease: The Scandinavian Simvastatin Survival Study (4S)." *Lancet* 344:8934 (November 1994): 1383–1389.

2. Guilland, J.C., A. Favier, et al. ["Hyperhomocysteinemia: An Independent Risk Factor or a Simple Marker of Vascular Disease? 2. Epidemiological Data."] *Pathol Biol (Paris)* 51:2 (2003): 111–121. Haynes, W.G. "Hyperhomocysteinemia, Vascular Function and Atherosclerosis: Effects of Vitamins." *Cardiovasc Drugs Ther* 16:5 (2002): 391–399.

3. Ridker, P., et al. "Inflammation, Aspirin, and the Risk of Cardiovascular Disease in Apparently Healthy Men." *N Engl J Med* 336 (1997): 973.

4. Pradhan, A.D., et al. "Inflammatory Biomarkers, Hormone Replacement Therapy, and Incident Coronary Heart Disease: Prospective Analysis from the Women's Health Initiative Observational Study." *JAMA* 288:8 (August 2002): 980–987.

5. "A Natural Anti-Cholesterol Dietary Supplement." *Life Extension Magazine* (June 2001). Available online at: www.lef.org/magazine/mag2001/june2001_cover_policosanol.html.

6. Jouven, X., M.A. Charles, M. Desnos, et al. "Circulating Nonesterified Fatty Acid Level as a Predictive Risk Factor for Sudden Death in the Population." *Circulation* 104 (2001): 756–761.

7. Ibid.

8. Charles, M.A., A. Fontbonne, N. Thibult, et al. "High Plasma Nonesterified Fatty Acids are Predictive of Cancer Mortality But Not of Coronary Heart Disease Mortality: Results from the Paris Prospective Study." *Am J Epidemiol* 153:3 (2001): 292–298.

9. Kelly, R.A., D.S. O'Hara, W.E. Mitch, et al. "Identification of NaK-ATPase Inhibitors in Human Plasma as Nonesterified Fatty Acids and Lysophospholipids." *J Biol Chem* 260 (1985): 11396–11405.

10. Davda, R.K., K.T. Stepniakowski, G. Lu, et al. "Oleic Acid Inhibits Endothelial Nitric Oxide Synthase by a Protein Kinase C-Independent Mechanism." *Hypertension* 26 (1995): 764.

## Chapter 19: Let's Talk about Cancer

1. Meropol, N.J., K.A. Schulman. "Cost of Cancer Care: Issues and Implications." *J Clin Oncol* 25:2 (2007): 180–186.

2. American Cancer Society. "Cancer Facts and Figures 2003." Available online at: www.cancer.org/downloads/STT/CAFF2003PWSecured.pdf.

3. University of Texas M.D. Anderson Cancer Center. "Decline in Breast Cancer Cases Likely Linked to Reduced Use of Hormone Replacement." *Science Daily* (December 15, 2006). Available online at: www.sciencedaily.com/releases/2006/12/061214142620.htm.

4. Brenner, D.J., and E.J. Hall. "Computed Tomography—An Increasing Source of Radiation Exposure." *New Engl J Med* 22:357 (November 2007): 2277–2284.

5. U.S. Environmental Protection Agency. "Radon." Available online at: www.epa.gov/radon/index.html.

6. Antony, S., R. Kuttan, and G. Kutta. "Immunomodulatory Activity of Curcumin." *Immunol Invest* 28:5-6 (1999): 291–303.

7. Balkwill, F., and A. Mantovani. "Inflammation and Cancer: Back to Virchow?" *Lancet* 357 (2002): 539–545. Coussens, L.M., and Z. Werb. "Inflammation and Cancer." *Nature* 420 (2002): 860–867. deVesser, K.E., L.V. Korets, and L.M. Coussens. "De novo Carcinogenesis Promoted by Chronic Inflammation is B-lymphocyte Dependent." *Cancer Cell* 7 (2005): 411–423.

8. Hijiya, N., M.M. Hudson, S. Lensing, et al. "Cumulative Incidence of Secondary Neoplasms as a First Event After Childhood Acute Lymphoblastic Leukemia." *JAMA* 297 (2007): 1197–1206.

9. Biello, David. "Chemotherapy Prompts Lingering Intellectual Deficit." Scientific American.com (October 5, 2006). Available online at: www.sciam.com/article.cfm? articleID=000C1484-6687-1524-A68783414B7F0000&sc=I100322.

10. Moss, Ralph, M.D. *Questioning Chemotherapy*. Brooklyn, NY: Equinox Press, 1995.

11. Hartmann, L.C., D.J. Schaid, J.E. Woods, et al. "Efficacy of Bilateral Prophylactic Mastectomy in Women with a Family History of Breast Cancer." *N Engl J Med* 340:2 (1999): 77–84.

12. Blakeslee, Sandra. "Better Odds; Faulty Math Heightens Fears of Breast Cancer." *The New York Times* (March 31, 2007).

13. CTV.ca News Staff. "Breast Cancer More Likely in Farm Workers: Study." October 12, 2006. Available online at: www.ctv.ca/servlet/ArticleNews/story/CTVNews/ 20061012/breastcancer_farming_061012/20061012?hub=TopStories.

14. People for the Ethical Treatment of Animals (PETA). "Got Breast Cancer?" Available online at: www.milksucks.com/breast.asp.

15. "Cadmium Exposure and Risk of Breast Cancer: Is There a Relationship?" *Medical News Today* (July 14, 2003). Available online at: www.medicalnews today.com/medicalnews.php?newsid=3946.

16. "Food, Nutrition, Physical Activity, and the Prevention of Cancer: A Global Perspective." World Cancer Research Fund and the American Institute for Cancer Research, November 2007. Available online at: www.dietandcancer report.org/.

## Chapter 20: The Plagues of Our Time—Diabetes, Osteoporosis, Alzheimer's Disease, and Multiple Sclerosis (MS)

1. Butler, A.E., J. Janson, S. Bonner-Weir, et al. "Beta-cell Deficit and Increased Beta-cell Apoptosis in Humans with Type 2 Diabetes." *Diabetes* 52 (2003): 102–110.

2. Health Scout. "Osteoporosis—Symptoms, Treatment, and Prevention." Available online at: www.healthscout.com/ency/1/48/main.html.

3. World Health Organization. "Osteoporosis: Both Health Organizations and Individuals Must Act Now to Avoid an Impending Epidemic." WHO Press Release (October 11, 1999).

4. Fackelmann, K.A. "Fluoride-Calcium Combo Builds Better Bones—Treatment for Osteoporosis." *Science News* (January 21, 1989).

5. People for the Ethical Treatment of Animals (PETA). "Why Dairy Products Won't Help You Maintain Healthy Bones." Available online at: www.milksucks. com/ osteo.asp.

6. Okinawa Diet. "The Evidence About Okinawa Coral Calcium Supplements." Available online at: http://okinawaprogram.com/coral_calcium/coral-calcium. html.

7. Abraham, G.E. "The Importance of Magnesium in Management of Primary Post-menopausal Osteoporosis." *J Nutr Med* 2 (1991): 165–178.

8. Fluoride Action Network. "Health Effects: Fluoride's Differential Effect on Bone Density." Available online at: http://fluoridealert.org/health/bone/density/ cortical-trabecular.html.

9. Pratt, W.B., J.M. Holloway. "Incidence of Hip Fracture in Alaska Inuit People: 1979–1989 and 1996–1999." *Alaska Med* 2001 43(1): 2–5.

10. "A First Step to Clearing up Memory Loss—Check Your Medications." *Johns Hopkins Health Alert.* Available online at: www.johnshopkinshealthalerts.com/alerts/memory/JohnsHopkinsMemoryHealthAlert_205-1.html.

11. Hebert, L.E., P.A. Scherr, J.L. Bienias, et al. "Alzheimer Disease in the U.S. Population—Prevalence Estimates Using the 2000 Census." *Arch Neurol* 60 (2003): 1119–1122.

12. American Health Assistance Foundation. "Alzheimer's Disease, About Alzheimer's." Available online at: www.ahaf.org/alzdis/about/adabout.htm.

13. Ernst, R.L., J.W. Hay. "The U.S. Economic and Social Costs of Alzheimer's Disease Revisited." *Am J Public Health* 84:8 (1994): 1261–1264. National Institute on Aging, National Institutes of Health. "2001–2002 Alzheimer's Disease Progress Report." National Institutes of Health, p. 2.

14. Evans, D.A., H.H. Funkenstein, M.S. Albert, et al. "Prevalence of Alzheimer's Disease in a Community Population of Older Persons. Higher Than Previously Reported." *JAMA* 262:18 (1989): 2551–2556.

15. Arvanitakis, Z., R.S. Wilson, J.L. Bienias, et al. "Diabetes Mellitus and Risk of Alzheimer Disease and Decline in Cognitive Function." *Arch Neurol* 61 (2004): 661–666.

16. Ott, A., R.P. Stolk, F. van Harskamp, et al. "Diabetes Mellitus and the Risk of Dementia: The Rotterdam Study." *Neurology* 53:9 (December 1999): 1907–1909.

17. "Alzheimer's is a Consequence of Inflammation." *Medical News Today* (April 29, 2004). Available online at: www.medicalnewstoday.com/medicalnews.php?newsid=7787.

18. Varner, J.A., K.F. Jensen, W. Horvath, et al. "Chronic Administration of Aluminum-Fluoride or Sodium-Fluoride to Rats in Drinking Water: Alterations in Neuronal and Cerebrovascular Integrity." *Brain Res* 784 (1998): 284–298.

19. Vitek, M.P., K. Bhattacharya, J.M. Glendening, et al. "Advanced Glycation End Products Contribute to Amyloidosis in Alzheimer's Disease." *Proc Natl Acad Sci USA* 91:11 (May 1994): 4766–4770.

20. Gorman, Christine. "Can You Prevent Alzheimer's Disease?" *Time* (January 8, 2006). Available online at: www.time.com/time/magazine/article/0,9171,1147142-3,00.html.

21. Pozzilli, C., P. Falaschi, C. Mainero, et al. "MRI in Multiple Sclerosis Dur-

ing the Menstrual Cycle: Relationship with Sex Hormone Patterns." *Neurology* 53:3 (1999): 622–624.

22. Hughes, M.D. "Multiple Sclerosis and Pregnancy." *Neurol Clinics* 22:4 (2004): 757–759.

23. "Estriol May Ease Relapsing-Remitting MS in Women." NeurologyReviews. com (November 2002). Available online at: www.neurologyreviews.com/nov02/ nr_ nov02_estriol.html.

24. Kim, S., S.M. Liva, M.A. Dalal, et al. "Estriol Ameliorates Autoimmune Demyelinating Disease: Implications for Multiple Sclerosis." *Neurology* 1999 52(6): 1230–1238.

25. "Testosterone Gel May Benefit Men with MS." MultipleSclerosisCentral.com (May 15, 2007). Available online at: www.healthcentral.com/multiple-sclerosis/ news-38988-66.html.

26. PRISMS Study Group and the University of British Columbia MS/MRI Analysis Group. "Long-term Efficacy of Interferon-beta-1a in Relapsing MS." *Neurology* 57:6 (2001): 1146.

## Chapter 21: Aging—It's Not Just for the Old

1. Kent, Saul. "BioMarker Pharmaceuticals Develops Anti-Aging Therapy." *Life Extension Magazine* (June 1993).

2. McFarland, G.A., R. Holliday. "Retardation of the Senescence of Cultured Human Diploid Fibroblasts by Carnosine." *Exp Cell Res* 212:2 (1994): 167–175. McFarland, G.A., R. Holliday. "Further Evidence for the Rejuvenating Effects of the Dipeptide L-Carnosine on Cultured Human Diploid Fibroblasts." *Exp Gerontol* 34:1 (1999): 35–45.

3. Yuneva, M.O., E.R. Bulygina, S.C. Gallant, et al. "Effect of Carnosine on Age-induced Changes in Senescence-accelerated Mice." *J Anti-Aging Med* 2:4 (1999): 337–342. Boldyrev, A., R. Song, D. Lawrence, et al. "Carnosine Protects Against Excitotoxic Cell Death Independently of Effects on Reactive Oxygen Species." *Neuroscience* 94:2 (1999): 571–577.

4. Quinn, P., A.A. Boldyrev, et al. "Carnosine: Its Properties, Functions and Potential Therapeutic Applications." *Molec Aspects Med* 13 (1992): 379–444.

5. Ibid.

6. Rosick, Edward R. "How Carnosine Protects Against Age-Related Disease."

*Life Extension Magazine* (January 2006). Available online at: www.lef.org/magazine/mag 2006/jan2006_report_carnosine_02.htm.

7. Hipkiss, A.R., C. Brownson. "A Possible New Role for the Anti-ageing Peptide Carnosine." *Cell Mol Life Sci* 57:5 (2000): 747–753. Brownson, C., A.R. Hipkiss. "Carnosine Reacts with a Glycated Protein." *Free Radic Biol Med* 28:10 (2000): 1564–1570.

8. Asif, M., J. Egan, S. Vasan, et al. "An Advanced Glycation Endproduct Crosslink Breaker Can Reverse Age-related Increases in Myocardial Stiffness." *Proc Natl Acad Sci USA* 97:6 (March 2000): 2809–2813. Liu, J., M.R. Masurekar, D.E. Vatner, et al. "Glycation End-product Cross-link Breaker Reduces Collagen and Improves Cardiac Function in Aging Diabetic Heart." *Am J Physiol Heart Circ Physiol* 285:6 (December 2003): H2587–H2591.

9. Preston, J.E., A.R. Hipkiss, D.T. Himsworth, et al. "Toxic Effects of Beta-amyloid(25-35) on Immortalised Rat Brain Endothelial Cell: Protection by Carnosine, Homocarnosine and Beta-alanine." *Neurosci Lett* 242:2 (February 1998): 105–108.

10. Re, O. "2-Dimethylaminoethanol (Deanol): A Brief Review of Its Clinical Efficacy and Postulated Mechanism of Action." *Curr Ther Res Clin Exp* 16:11 (November 1974): 1238–1242. Lewis, J.A., and R. Young. Deanol and methylphenidate in minimal brain dysfunction. Clin Pharmacol Ther 17 (1975): 534-540.

11. Swart, I., J. Rossouw, J.M. Loots, et al. "The Effect of L-Carnitine Supplementation on Plasma Carnitine Levels and Various Performance Parameters of Male Marathon Athletes." *Nutr Res* 17 (1997): 405–414.

12. Pettegrew, J.W., et al. "Clinical and Neurochemical Effects of Acetyl-L-carnitine in Alzheimer's Disease." *Neurobiol Aging* 16:1 (1995): 1–4. Carta, A., et al. "Acetyl L-carnitine: A Drug Able to Slow the Progress of Alzheimer's Disease?" *Ann NY Acad Sci* 640 (1991): 228–232.

13. Castorina, M., L. Ferraris. "Acetyl-L-carnitine Affects Aged Brain Receptorial System in Rodents." *Life Sci* 54:17 (1994): 1205–1214. Pettegrew, J.W., et al. "Clinical and Neurochemical Effects of Acetyl-L-carnitine in Alzheimer's Disease." *Neurobiol Aging* 16:1 (1995): 1–4.

14. Sima, A.F., H. Ristic, A. Merry, et al. "Primary Preventive and Secondary Interventionary Effects of Acetyl-L-carnitine on Diabetic Neuropathy in the Bio-Breeding Worcester Rat." *J Clin Invest* 97:8 (1996): 1900–1907.

15. Magnusson, Kathy R. "Aging of the NMDA Receptor Complex." *Frontiers Biosci* 3 (May 1998): e70–e80.

16. Rao, K.V., Y.R. Mawal, I.A. Qureshi. "Progressive Decrease of Cerebral Cytochrome C Oxidase Activity in Sparse-fur Mice: Role of Acetyl-L-carnitine in Restoring the Ammonia-induced Cerebral Energy Depletion" *Neurosci Lett* 224:2 (March 1997): 83–86.

# Index

# About the Author

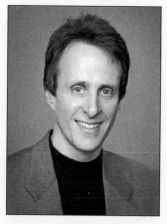

**Jon Barron** has been a pioneer in the study of nutrition, disease prevention, and anti-aging for the last 40 years. He is editor and publisher of the *Baseline of Health Newsletter* and the *Barron Report*, both of which are read by thousands of doctors, health experts, and nutrition consumers in over 140 countries. He is founder and director of the Baseline of Health Foundation and is also recognized as one of the world's leading formulators of nutritional products. His popular, award-winning health information website, www.jonbarron.org, receives thousands of visitors per day.